皮肤病光疗和光诊断学方法
Dermatological Phototherapy and Photodiagnostic Methods

第2版

主　编　Jean Krutmann　Herbert Hönigsmann　Craig A. Elmets
主　审　张锡宝
主　译　朱慧兰　王建琴
副主译　张三泉　罗　权　李振洁　李润祥　梁碧华　陈　荃
译　者（按姓氏笔画排序）
　　　　马少吟　王建琴　叶兴东　叶倩如　田　歆　朱慧兰
　　　　刘　清　江　娜　杨　艳　李振洁　李润祥　肖常青
　　　　张三泉　张尔婷　张倩雯　张锡宝　陈　荃　林　玲
　　　　罗　权　罗育武　周　欣　孟　珍　高方铭　唐亚平
　　　　黄茂芳　梁碧华　潘乔林
秘　书　陈　荃　孟　珍　周　欣

人民卫生出版社

Translation from the English edition:
Dermatological Phototherapy and Photodiagnostic Methods, 2nd edition, by Jean Krutmann, Herbert Hönigsmann, Craig A. Elmets
Copyright © 2009 Springer-Verlag Berlin Heidelberg
Springer-Verlag Berlin Heidelberg is a part of Springer Science+Business Media
All Rights Reserved

敬告

本书的作者、译者及出版者已尽力使书中的知识符合出版当时普遍接受的标准。但医学在不断地发展，随着科学研究的不断探索，各种诊断分析程序和临床治疗方案以及药物使用方法都在不断更新。强烈建议读者在使用本书涉及的诊疗仪器或药物时，认真研读使用说明，尤其对于新的产品更应如此。出版者拒绝对因参照本书任何内容而直接或间接导致的事故与损失负责。

图书在版编目(CIP)数据

皮肤病光疗和光诊断学方法/(德)吉恩·考特曼(Jean Krutmann)主编;朱慧兰,王建琴主译. —北京:人民卫生出版社,2016

ISBN 978-7-117-23920-2

Ⅰ.①皮… Ⅱ.①吉…②朱…③王… Ⅲ.①皮肤病-光疗法②皮肤病-光学诊断 Ⅳ.①R751

中国版本图书馆 CIP 数据核字(2017)第 008516 号

人卫智网　www.ipmph.com	医学教育、学术、考试、健康，
	购书智慧智能综合服务平台
人卫官网　www.pmph.com	人卫官方资讯发布平台

版权所有，侵权必究！

皮肤病光疗和光诊断学方法

主　　译：朱慧兰　王建琴
出版发行：人民卫生出版社(中继线 010-59780011)
地　　址：北京市朝阳区潘家园南里 19 号
邮　　编：100021
E - mail：pmph @ pmph.com
购书热线：010-59787592　010-59787584　010-65264830
印　　刷：北京汇林印务有限公司
经　　销：新华书店
开　　本：710×1000　1/16　印张：25
字　　数：490 千字
版　　次：2017 年 2 月第 1 版　2017 年 12 月第 1 版第 2 次印刷
标准书号：ISBN 978-7-117-23920-2/R·23921
定　　价：118.00 元

打击盗版举报电话：010-59787491　E-mail：WQ @ pmph.com
(凡属印装质量问题请与本社市场营销中心联系退换)

序

随着我国经济腾飞,科技水平进步,皮肤病的治疗已从传统的药物治疗扩展到理疗、激光治疗以及外科手术等。光医学是皮肤科学中诊断和治疗的重要部分,在皮肤病诊治中,光生物学、荧光、光疗、光化学疗法、光动力疗法、激光的知识和技能都是不可缺少的。对广大皮肤病的患者来说,光医学提供了更加精确的诊治方法,且全身副作用小。因此,了解和掌握光医学相关知识可以说是现代皮肤科医生的必备技能。

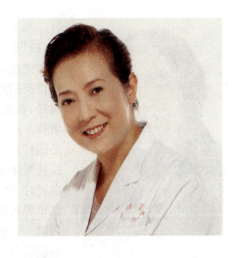

朱慧兰教授是广州市皮肤病防治所暨广州医科大学皮肤病研究所的副所长,多年来从事皮肤病光医学的研究,对光敏性皮肤病和光治疗都有着丰富的经验和深刻见解。我很高兴她组织翻译了Jean Krutmann、Herbert Hönigsmann 和 Craig A. Elmets 等欧美专家共同撰写的《皮肤病光疗和光诊断学方法》一书。本书全面综合地介绍了多种疾病适用的光诊断和光治疗方法,内容翔实具体,对广大临床皮肤科医师和技术人员有很强的指导意义。内容覆盖了银屑病、特应性皮炎、光敏性皮肤病、白癜风等常见病以及少见病适应证,探讨了传统的 UVB、PUVA 治疗,以及较新的光动力治疗、308nm 准分子光、UVA-1、体外光化学免疫疗法等,可以扩展我们的眼界和治疗思路。同时结合了最新文献综述和欧美专家的指导意见,把机制与光疗和临床问题紧密结合,可操作性强。值得推荐给广大皮肤科医师、研究生和光疗技术人员参考学习。祝大家阅读愉快,开卷有益!

何黎 教授
2016 年 10 月

译者前言

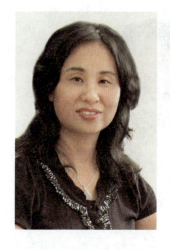

从事皮肤病学工作30年来，深刻感受到科技发展，特别是光医学的发展对皮肤病诊断治疗带来的巨大变革。紫外线治疗和光动力治疗是目前很多炎症性皮肤病、感染性皮肤病和皮肤肿瘤的最佳治疗选择，具有创伤小、副作用少和方便易行等特点，随着技术进步和广泛应用，治疗的性价比也逐渐增高，是现代皮肤科医生不可缺少的治疗手段。我国在皮肤病光医学领域一直走在前列，特别是前辈和同行在光疗、光动力治疗和荧光诊断方面的技术一直处在世界前沿，给广大患者提供了优越的治疗手段和环境。但我国地域广大，不少基层单位皮肤科缺乏相应设备和培训知识，限制了患者的治疗选择，在一定程度上也制约了光医学的发展。

一年前我有幸拜读了 Jean Krutmann、Herbert Hönigsmann 和 Craig A. Elmets 等欧美专家共同撰写的《皮肤病光疗和光诊断学方法》一书，受益颇多。本书详细阐述了欧美皮肤科专家对于光治疗、光化学疗法、光动力疗法、光生物学诊断和荧光诊断等方面的最新进展和治疗方案意见。全面具体地介绍了欧美光疗的选择与方案，可操作性很强，特别是对术前医患沟通以及治疗细节的全面解说确实是以往书籍较少提及而临床上至关重要的部分。虽然光疗对患者来说个体化的调整非常重要，作者也总结综述了大量最新文献，提供了其他治疗团队的意见。

感谢人民卫生出版社的支持，以及我所中青年骨干医师的努力，经过半年时间，我们完整翻译了《皮肤病光疗和光诊断学方法》一书，以飨读者。感谢昆明医科大学附属第一医院何黎教授百忙之中拨冗作序，感谢 Jean Krutmann 教授等人的优秀原著。希望广大读者，包括皮肤科医师、研究生和理疗护理人员都可以从中获益，促进我国皮肤科光医学的进一步发展。

朱慧兰

教授，主任医师

2016年10月

原著前言

在过去的几十年中,光疗对皮肤病的治疗概念产生了极大地影响。因此,光医学已经从经验论发展成为了生物医学研究中最令人振奋的领域之一。可见光和紫外线对皮肤影响的研究促成了基础科学家和临床工作者之间富有成效的合作。因此,光疗可被视为应用皮肤生物学中最好的例子。

近几十年来紫外线被用于治疗一些常见皮肤病,如银屑病和特应性皮炎。最近,引入了 UVB 和 UVA 的选择性光谱,如窄谱 UVB 和 UVA-1 光疗等,且增加了新的光疗适应证,极大地促进了光治疗学的发展。目前可见光结合光敏剂可用于肿瘤的诊断和选择性治疗。体外光化学免疫疗法并不只在皮肤病学中被证实有效,尤其在移植医学中同样有益。

大多数的光疗机制为经验性医学,而未涉及相关的生物学机制。对光生物学基础原理最新进展的认识将促使光疗更加有效,与此同时,更为重要的是将使之更为安全。

本书为第 2 版,将通过在目前光生物学原理的背景下来呈现临床资料。本书除了对一些选定的皮肤病的光化学疗法进行详细描述之外,还详述了光线性皮肤病的标准化测试共识和皮肤肿瘤的诊断。

光疗存在多种方式,临床医生可自行选择。对于某一特类疾病,可根据患者的特殊情况来选择其最佳的治疗方案。因此,本书的重点在于使用不同的治疗方式来治疗某一特类疾病,且将在临床章节中补充已被证实成功应用多年的光疗应用指南。

此外,各权威专家在这一项目中做出了巨大贡献,大部分作者不仅是临床经验丰富的光皮肤病学专家,而且也是光生物基础研究的国际知名专家。

我们非常感谢对本次出版做出卓越贡献的所有作者。我们希望这本专著能继续为日常操作、临床实践以及研究中的皮肤病光疗和光诊断学方法提供最新的参考。

J. Krutmann, H. Hönigsmann, C. A. Elmets
德国杜塞尔多夫,奥地利维也纳,美国阿拉巴马州伯明翰

原著作者

Christoph Abels
Medizinisch-wissenschaftliche Abteilung
Dr. August Wolff GmbH & Co.
Arzneimittel
Sudbrackstraße 56
33611 Bielefeld
Germany
Email:
christoph.abels@wolff-arzneimittel.de

Reinhard Breit
Theodor-Körner-Straße 6
82049 Pullach
Germany
Email: reinhard.breit@gmx.de

Piergiacomo Calzavara-Pinton
Chief of the Department of Dermatology
Azienda Spedali Civili di Brescia
Brescia
Italy
Email: calzavar@osp.unibs.it

Ponciano D. Cruz, Jr.
Department of Dermatology
University of Texas Southwestern
Medical Center
5323 Harry Hines Blvd.
Dallas, 75390-9069 TX
USA
Email:
ponciano.cruz@utsouthwestern.edu

Craig A. Elmets
University of Alabama
Department of Dermatology
SDB 67
Birmingham, 35294-0007 AL
USA
Email: celmets@uab.edu

James Ferguson
Head of Photobiology Unit,
Department of Dermatology
Ninewells Hospital & Medical School
Dundee, DD1 9SY, Scotland
UK
Email: jj.ferguson@dundee.ac.uk

Clemens Fritsch
Bankstraße 6
40476 Düsseldorf
Germany
E-mail: info@cf-derm.de

Kerstin Gardlo
Hauptstraße 108
53474 Bad Neuenahr-Ahrweiler
Germany
Email:
gardlo-jovic@derma-badneuenahr.de

原著作者

Werner Halbritter
OSRAM GmbH
Central Laboratory for Light
Measurements (QM CL-M)
Hellabrunner Straße 1
81543 München
Germany
Email: werner.halbritter@osram.de

Iltefat H. Hamzavi
Senior Staff Physician, Multicultural
Dermatology
Department of Dermatology
Henry Ford Medical Center
New Center One
3031 West Grand Boulevard, Suite 800
Detroit, 48202 MI
USA
Email: ihamzav1@hfhs.org

John Hawk
Department of Photobiology
St. Thomas Hospital
London SE1 7EH
UK
Email: john.hawk@kcl.ac.uk

Erhard Hölzle
Städtische Kliniken
Klinik für Dermatologie und Allergolgie
Dr.-Eden-Straße 10
26133 Oldenburg
Germany
Email: dermatologie@klinikum-oldenburg.de

Herbert Hönigsmann
Universitätsklinikum Wien
Dermatologische Klinik
Abt. Spezielle Dermatologie
Währinger Gürtel 18–20
1090 Wien
Austria
E-mail: herbert.hoenigsmann@meduniwien.ac.at

Werner Jordan
OSRAM GmbH
Central Laboratory for Light
Measurements, (I OSR QM CL-M)
Hellabrunnerstraße 1
81543 Munich
Germany
Email: werner.jordan@osram.de

Sigrid Karrer
Department of Dermatology
University of Regensburg
Franz-Josef-Strauss-Allee 11
93053 Regensburg
Germany
Email: sigrid.karrer@klinik.uni-regensburg.de

Robert Knobler
Department of Dermatology
Division of Special and Environmental
Dermatology
University of Vienna Medical School
Vienna General Hospital – AKH
Waehringer Gürtel 18–20
1090 Vienna
Austria
Email: robert.knobler@meduniwien.ac.at

Jean Krutmann
Universität Düsseldorf
Institut für Umweltmedizinische
Forschung (IUF) gGmbH
Auf'm Hennekamp 50
40225 Düsseldorf
Germany
Email: krutmann@rz.uni-duesseldorf.de

Michael Landthaler
Head of Department of Dermatology
University of Regensburg
Franz-Josef-Strauss-Allee 11
93053 Regensburg
Germany
Email: michael.landthaler@klinik.uni-regensburg.de

Percy Lehmann
Klinikum Wuppertal GmbH
Hautklinik
Arrenberger Straße 20
42117 Wuppertal
Germany
E-mail:
plehmann@wuppertal.helios-kliniken.de

Henry W. Lim
Department of Dermatology
Henry Ford Medical Center
New Center One
3031 West Grand Blvd., Suite 800
Detroit, 48230 MI
USA
Email: hlim1@hfhs.org

Bassel H. Mahmoud
Post-doctoral Research Fellow
Department of Dermatology
Henry Ford Medical Center
New Center One
3031 West Grand Boulevard, Suite 800
Detroit, 48202 MI
USA
E-mail: bmahmou1@hfhs.org

Renz Mang
Gemeinschaftspraxis für Dermatologie,
Venerologie, Allergologie, Proktologie
Hauptstraße 36
42349 Wuppertal
Germany
Email: mang@hautarzt-cronenberg.de

Hallie McDonald
Dept. of Dermatology
University of Texas
Southwestern Medical Center
5323 Harry Hines Blvd.
Dallas, 75390-9069 TX
USA
Email:
hallie.mcdonald@utsouthwestern.edu

Warwick L. Morison
Johns Hopkins at Green Spring
10753 Falls Road, Suite 355
Lutherville, 21093 MD
USA
Email: wmorison@jhmi.edu

Akimichi Morita
Department of Geriatric and
Environmental Dermatology
Nagoya City University
Graduate School of Medical Sciences
Nagoya 467-8601
Japan
Email: amorita@med.nagoya-cu.ac.jp

Norbert J. Neumann
Universitäts-Hautklinik
Moorenstraße 5
40225 Düsseldorf
Germany
Email: neumannt@uni-duesseldorf.de

Bernhard Ortel
Section of Dermatology
University of Chicago
5841 S. Maryland, MC 5067
Chicago, 60637-1470 IL
USA
Email: ortel@helix.mgh.harvard.edu

Vesna Petronic-Rosic
PDP Director, Section of Dermatology
University of Chicago
5841 S Maryland, MC-5067
Chicago, 60637-1470 IL
USA
Email:
vrosic@medicine.bsd.uchicago.edu

原著作者

Thomas Ruzicka
Universitäts-Hautklinik
Postfach 10 10 07
40001 Düsseldorf
Germany
Email:
ruzicka@mwed.uni-duesseldorf.de

Thomas Schwarz
Head of Department of Dermatology,
Venerology and Allergology
University Hospital of the Christian
Albrechts University Kiel
Schittenhelmstraße 7
24105 Kiel
Germany
Email: tschwarz@dermatology.de

Helger Stege
Chefarzt der Dermatologie
Klinikum Lippe-Lemgo
Rintelner Straße 85
32657 Lemgo
Germany
Email: helger.stege@klinikum–lippe.de

Rolf-Markus Szeimies
Department of Dermatology
University of Regensburg
Franz-Josef-Strauß-Allee 11
93053 Regensburg
Germany
Email: rolf-markus.szeimies@
klinik.uni-regensburg.de

Adrian Tanew
Division of Special & Environmental
Dermatology
Department of Dermatology
Medical University of Vienna
1090 Vienna
Austria
Email:
adrian.tanew@meduniwien.ac.at

Beatrix Volc-Platzer
Department of Dermatology
Donauspital/SMZ Ost
Langobardenstrasse 122
1220 Vienna
Austria
Email:
beatrix.volc-platzer@smz.magwien.gv.at

Peter Wolf
Research Unit for Photodermatology
Department of Dermatology
Medical University Graz
Auenbruggerplatz 8
8036 Graz
Austria
Email: peter.wolf@meduni-graz.at

Antony Young
Photobiology Department
St. Johns Institute of Dermatology
Guy's King/St. Thomas Hospital
London SE1 7EH
UK
Email: antony.r.young@kcl.ac.uk

目录

第1篇 光(化学)疗法的基本机制

1 紫外线照射、辐射和剂量学 ································· 3
   L. Endres, R. Breit, W. Jordan, W. Halbritter(审阅)

第2篇 光(化学)疗法的临床应用

2 光(化学)疗法的机制 ······································· 53
   J. Krutmann, A. Morita, C. A. Elmets

3 银屑病的光(化学)疗法 ····································· 66
   H. Hönigsmann, A. Tanew, W. L. Morison

4 特应性皮炎的光治疗 ······································· 87
   J. Krutmann, A. Morita

5 特发性光线性皮肤病的光疗和光化学疗法 ··················· 102
   A. Tanew, J. Ferguson

6 皮肤T细胞淋巴瘤的光(化学)疗法 ························· 115
   H. Hönigsmann, A. Tanew

7 白癜风的光(化学)疗法 ···································· 129
   B. Ortel, V. Petronic-Rosic, P. Calzavara-Pinton

8 移植物抗宿主病(GvHD)的光(化学)疗法 ··················· 159
   B. Volc-Platzer

9 少见适应证的光（化学）疗法 ·· 176
  T. schwarz, J. Hawk

10 光疗与 HIV 感染 ·· 197
  H. McDonald, P. D. Cruz, Jr.

第 3 篇　特殊光疗模式

11 光动力疗法在皮肤科的应用 ·· 209
  R-M. szeimies, S. Karrer, C. Abels, M. Landthaler, C. A. Elmets

12 体外光化学免疫疗法 ··· 246
  R. Knobler

13 UVA-1 光疗：适应证和作用机制 ································· 258
  J. Krutmann, H. Stege, A. Morita

第 4 篇　日常生活中的光防护

14 光（化学）疗法和日晒所致的急性和慢性光损伤 ············ 275
  B. H. Mahmoud, I. H. Hamzavi, H. W. Lim

15 光防护 ·· 293
  P. Wolf, A. Young

第 5 篇　临床实践中的光诊断学

16 光诊断学方法 ··· 323
  N. J. Neumann, P. Lehmann

17 光斑贴试验 ··· 332
  E. Hölzle

18 荧光诊断 ·· 341
  C. Fritsch, K. Gardlo, T. Ruzicka

19 宽谱 UVB、窄谱 UVB 和 UVA-1 的光疗应用指南，以及 PUVA 光化学疗法的建议·· 366
　　H. Hönigsmann , J. Krutmann

20 技术及设备·· 377
　　R. Mang , H. Stege

索引·· 382

第1篇

光(化学)疗法的基本机制

第1章 紫外线照射、辐射和剂量学

L. Endres, R. Breit,
W. Jordan, W. Halbritter(审阅)

内容

光辐射性质 …… 4
辐射特点 …… 5
辐射的光谱组成 …… 10
辐射的数量特点 …… 16
紫外线辐射器的显著特性 …… 19
灯光辐射的影响因子 …… 34
日光 …… 40
剂量学 …… 42
总结 …… 49

要点

> 光辐射的性质
> 光线和紫外线辐射的重要光生物学特性
> 剂量的定义
> 辐射器及灯的性能特点
> 分光仪基本原理及光谱分辨的数据表示

光辐射性质

19世纪初,人们才意识到光线中不可见射线的存在。1800年,弗里德里希·威廉·赫歇尔在七色光谱中邻近红色一方检测到不可见射线,该射线照射到可吸收物表面时能产生热量。紧接1802年,约翰·威廉·里特发现可见光谱另一端的辐射,即紫外线,能引发"强烈的化学效应。"

根据检测方法和频谱内几何位置,人们将这两种新发现的辐射命名为红外辐射(波长大于红光)和紫外辐射(波长小于紫光)。

目前尚无关于不同类型光辐射性质、传播方式、光效应产生方式的明确定义[16,20]。各种理论中,最有名的是1669年牛顿提出的流数理论及1667年惠更斯提出的波动理论。牛顿推测光由许多微粒组成,这些微粒被物质吸收从而产生已知的效应。惠更斯则认为光是一种波,像水波一样,其传播需要介质,他将这种介质命名为"光以太",其无处不在,但所用装置无法检测到该物质。

他们的理论能解释某一特定现象:如牛顿的微粒学说可解释光的辐射效应,惠更斯的波动学说能解释光的干扰现象,但并不能解释所有的现象。

因此这些矛盾引发了诸多讨论,人们试图尝试建立适用于所有现象的光学理论。然而,将近两个世纪以来该理论并没有太大进展。

1871年,詹姆斯·麦克斯韦提出光电磁理论,使得1888年海因里希·赫兹发现电气振荡。这些结果证明任何电磁辐射(包括可见光、紫外线、红外线辐射)都是以波的方式传播,不需要任何介质。所有电磁波,无论波长或频率,在真空中都是以光速传播。但是,仍不能清楚解释波的产生及吸收机制。

直到20世纪初其才得到进一步发展:1900年,普朗克发表光辐射定律,认为光是一种不稳定状态,由不能被进一步划分的不连续的低能量序列构成。1902年,在光电效应研究过程中,菲利普·莱纳德发现光的特性,从而建立光量子假说。1905年,爱因斯坦证实莱纳德的实验结果可完全由普朗克的量子理论来解释。

因此,以期完整描述电磁波的特性,有必要对两个理论进行研究。电磁波的产生、吸收、辐射效应、视觉过程、对热的感知、对紫外线辐射的反应,都可运用量子理论定律解释;而电磁辐射的传播过程及其在光学系统的反应仅可由波动理论解释。

直到20世纪下半叶量子物理学的新发现,将这两种理论联系起来,以数学方式呈现普遍有效的辐射理论[16]。然而,由于现代物理学的日新月异,对于这种理论解释的所有尝试,都超出了非专业人士的概念范围。虽然光无处不在,但其表现仍是未解之谜。

辐射特点

尽管电磁波表现的复杂性,但使用众多技术手段,能用公式对其精确描述[12,16,20]。一方面,涉及诸如波长、频率、光子能量和频谱是一种混合辐射,另外一方面,用定量方法记录了转移辐射强度及其空间分布。

波的特点

波长和频率

电磁辐射采用各种不同的形状以波动方式进行传播。傅里叶分析证明,任何可能的形状均由多个正弦曲线建立构成[16]。本章中关于这点的理解,仅需充分考虑简单正弦波的特点。

图1.1示一个可被创建的正弦波。旋转箭头形成了围绕中心点的圆,通过移动箭头的位置,产生不同的旋转角度,从而形成具有正弦形状的曲线图。箭头长度对应波的最大振幅。点的开始与结束之间的距离被称为一个周期。

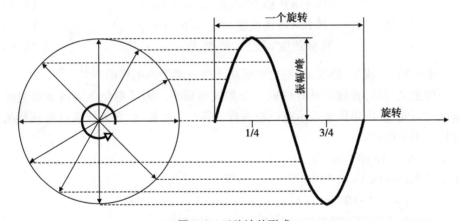

图1.1　正弦波的形成

如果箭头以恒定速度旋转,箭头可以在相同时间内到达。速度越快,在一定的时间内则会有更多的周期(图1.2a)。已知波的最小传播速度,可将坐标轴进行不同的长度分割(图1.2b)。如图1.2,我们能够推测正弦波的基本特征量:
- 频率指每秒的周期(cps)。图1.2a中分别表示频率为2、4、8
- 波长是指周期开始和结束之间的距离。图1.2b中分别表示波长为0.5m、0.25m和0.125m
- 传播速度是指在一定的时间内任意点移动的距离,单位为m/s(在图1.2中,所有三个波的传播速度均为1m/s)

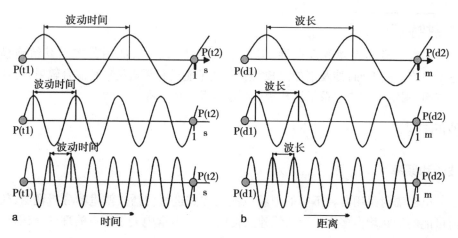

图1.2 a. 一定时间范围内正弦波的波长及频率。b. 一定距离范围内正弦波的波长及频率

这些变量相互之间的关系：

$$\text{频率} = \text{传播速度}/\text{波长}，即 \nu = v/\lambda \tag{1.1}$$

$$\text{波长} = \text{传播速度}/\text{频率}，即 \lambda = v/\nu \tag{1.2}$$

$$\text{传播速度} = \text{波长} \times \text{频率}，即 v = \lambda \cdot \nu \tag{1.3}$$

不论频率、波长、强度，这些公式适用于所有类型的电磁波[11,12,16,20,22]。

如上文所示，光辐射具有较短波长和较高频率。为了避免数字过大或过小造成的不便，常用单位来表示电磁波的数值特征。可见光、紫外线及红外线辐射波长常用单位如下：

- 1 埃(Å) = 1×10^{-10} m
- 1 纳米(nm) = 1×10^{-9} m
- 1 微米(μ) = 1×10^{-6} m

表示频率常用下列单位（cps 表示每秒的周期数）：

- 1 千赫(kHz) = 1×10^{3} cps
- 1 兆赫(MHz) = 1×10^{6} cps
- 1 千兆赫(GHz)的 = 1×10^{9} cps

传播速度

任何电磁辐射能量在真空中均是以光速传播。

$$\text{光速}(c) = 299792.458 \text{ km/s} \tag{1.4}$$

强调必须是在真空条件下，在所有其他情况下，如果辐射进入介质，传播速度降低,降低倍数与相关物质的折射率呈正比。(对于介质的传播速度,见表1.1)。

表1.1 光的速度

介质	折射率	符号	速度	占 C 的百分比
真空	n = 1	c	= 299 792km/s	
空气	n = 1.0003	c_{air}	= 299 690km/s	→99.9%
水	n = 1.33	c_{water}	= 225 410km/s	→75.2%
石英玻璃	n = 1.46	$c_{quartz\ glass}$	= 205 337km/s	→68.5%

指波长500nm的可见光在不同介质中的速度

通常情况下,对于普通测量这些是没有影响的。大多数情况下,在地球大气层中的传播速度与在真空中的传播速度间的差异可忽略不计。

公式1.3,传播速度等于频率和波长的乘积,也同样适用于介质传播。因此,需要降低速度时,频率或波长必须改变。物理学[16]认为在所有介质中频率恒定,波长变短,则对应速度越小。因此,频率是光辐射的显著特征。在可见光光谱范围内,通常用其在真空中的波长来描述辐射;然而在更长波长(例如无线电波)范围内,常用频率来描述辐射。

电磁波能量

单束光辐射如同图中的箭头所示(用数学方式表示,见图1.3的灰色直线),可被分解成红线的电波(E)和绿线的磁波(B)的正弦波[16]。

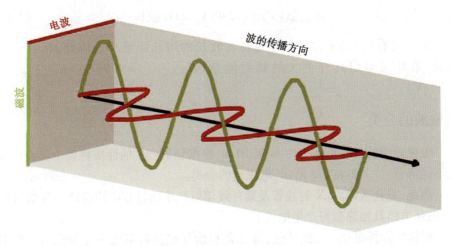

图1.3 光辐射束模式

基于电动力学理论,坡印廷矢量 S 是指电磁场中的能量密度矢量。其物理学上矢量方程如下:

$$\vec{S} = \varepsilon_0 c^2 \vec{E} \times \vec{B},\text{其中 }\varepsilon_0\text{ 为电离常量}。 \quad (1.5)$$

$S(J/m^2 s)$ 表示光束通过任意能量密度的时间间隔,依据其可推导出电离辐射强度常用单位见表1.3:

$$|\vec{S}| = \varepsilon_0 c^2 EB = \varepsilon_0 c E^2 \ (W/m^2) \quad (1.6)$$

注:所有用来解释辐射特征的学说(如高斯光学、光的直线传播理论)及许多其他的"宏观"推断,主要是以光学辐射波动理论为基础。

光子能量

电磁波能传播能量,量子力学认为,光子是能量传输的工具。根据爱因斯坦相对论,光子的能量 E 与其频率 ν 具有恒定关系[16,20]:

$$E_{photon} = h \times \nu \ (h = 6.626 \times 10^{-34} J \cdot s,\text{普朗克常数}) \quad (1.7)$$

根据真空中的波长,方程(1.7)可转换为如下公式:

$$E_{photon} = h\nu = hc/\lambda \quad (1.8)$$

能量辐射常用到的另外一个单位电子伏特(eV),1eV 表示在真空中一个电子穿过1V电压差所获得的动能。1 瓦特秒(Ws) = 1 焦耳(J) = 0.624×10^{19} 电子伏特(eV),也可表示为:

$$E_{photon}(eV) = (1240eV/nm)/\text{波长} \quad (1.9)$$

从上可看出:电磁辐射的能量随着波长的增长而减小。因此,相对于可见光,紫外线辐射具有更大的辐射能量($E_{photon,250nm} = 4.96eV > E_{photon,550nm} = 2.25eV$)。

电磁波的分类

电磁波谱的波长可从 10^{-16}m 至 10^7m,根据辐射产生的性质将整个光谱划分为不同部分[11]。如表1.2所示:电磁谱的分类。

因此,重叠区域内,X射线管及紫外线辐射产生的过程中均可产生X射线辐射,振荡电路及加热程可产生电波。

根据国际标准化[11],红外线,可见光和紫外线辐射形成光辐射范围。根据其化学和物理效应可将这些波长进一步细化。

表 1.2 电磁谱的分类

名称	波长	频率	来源
电波	$10^7 \sim 10^{-3}$ m	$10^1 \sim 10^{11}$ Hz	振荡电路
红外线辐射	$10^{-3} \sim 8 \times 10^{-7}$ m	$10^{11} \sim 4 \times 10^{14}$ Hz	散热器
可见光辐射	$8 \times 10^{-7} \sim 4 \times 10^{-7}$ m	$4 \times 10^{14} \sim 8 \times 10^{14}$ Hz	热激发 电子跃迁
紫外线辐射	$4 \times 10^{-7} \sim 1 \times 10^{-7}$ m	$8 \times 10^{14} \sim 3 \times 10^{15}$ Hz	电子跃迁
x-射线辐射	$5 \times 10^{-8} \sim 1 \times 10^{-13}$ m	$6 \times 10^{15} \sim 3 \times 10^{21}$ Hz	电子跃迁
核辐射	$1 \times 10^{-13} \sim 1 \times 10^{-16}$ m	$3 \times 10^{21} \sim 3 \times 10^{24}$ Hz	原子核反应

赫兹(Hz)是 SI 的国际通用单位,表示每秒内震荡的周期($1Hz=s^{-1}$)

红外辐射

长波红外线——IR-C(3μm~1mm) 该光谱范围内辐射能量低,具有极少生物学效应。

中波红外线——IR-B(1400nm~3μm) 这是发热玻璃(如灯泡)的主要发射范围。由于可被皮肤表皮层吸收,IR-B 并不被人体感知。强烈 IR-B 辐射可使人体体温调节失常,产生不适感。

短波红外线——IR-A(780~1400nm) 太阳辐射的主要范围。该辐射可深达皮肤,使人体产生舒适感。780~1400nm 范围内的波长具有治疗作用。

可见光辐射——光

视觉刺激和度不同,对绿色最敏感,对紫色、红色最不敏感。眼睛的灵敏度对于光源的经济学有着重要意义,一个标准的眼对于亮度敏感性是在试验研究的基础上确定。这种敏感性作为光谱光度因子,或 V(λ) 曲线被纳入国际标准化[6]。

人类心理与波长及颜色也是相关的。偏蓝的颜色可使人兴奋,偏红的颜色则会产生一种平静放松的效果。

尽管随着波长的增加,各种颜色逐渐融合到彼此,但对于每种颜色仍需要设定极限范围[1]。

---

1 在国际文献中,有不同的界限,经常被定义为:UVA-1(340~400nm),UVA-2(320~340nm),UVB(280~320nm)

紫外线辐射

长波紫外线辐射——UVA-1（340~380nm）：包括所有天然的、人工的、未过滤的及不被透明玻璃吸收的紫外光源。这一部分紫外线辐射具最低能量，其化学特性与短波可见光辐射（≥440nm）相似，因为它们具有相似的光生物效应，尤其是在对于眼的安全性方面（蓝光对眼睛有害）[6]。

表 1.3　不同颜色对应的波长范围

常见颜色	波长范围	常见颜色	波长范围
紫色	380~420nm	黄色	567~589nm
蓝色	421~495nm	橙色	590~627nm
绿色	496~566nm	红色	628~780nm

长波紫外线辐射——UVA-2（315~340nm）：表示 UVA 和 UVB 之间过渡的范围，同时具有这两种光谱的效应。

中波紫外线辐射——UVB（280~315nm）：由卡尔·豪塞尔威廉和威廉法勒根据大量基础研究所制作的红斑作用曲线得到的。

短波紫外线辐射——UVC（100~280nm）：波长最短，能量最高的一部分。在物理学上，紫外线可短至 15nm，接近于 X 射线。所谓短波紫外辐射是指小于等于 100nm，以避免与辐射防护规定冲突。当波长为 100~200nm 时 UV 辐射被空气吸收，因此，该波长范围内（也被称为真空-UV）的辐射不能发生在空气中[16,20,22]。

辐射的光谱组成

只有在特殊情况下，例如由激光器发出的，辐射才为单一波长构成。通常情况下，辐射是以不同强度波长的混合物形式发出的。辐射光谱的组成决定其效应，因此，为了评估辐射功效，一定要知道各种波长域发射的功率所占比例。代表波长相关的混合物辐射被程为频谱，用数学方式可表示为光谱功率分布（SPD）[1]。

1　光谱功率分布只能用光谱仪器进行分析（物理方法）。眼睛视网膜中一个点只能感知有一个印象。产生的印象主要取决于光的光谱分布，不能决定光谱的结构。不同的光谱功率分布可引起相同的印象即所谓的同分异构颜色刺激。

光谱仪

研究和分析光辐射混合物的仪器被称为光谱仪或摄谱仪[14]。原理及结构如图1.4和图1.6所示。

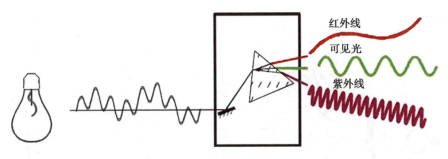

图1.4　光谱色散原理

按照功能,可分为以下几部分:

门区:光谱仪上用来收集待分析辐射的孔径,通常为一狭缝。

成像光学:经狭缝发射出的不同入射光经凹面镜转换为平行光。通过分散设备后,重新转换成光束聚焦在光谱仪的出射平面。

分散设备(棱镜或光栅):根据不同波长,棱镜以不同角度折射辐射。该基本原理可用一个简单例子说明。如果棱镜被置于日光下,同时一张纸被放置于出口面的后面,则在该纸张上可看到彩虹的颜色(见图1.5)。因此,彩虹是太阳光的光谱,但是眼睛不能分辨太阳光的光谱组成,近看是一片白色。

光栅能将辐射反射到不同方向(即光学衍射)。波长越短,方向改变越明显。蓝色偏转远超于红色,紫外线辐射被偏转远大于可见光。

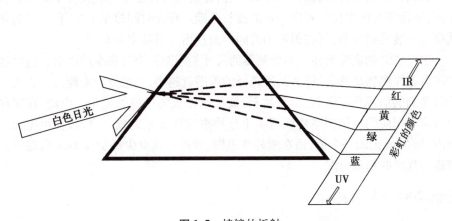

图1.5　棱镜的折射

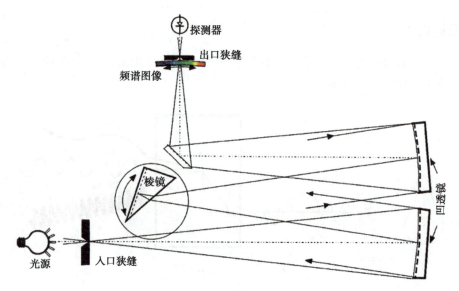

图1.6 单色光谱仪的光路原理

出口区：出口区是指聚焦频谱分散辐射的虚拟平面。

探测器的三个主要程序用来记录辐射强度：

照相检测器：感光材料经过曝光和显影后，可发现非常精细的光谱结构画面。变黑处通常为在该点的光谱强度。但不能定量地说明问题，因为该材料的黑化程度与光谱强度并不呈线性关系。

单探测器狭窄出口：打开分散设置按照时间顺序，全部光谱通过狭缝并按步骤被记录，如进行连续测量常需消耗大量时间。旋转棱镜或光栅具有较高精确度和稳定性，但其价格较昂贵。

像素探测器：像素探测器像阵列一样，密集分布在磁盘上直接置于光谱的像平面，使得每个像素位置对应一定的波长范围。曝光时间短至 1/20 秒。通过评估该电子装置的分布，可在很短的时间内测量出光谱功率分布。

出口狭缝的宽度及相应的检测器的尺寸是限制光谱分辨率的因素。该缝越窄或像素探测器越密集，那么其所选择的范围就越小，光谱分辨率越高。它主要受收集到的信号强度限制，信号越弱，波长所涉及的区域就越小。因此，在实践中对应于相应的应用程序建议留一个分辨率或任务来完成。通常，在可见光范围内，每 5nm 记录一个值；而在紫外线范围，频谱必须至少每步在 1nm 以保证光谱辐射强度的精确分配。

光谱功率分布的表示

光谱功率分布可用图表形式来表示。用波长（或频率）来描绘光谱分散辐射强度。光谱辐射的单位通常由辐射强度单位附加波长单位,对于紫外线部分通常是纳米(nm)[12]。例如,测量辐射强度,单位为 W/m^2;相应的频谱单位是则 $W/(m^2 \cdot nm)$,根据波长的表示方法。1

图 1.7 中的三幅图展示了光谱功率的不同分布。为了便于比较,选用波长范围为 295~405nm,功率为 100W 的辐射源,并且按步骤以每 10nm 测量一次。

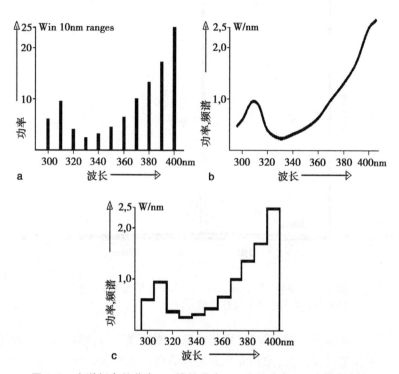

图 1.7 光谱频率的分布:**a.** 线性分布;**b.** 连续分布;**c.** 阶梯状分布

在第一个例子(图 1.7a)中,测得的强度被绘制为以波长范围为中心的直线(在 300nm 处的线包括了 295~305nm 的范围)。纵坐标单位是 W,附加有"范围为 10nm"。

如果可肯定被测量的光谱是连续的,那么可将线的顶端连接形成一条曲线(图 1.7b)。纵轴以 W/nm 为单位表示频谱功率。数值比图 1.7a 的还低 10 倍。

如果手绘光谱,更有利于绘制阶梯分布(图 1.7c)。

如图 1.7b 所示一种连续光谱,其特点是辐射在整个波长范围内发射。如果

1　在一些图中,频谱单位是 W/m^3。这是基于数学:将平方米和纳米结合,形成 $10^{-9} m$。

我们分析一个连续体,会发现分布的形状几乎完全相同,与所选择光谱分辨率无关。尤其是在处理低气压放电灯时,我们会发现光谱功率分布主要位于几个明确的波长范围而其附近无任何光谱发射。图 1.8 显示了一个使用不同光谱分辨率记录的线谱。

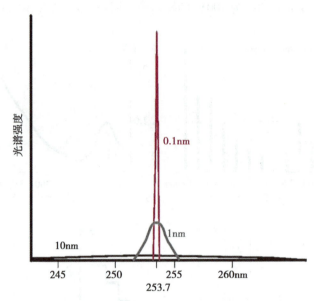

图 1.8 分别用 10nm、1nm、0.1nm 光谱分辨率记录了 253.7nm 处的汞谱的线性光谱

光谱分辨率越低,则其线性轮廓就越宽。线性强度与分辨率无关,如用该线性强度表示相邻部位波长,采用光化效应计算辐射效率能会导致错误。因此,不建议指定较小光谱波长来确定光谱仪的光谱分辨率。

通常有连续光谱、线谱,以及兼具两者特性的谱[1,3,8](图 1.9)。

日光和白炽灯的频谱分布是连续分布的典型代表,所谓连续谱是指:不论狭缝如何窄,以任何波长设定的辐射强度都可被检测到(图 1.9a)。此过程是典型的经高温激发使发射源产生发射的原理。

如钠灯和汞灯的气体或蒸汽被激发后,光谱功率分布于优选的波长,辐射发生时强度非常高,而邻近区域几乎没有发射可被检测到。这样的光谱被命名为线谱(图 1.9b)。

大多数人工辐射源发射的是 SPD,即连续性及线性谱的混合物。因为,现代灯厂家已越来越多地使用多种物理过程产生辐射。例如,荧光灯中汞的基本放电呈线性谱,其分布超出了 UV 和可见光范围。可见光线可直接产生光,而荧光的产生需紫外线激发灯泡内表面发光混合物材料。荧光体的 SPD 是近似于连

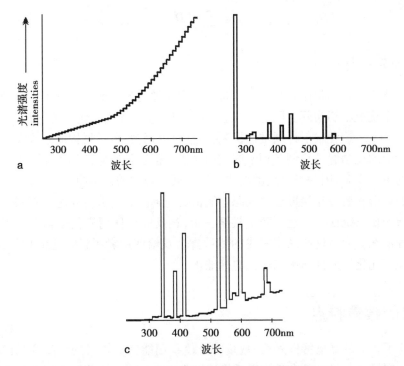

图1.9 连续光谱(a)、线性光谱(b)和混合光谱(c)

续及叠加的线性谱。这种类型的分布被指定为混合谱(图1.9c)。

光谱的真实特性受到众多物理学家和化学家的关注。由此,我们能够获得关于辐射体/散热器结构和/或组成元件的基本信息。连续辐射源分布的类型可表明辐射源的温度(如散热器);在线性和混合光谱下,线的位置以及连续体的表现形式可表明激发源的组成(频谱分析)。

如果是对特定辐射的效率感兴趣,可使用阶梯状SPD,其显示出特定波长范围内的强度。

光谱辐射分布对于所有有关辐射效应计算的研究是非常重要的[19]。为此,有针对辐射源的发射光谱,(对于一定时间间隔选择的波长绝对值),但也可用于单个波长范围内作用光谱定义的光谱灵敏度。作用光谱有许多已知的影响,部分已被纳入国家和国际标准。在可见光范围内,常被使用的作用光谱是眼睛的亮度及用于颜色计算的光谱值曲线;在光生物效应方面,作用光谱表现为红斑,色素沉着、灭菌作用[12]。

光化有效辐射可通过作用曲线的相关值乘以每个波长间隔(SPD)的强度值,最后将所得数值相加,得到结果,表示被研究对象的辐射混合物的效率及光化作用[12]:

$$SPD_{\text{effective actinic radiation}} = \sum_{\lambda} SPD_{\lambda} \times s_{\lambda,\text{action curve}} \times \Delta\lambda \tag{1.10}$$

光化学辐射计

光化学辐射测量昂贵且耗时。特别是在实地测量或测量控制工作的地方使用单色系统更不切实际。因此,在过去的十年中,手持式光化学辐射计,如照度计已被开发。这种辐射计通常由探测头、信号处理器、显示器构成。该探测器头通过相应的光学滤波片调节到不同作用光谱。但这种适应性作用光谱也是测量误差的主要来源,因为光谱灵敏度往往远远低于理想的作用曲线。因此,只有当所测的辐射光谱分布接近于校准源才能很好地解决光谱分析问题。不同光谱功率分布测量系统误差可达一两个甚至三个,相反简单使用光化学辐射计不会出现该种情况。为对这些系统完成的测量排名及给使用者提供一定的指导,尝试建立关于光化辐射计属性和功能的标准化[13]。

辐射的数量特点

除了辐射的光谱特性外,其数量特征使我们能够对辐射的强度及几何状态作出一定描述。目前已有 7 个定量指标被确立[12],这些定义符合国际标准且足以解决操作中的问题(表 1.4)。

表 1.4 重要的辐射及发光量单位的比较

辐射率		发光度	
量	单位	量	单位
辐射功率 φ_e	W	光通量	Lumen
辐射效率 η_e	W/W	照明效率	lm/W
辐射能 Q_e	J = Ws	光量	Lms
辐射强度 I_e	W/sr	光强度	cd = lm/sr
辐射率 L_e	W/m²sr	亮度	cd/m²
辐射度 E_e	W/m²	照度	lx = lm/m²
辐射曝量 H_e	J/m²	曝光量	lxs

注:通常索引中 e 表示电,V 表示光量。

光是评价光化学辐射最有名的例子。通过人眼的光谱发光效率对辐射进行评估。鉴于其重要性,在表 1.4 中,光的单位被添加,其与辐射单位相关。

在许多辐射源和照射系统的说明书中可发现关于这些定量描述,使得这些解释具有说服力。

这些量以简单方式构成,即在某一具体应用时,只需掌握四种基本类型的数学运算。

瓦特是任何类型能源常用的单位。它不仅适用于辐射,也适用于电力系统或汽车发动机的功率。

因此,对所有物理辐射进行测量时,必须对所测能源的特点进行详细说明。对于未加权的辐射,必须指出波长范围,例如,300~400nm 辐射(或 UVB 辐射);通过参考作用曲线进行评估时,必须说明作用和评价的特点,例如,有效红斑辐射功率。

辐射量及其单位

辐射功率 ϕ_e:表示发射源发出的辐射总量。与能源是否均匀发射或定向发射无关。

辐射效率 η_e:表示辐射源发射的辐射通量与消耗功率之比,包括一些辅助设备如镇流器,所消耗的功率。

辐射能 Q_e:表示是在一定时间间隔内发射的辐射功率。

辐射强度 I_e:表示是在一个特定的方向发出的辐射功率。其单位为 W/sr。其中"sr"表示立体角,被称为球面度(图1.10)。A 面角度可采用从圆中切割出的角度或长度来表示。如果此长度等于圆的半径,那么该角度具有 1 个弧度值。

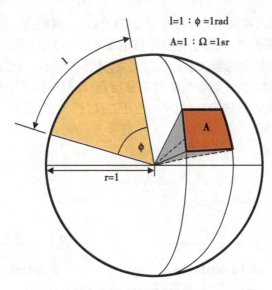

图 1.10 弧度和球面度

这一原则被采用定义几何立体角。如果圆锥或棱锥切出的区域等于一个球体的半径的平方,这个立体角为 1 球面度(sr)。在此图中 A 的形状并不重要。整个球的表面积为 $4\pi r^2$,也可表示为 $4\pi sr$。

对于灯,其能量辐射朝不同方向,灯周围的能量分布很少对称,其特点在于空间强度分布(图 1.11)。

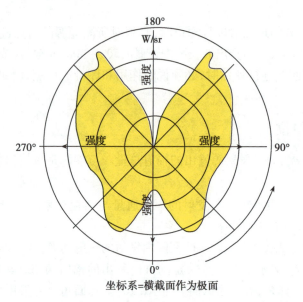

图 1.11 举例:灯光的空间分布

另外,反射器或其他光学设备常常被定向标记。因此,这种定向辐射在灯的总输出中具有重要意义。因此,能量分布用每单位立体角表示。

辐射率 L_e:与辐射通量及辐射强度无关,光源仅表示一个数值,无任何尺寸大小。从辐射率定义可了解辐射源的部分特点:辐射率指某一确定区域发射出的辐射强度。在光度测量中,辐射率对应于亮度(图 1.12 表示强度与辐射范围 f 和辐射率 L 的关系)。

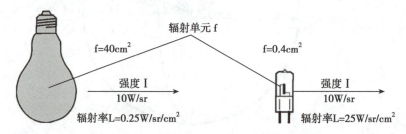

图 1.12 强度与辐射范围 f 和辐射率 L 的关系

辐照度 E_e：表示入射在物体表面的辐射功率。它与辐射源的数量及入射方向无关。因此,辐照度是一个仅涉及接收表面的量,与先前所描述的辐射源相关量相反。表示每个接收器表面接收的入射光的辐射功率 Φ,单位为 W/m^2。

只有在某些情况下,单束光的辐射强度与平面的辐照度相关。如果从光源到平面的距离大于 10 倍光源大小,此时辐照度等于辐射强度 I 乘以入射角 ε 的余弦值再除以距离 r 的平方(图 1.13)。

$$E = I\cos\varepsilon/r^2$$

辐射曝量 H_e：表示入射在表面上的辐射功率乘以时间。在光化学、光疗、光生物学中辐射曝量也被称为"剂量"。

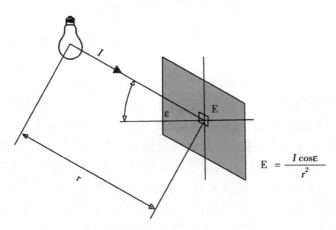

图 1.13　辐射量 E 的定义

紫外线辐射器的显著特性

对于所有已知的天然及人工光源,紫外线,可见光以及红外辐射,它们常常同时发生,虽然在各自范围内其辐射强度也可表现出较大差异,这取决于灯的类型[1-4,21]。通常将其分为紫外线辐射、可见光辐射、红外辐射;因为它给人以该光谱中心的初步印象或揭示其应用的主要领域。这些类型的辐射器之间的过渡是连续的,因此,其数值不可能是指定数值或其他极限值。

进一步分类,按照其物理结构和辐射器的设计,决定所产生辐射的性质,独立于其应用领域。依据该标准,辐射器设计的各个细节均要被充分考虑到,无论是在外部尺寸和内部结构,多个实例表明,可将其分为三类(图 1.14)。

第一类包括热辐射,固体和一些特殊情况下气体被加热直到它们产生有效辐射。大多数情况下它们发出与温度相关、具有物质特异性的连续光谱。该热

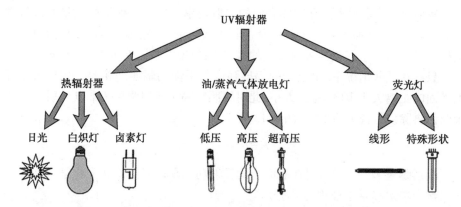

图 1.14 可产生辐射的物质

辐射最重要的代表是阳光。人们可以把太阳表面看作为具有大约 6000℃ 的散热器。

最普遍的人工热辐射器是白炽灯,其中的钨丝可被加热至约 2800℃,它的辐射发射主要是通过在线圈中产生的温度来决定[1,3]。家用的热辐射器还包括蜡烛(其中发光碳粒子代表辐射光源)及弧光灯中加热的碳插头。

第二类包括放电灯,通过电流或电场辐射将其中的气体或蒸汽激发[1,3]。在大多数情况下,该光谱呈线状或带状及典型的激发物质。灯泡内压力越大,其光谱越接近连续形状。包括大部分紫外线辐射器,通过选择合适的物质,在所需光谱范围内设置发射光谱的的中心是可能的。根据其产生的辐射类型,人们将其区分为气态,金属蒸气及金属卤化物放电灯。例如气体填充灯包括二氧化碳、氦、氖、氪、氮和氙。金属蒸气可通过铁、汞或钠产生,金属卤化物蒸气基于稀土元素钴、铟、镍、锡。近年来也有将气体和蒸气混合物作为辐射源(如氙和钠)。

第三类包括由荧光产生辐射的灯。首先气体放电产生高能量(短波长)的紫外线辐射,入射在荧光体层,然后被转换成较长波长的辐射例如可见光或紫外线辐射。其光谱形状可以是线型或带型。

按照初级辐射产生的类型,气体放电灯应包括荧光灯,但因特殊技术和经济原因,厂家将这些灯归为特定类。

根据产生机制,进一步细分其特征:
- 电气工作条件
- 几何尺寸
- 平均寿命
- 辐射输出
- 光、紫外光、红外光的特点

第1章 紫外线照射、辐射和剂量学

- 辐射场的辐射率及大小
- 燃点位置
- 色温[1]

由于辐射器形式及设计的多样性,使得找到正确的类型或评估其适用性往往很困难。在紫外辐射范围内寻找合适的辐射器较容易,因为在某些情况下,厂商将这些类型的灯整合在单独的列表中,或至少在其产品说明书中用独立部分说明[4]。

在经济方面,辐射器的选择要考虑操作成本和使用寿命。若想进一步了解,建议咨询相关厂家的工程师,因为凭借他们的经验,会提供更多信息,关于该灯的性能和工作条件[2]。

以下各段分别描述了市场上主要销售的紫外线辐射器及其特征。其中个别被提及的厂家名仅仅是为了便于寻找合适的类型,并不意味着其他没有被提到的厂家不具有该种类型的辐射器。

同类产品按照辐射产生的方式分类,可在产品列表中找到。因此,在本汇编中灯的技术数据参考仅以语句描述的形式表现[1,3,4,8]。

热辐射器

任何高于绝对零度温度(开尔文=-273°C)的物体均可发射电磁辐射。温度越高,辐射越强,短波辐射所占比例越大。在理想的情况下,全黑色物体表面不能反射任何光线,其强度和光谱分布只依赖于它的温度。因此,这些黑色物体或空腔辐射器的发射可用两种定律描述。

斯特藩-波尔兹曼定律(公式 1.11)指出物体总电磁辐射量与其温度的四次方呈正比。在这种情况下,总辐射表示零到无穷大之间的波长范围。

$$总辐射\ L=\sigma T^4,其中:\sigma=5.67\times10^{-12}\mathrm{W/cm^2K^4} \quad (1.11)$$

在此基础上,若温度加倍则产生的辐射能将增加 16 倍,如果温度增加 3 倍,则辐射能增加 81 倍。

表 1.5 所示:多种温度下,按照斯特藩-波尔兹曼定律计算所得黑体表面的辐射总量。

---

1 普朗克辐射器的典型光谱分布取决于它的温度,同时产生一种典型颜色。颜色是可见光的属性,并不能说明紫外辐射特性。

2 在一般情况下,现代灯具适用于普通照明,不像紫外线辐射可用于光学应用。一般照明用,其目的是使中短波紫外线成份最小化,以排除 UV 对健康造成危险的可能性。在某些情况下,也能防止辐射对材料的损伤,主要是塑料和着色颜料。为了实现这一目标,该灯的内部直接改变,在多数情况下,具有降低紫外线透射率的灯泡(关键词"停止紫外")都可以使用。通过这种方式,可以以数量级方式减少短波范围。

表 1.5 黑体表面的辐射总量及近似最大波长处的发射

温度 T(K)	总辐射量 L_e (W/cm²)	最大波长处的光谱发射 (nm)
1000	5.7	2890
1500	29	1930
2000	91	1450
2500	224	1150
3000	459	960
3400	765	850
4000	1465	725
5000	3580	580
6000	7420	480

空腔散热器 $S_{\lambda T}$ 的光谱强度根据普朗克定律计算。该方程(公式1.12)再次表明光谱分布仅由温度决定：

$$S_{\lambda T} = (c_1 \times \Delta\lambda) / [\lambda^5 \times (e^{c_2/\lambda T} - 1)] \quad (1.12)$$

其中 $c_1 = 3.72 \times 10^{-12}$ W/cm² 和 $c_2 = 1.438$ W·K

如果空腔辐射器(即普朗克辐射器)的光谱分布按照普朗克公式计算,则会出现以下关系:随温度升高,最大光谱辐射分布出现在较短波长处;在这种情况下,温度与最大辐射波长之间呈简单、线性关系:

$$\lambda_{max} = \nu/T \,(\nu = 2.898 \times 10^6 \text{ nm K}) \quad (1.13)$$

在普朗克阐明普朗克公式之前,上述关系已经被威廉·维恩发现。因此,方程1.13又被称为维恩位移定律(数值见表1.5)。

随温度上升,短波增加更为明显,长波所占总辐射越少。表1.6所示一定数量的波长范围内,辐射条带随温度增加而增加。表明达到3000K的紫外线强度即可应用于实际。

目前,钨丝白炽灯达最高可达3400K,碳弧的沟槽可产生4000K,可见光、UVA范围内,太阳表面可以被视为近似6000K的热辐射器。

表 1.6 空腔辐射器(黑体)-不同光谱范围所占辐射百分比

温度(K)	波长范围					
	220~280	280~315	315~400	380~780	780~1400	1400~3000
1000	10^{-15}	10^{-14}	10^{-9}	0.001	0.78	26.2
1500	10^{-9}	10^{-8}	10^{-5}	0.17	8.1	47.0
2000	10^{-6}	10^{-5}	0.002	1.70	21.0	48.8
2500	10^{-4}	0.001	0.033	5.94	32.0	42.1
3000	0.004	0.015	0.21	12.7	38.1	33.8
3400	0.019	0.058	0.59	19.0	39.7	27.8
4000	0.11	0.25	1.72	28.5	38.6	20.5
5000	0.74	1.14	5.12	40.6	32.3	12.5
6000	2.35	2.73	9.35	46.6	25.3	7.8

传统白炽灯

传统白炽灯是具有圈状钨丝的热辐射器。线圈-白炽灯泡发光电流通过之处,被安装在一密封真空或惰性气体玻璃灯泡内。常用钨丝作为线圈材料,因为它是所有金属中熔点最高的为 3653K。

同空腔辐射器一样,钨的光谱分布也取决于其温度,并遵循普朗克定律。但当计算其在紫外线区域内的能量分布时,往往会忽视以下两方面,从而导致问题产生:一是灯泡光谱的影响,二是钨表面的光谱特性[1]。

相比空腔辐射器,钨的发射率约为 0.40~0.45,由温度和波长决定。因此,在相同温度下,钨线圈的辐射率仅为空腔辐射器(黑体)的一半。

传统白炽灯,旨在光输出的良好结合,即高线圈温度和较长使用寿命。然而,这两个要求往往相互矛盾(见图 1.15),因此,一般普通照明灯的设计温度低于 3000K,寿命约为 1000H。如表 1.6 所示,这种温度下,紫外线辐射的输出很低,这种类型的灯不适合在实际应用中作为 UV 辐射源。

摄影等技术应用中的灯具,拥有高达 3400K 的色温和能透射 UV 的厚玻璃

---

1 基尔霍夫定律,吸收率 α=ε 发射。这意味着,只有一个全黑的表面(吸收率=1)能够生产全辐射功率。
另一极端是全白色表面(吸收率=0),无论温度高低,它都不能辐射。

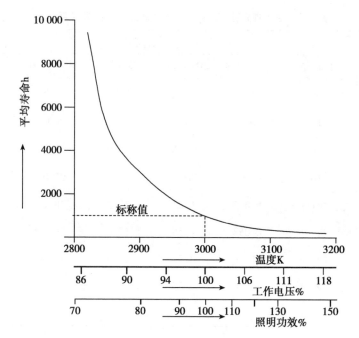

图1.15 白炽灯的平均使用寿命与温度、工作电压、照明功效的关系

灯泡。而其使用寿命仅为几个小时,因此,它们不能被用于紫外治疗。

科学应用方面,例如光谱仪器的校准,使用的是具有高度稳定性的灯,用钨条代替线圈及耦合的石英窗,将其发送到UV-C范围内。这些灯,商品名为WI17/G(商标OSRAM),其强度并不大,可用于250nm以下的光谱仪校准。

卤素白炽灯

在高温下,钨蒸发并在灯泡的内壁沉积。这导致灯泡发黑,并可以通过高填充气体而使压力降低;但限制设置为任何可能增加的、限制的机械强度的"梨形"标准的白炽灯灯泡。

为了减少这种灯泡发黑,可以添加少量的卤素(氟,溴,碘)作为填充气体。在较低的温度下,在灯泡壁附近发生聚合,然后又在附近的温度高的线圈处分解,形成钨卤素气态卤化物分解。在这一过程中,钨沉积在线圈,和卤素可再次重复这个过程(卤素电路工艺)。

通过这种技术进一步的优点是:灯泡可以大大缩小,在那小的、重的灯泡,充气时压力可能急剧增加;相反导致钨的蒸发明显减少。因此,对于相同温度的线圈,卤素白炽灯比标准白炽灯持续更长的时间。相反,线圈的温度可以提高紫外发射,因此较短的寿命仍然是可以接受的。根据目标应用领域的需求,这些灯都配有石英玻璃,信封硬质玻璃,或掺杂玻璃灯泡[1]。

卤素灯的小尺寸使其适合装在反射装置中。低压可达24V的卤素灯已经安装并准备使用,他们具有不同的光谱反射面,包括抛物线和椭圆的轮廓,在抛物面进行辐照的任务,在椭球面注入光波导。

在医疗行业中,卤素白炽灯的紫外线辐射目前在牙科用于硬塑材料。这个"紫外线"的特殊设计,主要反映了400~500nm的可见光和红外辐射。因此,强光和热负荷减少辐射场。

卤素白炽灯的最重要的技术性能列于表1.7。

表1.7 卤素白炽灯的主要技术性能

属性	值
工作电压	6~240V
功率,低电压型	5~150W
功率,高电压型	25~20000W
色温	2600~3400K
平均寿命	25~400小时
低电压操作	使用传统的或电子变压器
高电压操作	直接在线路电压

放电灯

放电灯产生辐射时,电流通过气体或金属蒸气。将最初不导电的气体变为导电状态,需要点燃每个灯。这是通过高电压的手段,它的应用作了简要的介绍和所产生的特殊设计的初学者或点火系统。电弧管中高的蒸汽压力,则更长的热身时间。这个预热时间可长达15分钟;在技术规格中可以找到精确的信息。

与白炽灯相比,随着电流的增加,钨电阻增大,从而在任何电压中变得稳定,灯有负电流-阻力的特性。也就是说,灯电流变大,放电路径的电阻变小。反过来,灯电流进一步变大。因此,无需外部电流控制,过热时放电灯被毁,甚至在操作初期。为了限制电流,所有的放电灯都必须与控制装置操纵。压载系统电阻

---

1 在卤素白炽灯尽管优势,即使这类"死"按照经典的老化机制:白炽线圈在中心最热和钨蒸发。然而,高蒸发导致的钨丝截面减小,这反过来又导致温度上升,直到线圈最后燃烧过这个位置。不幸的是,即使是卤素电路仍不能阻止这个过程,用于蒸发的钨实际上不是存放在其起点,但优先在冷线圈两端的电流引线,那里是没有受益或者辐射产生或线圈再生的。

是以其最简单的形式,预定电流流动成为了灯内的设计。

如果这是由欧姆的电阻来实现的,那么在消耗大量电力的过程中,甚至可能延长灯管的功率。此外,这种运行方式的经济性差,大量热量的产生也是一个令人不安的影响。这种类型的电流限制仅用于与功率低于5W或用于特殊应用的灯。例如,用于美容和治疗的ULTRA VITALUX®反射灯应用散热器的目的是同时产生紫外线和短波红外辐射。紫外辐射源是一个高压汞弧管;红外辐射是由钨线圈产生,同时也能产生镇流电阻的作用(图1.16)。

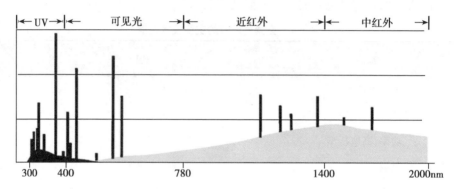

图1.16 ULTRA-VITALUX®紫外/红外辐射器(汞管;黑体辐射白炽线圈灰辐射)的光谱分布

然而,在传统的系统中,感应线圈或电容器作为镇流器,因为在交流阻抗的情况下,灯的功率的损失可以降低到15%~30%。

在长达15年的时间里,电子适配器系统也已商业化,减少功率损失也已进一步下降到3%~10%。此外,这些系统本质上也变得较轻,铁夹套的扼流圈,他们点燃灯更迅速,自从不在行频率上操作这些灯,他们具有无闪烁而更稳定的灯光,但有几千赫兹的频率或矩形电流的特性。

放电灯有多种尺寸和设计。主要的分类标准是产生的辐射和光谱输出的优势。以下类型用于商用:
- 低压水银灯(无磷)
- 高压水银灯
- 低压钠灯
- 高压钠灯
- 金属卤化物灯
- 高压氙气灯
- 高压氘灯

钠灯是个例外,具有低紫外排放,因此将不被考虑,以下各节描述的所有的灯和紫外线灯也可以作为紫外辐射源。

低压水银灯（无磷）

低压汞蒸气灯是管式散热器。它们可设计为条形灯、双灯管的和紧凑型荧光灯（发夹灯）。他们给一个纯粹的谱线,只有纳米级的宽度。这些灯的典型特征是在紫外线范围内的高辐射输出；254nm 线发射了高达 30% 的电力。低强度线出现 240nm 和 200nm 之间,其次是汞的共振谱线波长为 185nm,其强度达 10%~20% 的 254nm 的辐射,负责产生臭氧,因为它是由空气中的氧吸收。

灯是由无臭氧（OFR）（灯泡传输是 220nm）和臭氧（OZ）版本（灯也发射 185nm）提供设计。对于 OZ 类型主要的应用领域是水的消毒。水也传输 200nm 以下的辐射,使微生物在水中的分散性可由短波紫外线提供高能量辐射灭活。

这些灯的亮度低。因此,它们不适用于反射镜。然而,他们只产生少量的热量,因此可以在很短的距离产生高辐照度。

除了水的消毒其他的应用领域是空气消毒,除臭的空气,和医药产品的表面消毒。

低压汞蒸汽散热器的技术性能列于表 1.8。

表 1.8 低压汞蒸汽散热器的性能

属性	值
功率,紧凑型节能灯	5~24W
功率,L 形灯	4~115W
灯长	7~12cm
254nm 的辐射功率	1~35W
电源电压	125~240V
操作	使用电感镇流器或电子适配器系统。启动器是必要的点火装置
品牌名称	TUV 散热器,HNS 散热器

高压水银灯

这些是紧凑型灯,在大多数情况下,有一个椭圆形的球,含有水银称所谓的燃烧器。就像所有的气体放电灯一样,由于负电流-电压曲线这种类型的灯也必须在限流适配器系统下进行工作。点火后,将自动通过内置点火探头,几分钟内汞就完全蒸发并且形成了蒸汽压。这种高汞压力有两个作用:流量限制在放电管的中间,这样可产生高辐射(即,高亮度)。与低气压放电相比,发射光谱的中心转移,从 254nm 的光线到 365nm,以及 405nm、436nm、546nm、578nm 的 UVA。因此,相对于白炽灯,以其简单的工作原因,它的光输出高,高压水银灯的首要任务是照明。这种灯经济实惠,有几千小时的使用寿命,因此,目前还用于银屑病的治疗。HOK 或 HQA 是市场上现有的品牌,功率在 125~1000W。

一种特殊的高压水银灯是前面已经提到的 ULTRA VITALUX 散热器,其燃烧器是整合成一个蘑菇状的反射器。总功率为 300W 线可以拧在任何正常的灯(E27)上,因为这个简单的操作原理,现在仍广泛的在家庭系统治疗和化妆品的得到应用。

高压水银灯有 125W 的功率,也就是所谓的黑玻璃球,可吸收可见光和发射波长只在 365nm 的紫外线。不可忽视的是,由于这种灯对荧光强度的影响,它们也用于诊断。

汞高压灯照明用的灯作为 UV 的发射源是不合适的,由于他们的外壳在某些情况下还覆盖有荧光粉,可转换紫外光,因此只允许在一个微不足道的数量下发射紫外辐射。表 1.9 详细地描述了高压水银灯的技术属性。

表 1.9 高压水银灯性能表

属性	值
功率	125~1000W
灯长	130~39mm
功效 UVA、UVB、UVC	各 5%(最大)
电源电压	125~230V
操作	使用扼流圈,低于 220V 的电压,结合变压器和电感镇流器是必需的
品牌名称	HOK,HQA,HQS,HQV 散热器

金属卤化物灯

这种灯也是高压水银灯,但是增加了金属卤化物(图 1.17)。这些散热器不仅释放汞光谱,也是前面介绍的典型性能(表 1.10)。

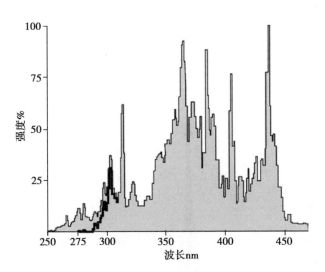

图 1.17 ULTRAMED® 金属卤化物灯的紫外线辐射器在 UVA、UVB 和 UVC 的光谱。粗线显示 UVA 和 UVB

表 1.10 金属卤化物灯的典型性能

属性	值
功率	150~2000W
灯长	50~200mm
电源电压	125~400V
光照的面积	0.5~5cm^2
操作	可能只能使用特殊的控制装置
点火	提供两种方法：冷点火（只有灯冷却后才能点燃）和热点火（在关掉灯后，可以立即再次点燃）。因为在这种情况下，高频点火的电压达几千伏电压，适当的筛选防漏电脉冲是必需的
品牌名称	ULTRAMED，ULTRATECH，HMIs，MsR，HPA，HPI

短弧汞灯（压力最高的灯）

这种灯的电弧管很小，他们几乎为点辐射源。他们在某些范围内相当于太阳紫外的范围。这种特性使它们也适合作为荧光显微镜和荧光内镜的辐射源。他们还成功地采用了单色的辐射源，具有高光强足够高的频谱纯度可用于光生物研究。

这种灯需要从水银蒸发开始工作，需要几分钟。事实上，这种灯的光谱的最大强度是显示在汞线的光谱区域的辐射值。然而，在几百条灯中线轮廓承受着普遍的压力，扩大到这样的程度，它可能是一个几乎连续的光谱。这些线的尾端重叠，所以与高低压灯相比，在整个范围内，每个波长都含有用的辐射，且主导线之间是低辐射地区(图1.18)。

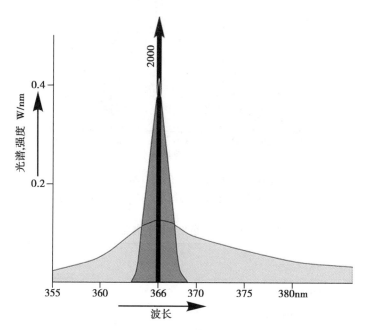

图 1.18 紫外汞线在 366nm 的低(黑色)、高(灰色)和最大(浅灰色)压力灯

一些功率低的灯的典型弧长是 1mm(照明领域只有 $0.25 \times 0.25 mm^2$ 的最小幅度)，即使在较大的物件中不超过 4mm 弧长度。

这些灯具有高辐射强度的特性，从而为光引导小直径。内置的椭球面镜，灯的亮度的总电场可印制在入口面，如果反射器利用孔径角及导光按 1∶1 的比例合理设计，仅略减强度且传输低损耗，这样的组装配件已有供应。

没有特殊类型的紫外线，但所有类型的紫外在使用 UV-AB 能提供足够的能量。灯的典型性能见表 1.11。

表 1.11 短弧汞灯的典型性能

属性	值
功率	50～8000W
灯长	5～45cm

属性	值
辐射面积	0.06~4mm^2
电力供应	根据不同的类型使用直流或交流电
操作	使用特殊的系统
品牌名称	CS,HBO

氙短弧灯

这种辐射源提供高亮度的可见光谱范围与在白天一样的。在工业应用中，它们主要用于电影放映和模拟太阳能。在科学领域，它们用于光化学反应，分析测量，并在光生物学研究中作为单色器照射源。像太阳光谱，灯发射的强度几乎同样覆盖整个可见光范围；仅在450nm和500nm之间的范围内有几个带状的峰。这表明色温的氙气辐射和太阳几乎是相同的(5800K)(图1.19)。

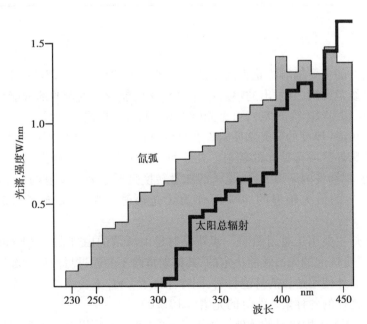

图 1.19 短弧氙灯和全球太阳辐射(太阳+天空)的光谱功率分布，两者的光度值相同

同样在紫外范围内，氙气放电显示在可见光范围内纯粹的连续光谱的强度比太阳光谱中的更大。较短的波长强度缓慢下降，但只受到灯泡所用材料的限

制。使用石英作为灯泡的材料，仍然可以检测到170nm的波长。

放电管中只含有稀有气体氙。因此，就像白炽灯一样，氙气灯点火后的几秒内达到辐射功率。

这种灯有一个更重要的特性是具有高度稳定性的光谱辐射分布，且在灯的整个寿命中辐射功率只有轻微的下降。这些特性和高辐射强度使氙短弧灯在紫外区具有良好的参考辐射源。然而，部分原因是由于成本，但也由于寿命（约3000小时最高），他们只有在特殊情况下用于照射治疗。

在一个类似的结构设计中含有氪灯，辐射中心的波长为220nm。表1.12集锦了氙短弧灯的一些重要性质。

表1.12 氙短弧灯的典型性能

属性	值	属性	值
功率	75～12 000W	电源	直流
灯长	8～48cm	操作	使用特殊的系统
光照的面积	0.25～40mm^2	品牌名称	XBO, CsX

荧光灯

荧光灯的主要辐射源是低压汞放电。该放电的谱线在185nm和254nm的短波紫外线范围内，其发出的辐射包含约50%的能量。剩余的部分能量分布范围在UVA和UVB（约20%），可见光（约20%），以及弱的红外线。

20～30μm厚度的荧光物质附着在灯泡壁的内表面，转化短波长紫外线、较长波长的紫外线或可见光的辐射。几乎每一个光量子都转换为波长较长的光子。然而，根据爱因斯坦关系，光子的能量转换是低于激发辐射的。一般来说，汞放电产生的最大辐射的50%可作为荧光辐射。然而，荧光灯却是最经济的灯。

荧光灯主要用于通用照明。紫外辐射是由所谓的白灯在约300nm强度低处发射，是由灯泡的光谱性能决定的，其辐射危险不会超过目前保护健康所规定的限值。另外使用适当的灯泡材料，同样保证了UVC不会渗透到外界。

用于光疗的各种紫外线灯的光谱（图1.20）。

位于UVA范围辐射的紫外灯用于光化学疗法、光疗以及日光浴和日光浴等大型场所。这些灯，最大发射波长在350～370nm之间；也有一些灯延伸到UVB范围的下限，但仍然有残余的紫外线和蓝光，因此在白色荧光灯中清晰可辨，甚至视觉上可见蓝色光的颜色。

灯的形状有线形、环形和U形灯。近年来，U形荧光灯已发展成为紧凑型节

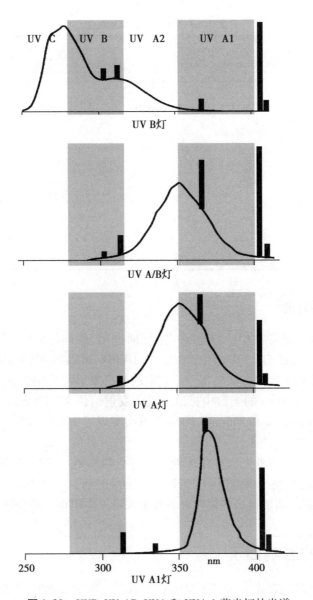

图 1.20　UVB、UV-AB、UVA 和 UVA-1 荧光灯的光谱

能灯,这些与白炽灯的尺寸相同;因其高光输出和更长的寿命,他们正越来越多地保留了白炽灯。这些紧凑型荧光灯也应用于特殊的紫外,例如,用于治疗头皮银屑病。表1.13列出了一些荧光灯的特点。

表1.13 荧光灯的典型性能

属性	值
功率,紧凑型节能灯	7~120W
功率,管形灯	40~100W
灯长,紧凑型节能灯	14~24cm
功率,管形灯	60~180cm
电源	125~230V
操作	使用电感镇流器和启动器或电子适配器系统。每种型号有其对应的系统
品牌名称	Light color 78 and 79, EVERSUN SUPERTL/10, 12, TL/09 CLEO

固态紫外辐射源

由于发光二极管(LED)的开发用于照明应用,紫外固体发光器件(这里命名为"UVED")也已自2001起生产。这些UVEDs可以用AlInGaN材料采用先进的半导体外延生长的方法制备[4]。它们的光谱发射特性相似,可见LED呈现钟形曲线在大约20nm的光谱中扩散。最大发射值位于247nm、254nm、264nm、280nm、304nm、338nm和365nm。2004年首次实现了UVED发射280nm的波长和1mW以上的辐射功率。

由于惯例使用紫外光源就意味着紫外辐射功率更小,但这种技术的典型优势是小而更坚固,快速调制时间(纳秒级的响应时间),由于非常小的产热使得表面接触射线,从而使得这些辐射源的在未来可以应用在一些特殊医疗技术中。

灯光辐射的影响因子

灯的规格包括在正常条件下灯的运行数据。但是根据时间、温度或机械和电气的调整,导致灯发射有变化。有时,灯泡材料改变的后果会不在可见光范围内,但是由于这种构造上的测量会导致紫外线辐射改变。

这些影响可以被否定,例如,通过照射时间延长或更好的冷却。与其他的影响相比,没有什么改变。因此,以下的章节提供一些可以承受的影响[1,3,8]。

灯泡材料对紫外发射的影响

滤波器中有未经处理的玻璃灯泡,即一切形式的透射光谱曲线,它不影响短波长的辐射。它在典型材料发射一个波长范围内的辐射且能透射到短波红外。图 1.21 显示关于这个的一些典型的例子。

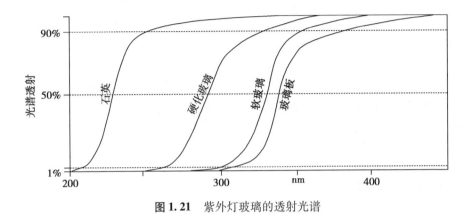

图 1.21　紫外灯玻璃的透射光谱

根据玻璃的成分,在可能在一定范围内削减 180nm 以下的真空紫外,而且在 315nm 的中波紫外线范围内,未经处理的灯泡眼镜和宽边眼镜总是在 340nm 的长波紫外线范围内透射。

对应于 1%、50% 和 90% 的表征截止滤光片它可以通过三个波长。在表 1.14 中,列出了常用灯泡的玻璃类型。

表 1.14　一些灯泡玻璃的光谱透射

玻璃的类型	光谱传输的波长(nm)		
	1%	50%	90%
宽玻璃 $d=2.5$mm	295	330	360
宽玻璃 $d=5$mm	310	340	380
软玻璃/钠玻璃	290	330	350
硬质玻璃/硅酸盐玻璃	260	290	340
高硼硅玻璃	210	230	250
石英玻璃	175	190	240
透明石英	165	175	220

挑选灯泡材料的热稳定性和耐化学性是其主要的过程。只有当进一步的选择标准依然存在时,光谱的透过率也被纳入评议。然而,在许多情况下,达不到技术和光学的要求,因此有必要对玻璃采取一些特殊的处理。

评估灯泡玻璃的透射光谱值时,有必要考虑它的温度依赖性。通常的目录仅指在室温下测定的值,而在工作温度下的性能对用户来说是十分重要的。所有的灯泡玻璃都有一个特性,随着温度上升,灯泡将向长波方向传输。

该位移的大小取决于材料性质,并且温度每升1℃,移动0.03~0.15nm。在800℃时,卤钨白炽灯和高压燃烧器的位移可能高达100nm[1]。

位移对于解决灯是否能发出 UV-C 或 UVB 的问题有帮助。根据记灯泡玻璃细节问题的手册上的记录,有这种可能性。然而事实上,如图所示,通过灯的光谱,紫外成分基本上是小于这些曲线的预期基础。

通过薄层改变灯泡的透过率

采用独特的技术:
- 改变玻璃的壁厚
- 染色
- 着色表面

灯泡材料的传输可被改变。这些过程主要应用在可见光范围内。与温度上升的原因有关,这些技术只能用于灯在不过高的负荷下。

通过涂层薄、干扰层等过各种方式可以改变灯泡的传输性。不是通过吸收而是通过选择性反射来达到效果,由于其高热稳定性的原因,因此当灯在高负荷的情况下,它不会使灯泡的温度直接上升。减少更换的可能性同时达到指定光谱范围的选择。

除了改变光的颜色,目前还有对涂层应用的技术。在第一层应用于白炽灯泡致反射红外线(红外反射涂层;IRC 层),使热辐射保留在灯泡内。这提高了灯的辐射输出,因为提供相同的辐射功率却需要更小的电能。目前能源节约约30%。

在第二层反射一个的高八度波长范围且能透射相邻的范围。应用于反光板时,所需的光谱范围只在主光束路径上反射,而其余的辐射由玻璃内部发射或吸收。首选的辐射可能在 UVA(图 1.22)、可见光或在红外线附近的范围内。

---

[1] 温度上升对移大小的影响,甚至可能没有对石英玻璃-超促进剂氙气灯进行测量的设备。氙气灯有一个很短的预热时间,在开灯时已经发射全光谱的光。根据表 1.14,Ultrasil 在室温下可发射 200nm 以下的光,由于氙气也在此范围内,臭氧必须在点火之后才能发射。这一过程迅速被典型"臭氧味"识别,然后在短暂的时间内再次消失(臭氧是一种无味的气体,刺鼻的气味来源于它们与臭氧结合形成氮氧化物)。然而,由辐射产生臭氧的上限约为 240nm,透射率必须被被超出此范围的灯泡材料加热后才能转换。

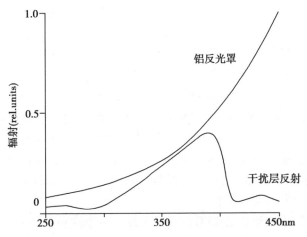

图1.22　反射镜通过光谱选择性的作用可以改变光谱

通过掺杂改变灯泡的透射率

可通过掺杂的玻璃进一步降低灯泡对紫外线过高的透过率。掺杂可以在制造过程中加入，加入少量的添加剂，以增加氧离子的键合强度，这对于辐射透射率是必不可少的（图1.23）。

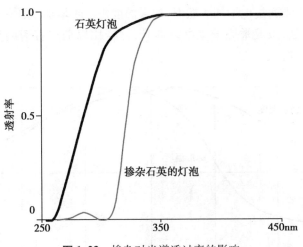

图1.23　掺杂对光谱透过率的影响

这项技术用在卤素白炽灯在普通照明时可以避免不必要的短波紫外线的辐射。

环境温度的影响

空气的温度对各种类型的灯的意义是不同的。所有类型的灯都产生少量的辐射,有些灯泡可以产生几百度的温度。因此,当使用这些类型的灯时,必须确保温度不超过安全水平,否则灯就会损坏。最常见的损害包括插座松动和灯泡爆炸。两者都会导致灯立即坏掉。

所有的高压放电灯和高功率的白炽灯都存在这些危险,而这些类型的辐射通量在很大程度上是独立于环境温度的。

低压放电灯(最重要的例子是荧光灯),对环境温度的辐射通量是明显相互依存的。这其中的原因可以在汞蒸气压力与温度的关系中被发现。

在较低的温度下,汞的数量不足以至于存在极少的电荷放电。随着温度的升高,激发的汞原子数量增加,却可以吸收自己的紫外辐射(自吸);因此,这种辐射不再是可激发的荧光材料。

标准的灯的最大辐射是25℃的环境温度。由于这种设计,最大光通量可在15~35℃之间被替换,所以户外作业时,灯可在15℃时可被优化,而35℃时的最大发光灯可以在封闭的室内用于照明系统。

根据现有的研究结果,蒸汽压力可以通过如扩大影响等物理的方法使表面的扭曲或通过对灯使用附加性手段,或用化学方法将汞合金是添加到灯中。在这一过程中"银汞合金技术"——在同一温度下形成较低的压力,所以,最大光通量只出现在更高的温度中。

这可能不是新的,但是,由于一些汞合金和相应设计修改的组合,如图1.24所示,温度同样光通量也增加。然而,如果温度进一步增加,汞原子增加,却不能激发它们。但是,激发汞原子也可以提升,这样比以前更普遍的灯可能被制造出来。

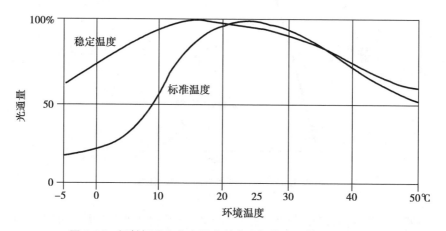

图1.24　辐射标准和稳定温度的荧光灯作为环境温度的函数

时间的影响

开灯后,需要一定的时间才能使灯达到全发射的状态(燃烧或升温)。根据不同灯的燃烧时间的范围,取决于电气和环境条件的变化而变化。为此,燃烧次数如表 1.15 中所列出的,仅提供翔实的参考值。

表 1.15 一些灯的燃烧时间和平均寿命

灯	燃烧时间	平均寿命
GLS 白炽灯	5 秒	1000 小时
卤素灯低电压		
$T_f = 3000K$	20 秒	3000 小时
$T_f = 3200K$	15 秒	200 小时
$T_f = 3500K$	10 秒	25 小时
卤素灯高电压	20 秒	1500 ~ 3000 小时
卤素灯红外涂层	15 秒	3000 小时
荧光灯:		
标准	5 分钟	10 000 小时
银汞合金	15 分钟	10 000 小时
无电极	5 分钟	60 000 小时
紫外荧光粉	5 分钟	300 ~ 1000 小时
紧凑型荧光灯	15 分钟	10 000 ~ 15 000 小时
低压汞(HNS®)	10 分钟	6000 小时
高压汞(HQL®)	15 分钟	15 000 小时
金属卤化物灯(HQI®,HMI®)	15 分钟	6000 ~ 8000 小时
氙气灯(XBO®)	10 秒	400 ~ 1200 小时
ULTRA-VITALUX®	5 分钟	1000 小时
ULTRAMED®	3 分钟	500 小时

灯在完成总的工作时间后或根据指定的标准会变为废弃品。可以用不同的方法或在使用中确定灯的寿命或平均寿命。不幸的是,大部分的灯具制造商没有说明这一点。因此,为了更好的比较,表 1.15 只使用了一个制造商的数据(欧司朗)。因此,只比较灯寿命特性而不是用不确定的方法来比较灯的寿命。

对于某些类型的灯,常用的开关周期对灯寿命的影响很大。例如,金属卤化物灯,每次燃烧8小时,当达到1小时循环切换应用时,6000小时的寿命降低到1200小时。另一方面,白炽灯的开关对灯的寿命没有任何影响。

进一步的影响

当灯运行时,还受到许多其他因素的影响,这些因素可以改变辐射的性质和灯的使用寿命。

- 工作电压应不超过5%的额定值;甚至低电压可以缩短灯的寿命。
- 镇流器必须是在有电源频率下使用。
- 电子镇流器是延长灯具寿命的首选。
- 通常燃烧的位置是由灯具制造商选择的。如果可能的话自己选择位置,以确保最高的辐射输出。

粒径较小的荧光灯具有更高的亮度,从而反射辐射强度更高多,辐射强度更高,发光效率更好(图1.25)。

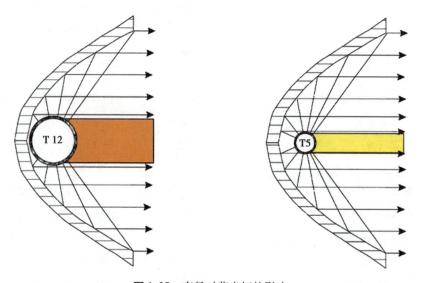

图1.25　直径对荧光灯的影响

日光

阳光与相邻波段的紫外线和红外线是地球生命的基本要求。我们总是有意或无意受其影响,其治疗作用人类自古以来已是众所周知的。然而,由于可用的人工辐射源可以在任何时间使用,自然光作为一种治疗剂在很大程度上已被取代。人工辐射源的强度和光谱分布可以用于也有不同的治疗功能。然而,日光也包含在用于医疗领域的紫外线,主要是用于比较人工光和自然辐射的性能。

特别要注意日光的光谱在日常和季节周期性的变化。

大气的地外辐射的光谱

光辐射从太阳到光球的总量,也就是太阳的最外层,其厚度约300km[5,23]。在色球层的上方,气态的日冕,辐射的选择性衰减是通过吸收来实现的。虽然在100万℃的温度以下,但因日冕的自辐射的光学密度较小,只占总太阳辐射谱的极小部分。

就其光谱辐射分布而言,太阳辐射并不表现为黑体。根据普朗克规律仅可能在一个指定温度的局部地区发展。在可见光和近紫外线,分布对应于5800K的黑体辐射。然而在这个温度的基础上,那些波长较短的区域可以预期的增加强度。在短波紫外线的范围内,光谱的分布对应只有4700K的黑体温度。

地面太阳辐射

当太阳光谱穿过地球大气层时由于空气分子出现散射和悬浮物的变化(悬浮颗粒)以及吸收大气中的气体和水蒸气[5,23]。紫外线的范围,在低于300nm范围内的波长被臭氧吸收,且其散射性极强。因此,太阳发出的短波长的辐射几乎没有到达地面,而较长的波则穿过大气层。相反,当太阳的高度越低,因其已渗透到更大的气团中,由于散射出现了可见的蓝天。

在紫外范围内,如图1.26所示,太阳高度角为45°对大气光谱的影响:太阳

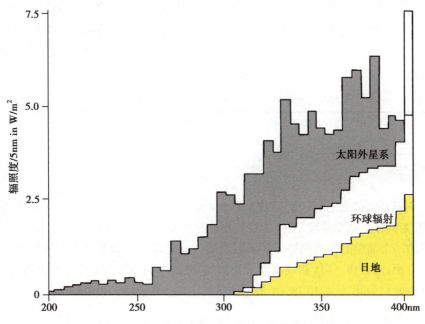

图1.26 太阳高度角为45°时地面光谱辐射全球

辐射、辐射全球和太阳辐射。全球辐射是太阳直接辐射和天空辐射的总和。

表 1.16 和表 1.17 表明,不同太阳高度角的光谱范围以及太阳直接辐射和天空辐射间接关系。

表 1.16 根据太阳高度角度计算出的太阳光照度和照度

太阳高度 (°)	照度 E (KL)	辐照度 E_e (iW/m²)			90°时太阳高度的比较(%)			
		总量	UVB	UVA	总量	可见度	UVB	UVA
90	120	1150	2.48	43.7	100	100	100	100
60	105	980	1.84	36.3	88	85	74	83
45	80	720	1.18	28.0	67	63	48	64
30	55	510	0.54	17.7	46	44	22	40
15	25	230	0.10	7.7	21	20	4	18

表 1.17 根据太阳的高度,天空和太阳直接辐射

太阳的高度 (°)	可见			UVB			UVA		
	太阳 W/m²	天空 W/m²	太阳/天空 %	太阳 W/m²	天空 W/m²	太阳/天空 %	太阳 W/m²	天空 W/m²	太阳/天空 %
90	510	90	570	0.87	1.61	54	26.2	17.5	150
60	450	97	460	0.55	1.29	43	20.0	16.3	120
45	345	86	400	0.24	0.94	26	12.6	15.4	85
30	200	78	260	0.06	0.49	12	6.2	11.5	55
15	70	50	140	0.01	0.09	10	0.8	7.1	13

紫外线辐射很大程度上取决于太阳的高度角。较低的太阳高度,紫外辐射的区域越少。

剂量学

剂量是尝试确定与计量[19]光辐射影响的方法。术语"尝试"已经重新被使用,因为,尤其在生物学领域,反应的是其复杂的性质(本书其他章节将介绍),精确的计算由一个简单的精准的描述是不可能的。只能提供典型紫外线影响的近似值。另一方面,随着30年代初现代人工光源的发展,人们寻找一个程序来比较光源的紫外性能。为此,活动相关的函数来测试预定任务中光源是否合适[1]。

---

1 辐射,"剂量"的标准化,是指一种光化辐射照射、照射时间和相应的产品。

现在,这些程序已经包含在 CIE[19] 国际建议或在德国标准 DIN 5031-10 中。它们中的一些也成为后继相关出版物的构成,例如在联邦健康公报中,美国食品和药物管理局报告或国际电工委员会(IEC)程序。在美国,由于紫外线辐射,在工作场所,规定辐照系统必须有已正式批准的有可能的有关健康风险已在 2006/25/EC 2006 年 4 月 5 日前完成,这同样也是欧盟指令。

计算活动相关的剂量,下面的量是已知的:
- 一个足够精细的光谱分辨率的 $E_{e,\lambda}$ 辐照度光谱分布
- 光谱依赖 $S_{actinic}(\lambda)$ 的活动相关的功能
- 照射时间 T

在数学上,根据以下公式得出照射 H 的定义:

$$H_{actinic} = \left(\int_\lambda E_{e,\lambda} \cdot s_{actinic}(\lambda) \cdot d\lambda \right) \cdot t \tag{1.14}$$

通常 $H_{actinic}$ 由 $\Delta\lambda = 5\,\text{resp.}\,1\,\text{nm}$ 计算总和:

$$H_{actinic} = \left(\sum_\lambda E_{e,\lambda} \cdot s_{actinic}(\lambda) \cdot \Delta\lambda \right) \cdot t \tag{1.15}$$

作用谱

通过光辐射产生的活性的中心光谱具有高效性,其中的一个或多个区域具有不同灵敏度,其活动性仍然可以被检测到。这个光谱依赖被命名为"动谱曲线"或对相关反应的"作用谱"[12,13,19]。

动作信号的频谱这可能与物理、化学或生物性相关,这一点已通过我们的实验研究确定。因此,由于个体敏感性的差异,以及由于不同的实验条件,也可以理解成在较大范围传播时产生了光谱的级数。因此,标准化的目的,往往使这些结果平均或简化。图 1.27 显示了产生红斑时根据作用光谱修改其大小[9,10,17,18]。

结合有关光辐射活动,应参考标准化的作用谱[6,7,12]。

图 1.28 中绘制了一些作用曲线。

光生物作用在许多情况下,只始于一个小的波长范围内,因此,在许多情况下,它们的坡度非常陡峭。但是,活动曲线不应与吸收光谱图混淆,这是依靠的有效证据。根据 Grothus-Drape 定律,只有吸收辐射才能引发反应,而相反的结论是,即任何吸收辐射量子也不可能出生特殊的作用。

光生物作用不仅限于紫外还发生在可见光谱范围内,例如,眼睛的亮度知觉活动曲线(即所有光学工程,是所有的测量系统照明工程的基础),颜色的感知,眼睛的蓝光危害,或植物生长所需。

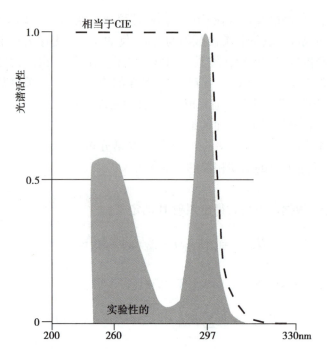

图 1.27 红斑的作用光谱:实验测定(安)和根据 CIE 推荐的标准化的红斑

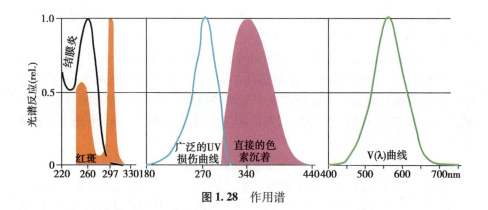

图 1.28 作用谱

作用相关量的计算

作用相关量的测定从量的光谱辐射分布的照射系统和作用谱开始的,归一化的值最大为 1。用于确定一个所谓的积分,这意味着这两个量,是非无穷小的符号,在小的波长范围内的辐射强度乘以谱相关的敏感性,再把这些单个的价值加到一起形成总数。

第1章 紫外线照射、辐射和剂量学

在图 1.29 和表 1.18,计算过程是通过参考数例来说明;为了保持数量在一定的范围内,只用一盏水银灯的中波紫外线光谱的最密集的光线作为辐射源。

$\sum Xe\lambda \cdot S_{eryth}(\lambda) \cdot \Delta(1)=100$

$\sum Xe\lambda \cdot S_{eryth}(\lambda) \cdot \Delta(5)=126$

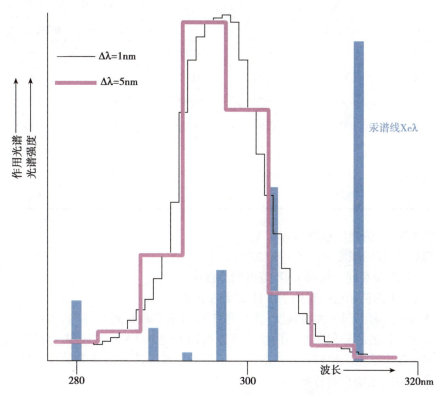

图 1.29 根据科布伦茨不同的权重在 UVB 范围,低压汞灯的光线致红斑的作用曲线(代表 5nm 的步骤和逐步演示 1nm 的步骤)

在图 1.29 中可见:
- 红斑的作用曲线逐渐到 5nm,作为已公布的标准表
- 红斑作用曲线插值逐渐到 1nm
- 低压汞灯 UVB 辐射线的辐射值

在表 1.18 中,你会发现:
- 第 1 列:线的中心波长
- 第 2 列:线的强度
- 第 3 列:在 5nm 的步骤红斑活动 Seryth(λ5)
- 第 4 列:在红斑活动 Seryth(λ1-nm 的步骤 1)

表 1.18　红斑作用的加权辐照度

1	2	3	4	5(列 2×3)	6(列 2×4)
汞线,发射	辐照度值	红斑光谱作用 $S_{eryth}(\lambda)$		红斑加权辐照度 E_{eryth}	
		5nm 步骤	1nm 步骤	5nm 步骤	1nm 步骤
				$S_{eryth}(\lambda) \cdot E_e$	$S_{eryth}(\lambda) \cdot E_e$
nm	mW/m²			mW$_{eryth}$/m²	mW$_{eryth}$/m²
280	300	0.06	0.06	18	18
289	160	0.31	0.18	50	29
292	40	0.99	0.87	40	35
296	450	0.99	1.00	450	450
302	960	0.19	0.37	182	355
313	1560	0.01	0.03	16	47
总计	3470			756	934

- 第 5 列:线的强度乘以 Seryth(λ5)
- 第 6 列:线的强度乘以 Seryth(λ1)

第 2、5 和 6 列已概括 UVB 范围的总强度。

这么小的例子已经说明了三件重要的事情:

- 非加权辐射不同于加权强度(比较第 2 列与第 5 和 6 列)。这些数量的差异取决于光谱的分布和作用曲线。所以我们不能从 UVA 和 UVB 内容加权作用中得出结论。比较不同光谱的作用仅基于波长范围可能会导致强烈的差异(例如,未加权的特殊作用光谱)。
- 光谱分布有不同的分辨率,光源以及作用曲线也可能导致差异。在这个例子中,可以发现 25% 的差异,光谱分辨率从 5 变化到 1nm。
- 陡峭的梯度作用曲线,大多只有一小的面积决定作用。在我们的例子中,在 296nm 光线的强度是总数的 13%,但当红斑作用曲线加权时,UVB 辐射达 50% 的总效应。

这些说明也适用于连续或混合光谱,对几百个人的计算可能有必要[1]。

在大多数情况下,紫外辐照系统操作员不知道光谱辐分布在物体表面上强度的绝对值,在大多数情况下,它也不可能为用户进行这些昂贵的测量。但这些值是确定活动相关数的前提。下面的过程是通过简单的测量来推荐确定的辐

---

[1] 以前这是一个艰苦的过程,但现在,它是一个自动数据处理程序。因此,最重要的生物作用的加权辐射量可用于所有的散热器,包括那些要求生产厂家印刷在产品规格中但却没有印出来的散热器。

射值。

为此,有必要要求生产商生产待遇光谱分布和可见光范围的特定紫外线。纵坐标值现予以规范,1000lx 照度产生图像评估。它甚至更好,因为这样可以节省计算工作量,如果直接给出所需活动有关的量,如 1000lx 相关。在第一种情况下,纵坐标必须在 $mW/m^2/1000lx$ 上,并在第二种情况下,必须是活动量/1000lx。

该测量仪采用目前市售的照度计,用来确定被照区域的照度。实测照度再除以 1000lx,再乘以输出值。因此,当测量值是 500lx 时值应减半;当 4000lx 时应插入 4 倍值。

这个过程有一个渐进的控制优势,其中由于老化和污染导致辐射下降的过程也被记录下来,在适当的地方,可以纠正。但在可见光和紫外范围的不同变化对测量精度有不利影响,因为在所有的情况下,参考是可见的。根据经验,这种情况可能会导致产生约 15% 的错误,但这在绝大多数情况下可以忽略不计。

剂量的测定

用物理公式,剂量可以写成:

$$剂量\ H = 辐射\ E_{actin} \times 照射时间\ t$$

单位:$(W/m^2 \cdot s)$ 或 (J/m^2)。

这个公式对所有的数量关系都是有效的。但在评价剂量造成的效应时必须指定范围,原因(辐照,辐照时间)和存在的效应之间关系的真实性。在此范围内,必须符合以下条件:

在 Bunsen-Roscoe 定律必须是有效的。这个定律是非物质,是否为同一剂量产生短暂的高辐照度或在长期内产生低照度。1000 单位的剂量是在时间 1 内产生 1000 的辐射和在 1000 的时间内产生 1 的辐射。

活动的可加性是有效的。在宽带辐射的情况下,不同波长的辐射参与活动的产生。必须确保所有的光谱范围产生影响,且可箱另一个方向移动,而且,根据其强度,这些个体的效应可能会线性相加后作为总的作用。如果 λ1 和 λ2 作用等于 1,同一时间内受到影响,那么两者的作用一定是 2。

放射活性的比例是有效的。一个光谱范围内的个体活动区别于另一个体时只能用比例因子。加权辐射,这个因素是相关波长活动曲线的值预定的。因此,任何可选择的波长强度为 1 和光谱加权为 1 的辐射必须产生相同的活动,同样的另一个波长的辐射强度为 5 和光谱加权为 0.2。

光生物复杂的反应过程和反应链形成光化作用的基础,这些条件只能大致完成辐照度水平以下的测定。三个例子可以验证这个概念:

众所周知，在紫外线导致红斑的情况下，没有泛红的皮肤甚至可以接受任意长时间的照射，由于反应结果与产生相比能更迅速的分解。在红斑的情况下，有必要把照射的时限定为 1 小时以上才能达到最初的反应。

产生所有等级红斑的剂量都不是零。如果光化辐射超标是指皮肤出现红斑潜伏期后（图 1.30）。

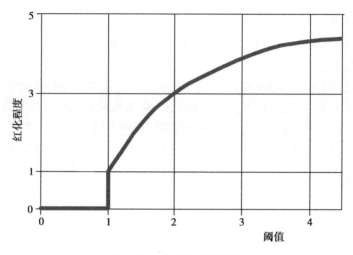

图 1.30　出现红斑的剂量

早在 1927，Hauβer 和 Vahle[17] 建立的皮肤发红曲线梯度是高度依赖于波长的（图 1.31）。在此基础上，级配变平的辐射波长缩短。这样做的结果是，250nm

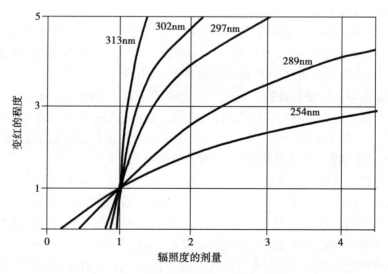

图 1.31　不同照射波长出现的红斑等级

的波长时皮肤发红的程度从 1 增加到 2,同时有必要再次进行 1.5 的剂量,为实现这一结果可采用波长 300nm 得辐射,只有 10% 的剂量达到 1。

此外,必须对皮肤类型进行测试,考虑到血液中的营养物质或药物产生的光感剂,能够增加特定波长的效果,在某些情况下甚至扩大整个作用谱。众所周知的例子是呋喃香豆素、补骨脂素。

阈剂量

表达"剂量"或"阈限"用于初始反应出现光化作用时需要的最小照射量。在医学上,这些主要是紫外线红斑,眼部的皮肤色素沉着、结膜炎、角膜炎的各种类型。如果响应辐射在延迟一段时间后不出现,照射和评估之间的时间间隔确定与阈值剂量也有关。

总结

测定阈值的实验条件和评估过程是标准化的或者至少目前在很大程度上得到认可的。但在几乎所有情况下,光化作用通过特定的照射产生的预测计算一个大的不确定的,且假设或物理性质的应用不能解释的光生物的过程。

甚至在仔细应用程序的情况下,相当数量的不确定性(测量和再生产)必须测定预期的阈值剂量。对于此评估的目的,不仅仅说明规范辐射源是必需的,例如,计算必须通过实验证明。

在某些情况下,它可以在文献中找到,在指定红斑阈剂量之前会就会出现典型的晒伤。这也就是说是光和时间的乘积是指定的多个红斑的阈剂量。

级数不同的波长有不同的级配曲线,它不再是可以简单的描述为光化反应为多的红斑阈剂量所需的剂量。首先辐射活性的比例必须先评估每个单独的波长。因此,在这种特殊情况下关于晒伤程度的平均辐照度的变化是无法通过根据照射时间与 Bunsen-Roscoe 定律计算后抵消的。

下面的描述在这些情况下是正确的:随着 X W/m^2 和照射时间 y 秒的红斑,在照射结束后的 Zh 观察到典型的红斑。然而,这样的声明才有意义,在这种情况下,这涉及一个经常发生的辐射水平,例如,正午的阳光;然而,这必须是指定的。

如果,然而,关于辐射范围已辐射这样的细节是不可用于观察晒伤的评估的目的,然后有关照射时间的数据,发生皮肤反应通过实验可以用公式表示。在这种情况下,对方程照射 H 的测定先决条件是不再满足于超越红斑阈反应的皮肤反应。

(刘清　江娜 译,罗权　林玲　孟珍 校,朱慧兰 审)

参考文献

1. Anonymous (1987) Pocket book of lamp engineering. OSRAM, Berlin
2. Anonymous (1987) International lighting vocabulary. International Commission on Illumination, CIE Publication No. 17.4
3. Anonymous (1993) Technical information—Principles of optical radiation. Philips Light, Hamburg
4. Anonymous (2006) Licht Programm 06/07. OSRAM, Munich
5. Bartels J (1960) Geophysics. Fischer, Frankfurt
6. CIE S010/E:2004 / ISO 23539: 2005 (E) Photometry—The CIE system of physical photometry, Commission Internationale de L'Eclairage, 01-Aug-2005
7. CIE S009/E:2002 (2002) Photobiological safety of lamps and lamp systems
8. Coaton JR, Marsden AM (eds) (1997) Lamps and lighting. Butterworth & Heinemann, Oxford
9. Coblentz WW, Stair R, Hogue JM (1931) The spectral erythemic reaction of the human skin to ultra-violet radiation. Physics 17:401–405
10. Coblentz WW, Stair R (1934) Data on the spectral erythemic reaction of the untanned human skin to ultraviolet radiation. U.S. Department of Commerce, Bureau of Standards, Research Paper RP631
11. DIN 5031 Teil 7 Strahlungsphysik im optischen Bereich und Lichttechnik—Benennung der Wellenlängenbereiche
12. DIN 5031 Teil 10 Strahlungsphysik im optischen Bereich und Lichttechnik—Teil 10: Photobiologisch wirksame Strahlung Größen, Kurzzeichen und Wirkungsspektren
13. DIN 5031-11 Strahlungsphysik im optischen Bereich und Lichttechnik—Teil 11: Radiometer zur Messung aktinischer Strahlungsgrößen—Begriffe, Eigenschaften und deren Kennzeichnung (draft standard)
14. Endres L, Fietz H (1989) Radiators. In: Erb W (ed) Introduction to spectroradiometry. Springer, Berlin
15. Gaska R, Zhang J, Yang J, Shur MS (2007) Solid-state ultraviolet light sources. Light Eng 15(4):51–52
16. Gobrecht H (ed) (1987) Bergman Schaefer Lehrbuch der Experimentalphysik Band III Optik. Walter de Gruyter, Berlin
17. Hausser KW, Vahle W (1927) Sonnenbrand und Sonnenbräunung. Wissenschaftliche Veröffentlichung des Siemens Konzern 6, p 101–120
18. ISO 17166 CIE S007/E (1999) Erythema reference action spectrum and standard erythema dose
19. Kockott D (1997) Second draft for a technical report of the CIE (CIE TC 6.08). Guidelines for determining action spectra
20. Koller LR (1952) Ultraviolet Radiation. Wiley, New York
21. Lompe A (1969) Technical-scientific proceedings of the OSRAM company, vol 10. Springer, Berlin
22. Meyer AEH, Seitz EO (1949) Ultraviolette Strahlen—Ihre Erzeugung, Messung und Anwendung in Medizin, Biologie und Technik. Walter de Gruyter & Co, Berlin
23. Schulze R (1970) Strahlenklima der Erde. Steinkopf, Darmstadt

第 2 篇

光(化学)疗法的临床应用

第2章 光(化学)疗法的机制

J. Krutmann, A. Morita, C. A. Elmets

内容

引言	53
历史观点	54
光免疫学的治疗	54
光(化学)疗法的光生物学作用	61
展望	62

要点

> UVB、UVA 和 UVA 联合补骨脂(PUVA)治疗对人类皮肤所产生各种免疫调节作用。
> 诱导皮肤浸润的 T 细胞凋亡是 UVA 治疗特应性皮炎的基本作用机制。
> UVA-1 和 UVB 诱导 T 细胞凋亡的作用机制有显著差异。

引言

紫外辐射(UV)成功用于皮肤病治疗已有几十年的历史并且呈一定比例持续增长,已成为现代皮肤病治疗中重要的一部分[28]。UV 的成功使大家开始研究 UVA 和 UVB 光疗的作用机制。该项工作所获得的知识对于治疗的决策是必不可少的前提条件,而不是凭借经验。现代皮肤病光疗才刚刚开始从这项工作中获益,很有可能将继续发展,帮助皮肤病医生改进光治疗方式,建立新的适应证。本章提供了关于当前的皮肤病光疗作用模式概念的概述。特别强调的是,我们已经确定了先前未认识的光(化疗)治疗的免疫抑制/抗炎原理。

历史观点

皮肤病中对 UVB 治疗反应良好的疾病是银屑病,它是以角质形成细胞过度增殖为特征的炎症性皮肤病。最初认为 UVB 光疗的抗增殖作用是通过 UVB 诱导 DNA 损伤而实现的[1,2]。然而,除了银屑病之外,其他许多皮肤病均对 UVB 和 UVA 治疗有效,这些不是过度增殖模式的疾病,而是免疫性疾病[51]。20 世纪 70 年代,经过大量研究首次发现 UV 辐射可影响机体的免疫功能。目前的普遍观点是 UVB,UVA,UVA 联合补骨脂(PUVA)治疗对人类皮肤产生各种免疫调节作用,这也对 UV 光疗的疗效至关重要。

光免疫学的治疗

迄今为止,所报道的免疫调节作用并非通过具体的某种单一方式而发挥。至少在体外实验中,UVB、UVA 和 PUVA 具有相似甚至相同的免疫抑制作用。而实际上,其治疗相关的免疫抑制作用是由 UV 类型的物理特性所决定的[3]。UVB 主要作用于表皮角质形成细胞和朗格汉斯细胞,而 UVA 可穿透至真皮层,可作用于真皮成纤维细胞、树突状细胞,血管内皮细胞以及浸润的炎症细胞,如 T 淋巴细胞、肥大细胞及中性粒细胞(图 2.1)。所有这些作用均能通过动物实验或体外培养人类皮肤细胞得到证实。对光免疫学的综合评估已经超出了本章讨论范围,读者可阅读对光免疫学作用讨论的更广泛的专著[23]。本章的重点是讨论和光疗相关的光免疫学作用,尤其是采用原位合成技术分析光(化学)疗法对患者皮肤所产生的免疫调节/抗炎作用。

总而言之,光疗相关的光免疫学作用分为以下三个方面:
1. 影响可溶性介质的产生
2. 调节细胞表面相关分子的表达
3. 诱发疾病相关细胞的凋亡

对可溶性介质的影响

光(光化学)治疗的治疗作用是由于诱导产生的介质具有抗炎、免疫抑制或二者均有来实现的。也有证据证明,光疗可抑制促炎细胞因子的产生。此外,UVA-1 治疗硬皮病的作用是通过产生可调节基质金属蛋白酶表达的因子而实现的。除了 UVB,UVA 和 UVA-1 均可调节可溶性免疫调节介质的产生[32,36],但 PUVA 对细胞因子、神经肽、前列腺素释放的影响目前还不太清楚。

第2章 光(化学)疗法的机制

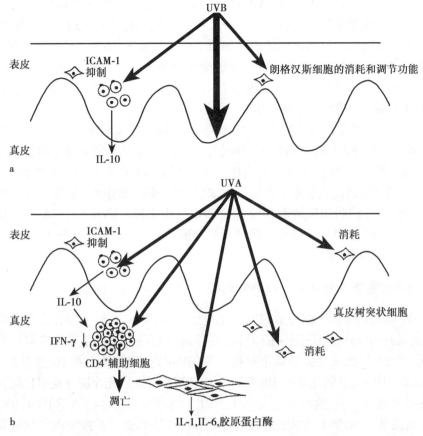

图2.1 UVB诱导的光(化学)疗法的免疫调节作用机制(a)或UVA-1诱导的光(化学)疗法免疫调节。ICAM-1,细胞间黏附分子-1;IFN-γ,干扰素γ;IL-10,白介素-10

对抗炎/免疫抑制因子的诱导

UVB或UVA的治疗作用一部分可归因于其可诱导分泌具有抗炎/免疫抑制作用的介质。体外培养人类角质形成细胞实验证明UVB,甚至UVA辐射可以诱导其产生细胞因子、神经肽、前列腺素。例如,IL-10是角质形成细胞来源的具有特殊治疗作用的细胞因子,它能够抑制辅助Th1淋巴细胞分泌干扰素(IFN)-γ。人类角质形成细胞能否分泌IL-10曾有争议,但最近的体内外研究指出,经UVB,特别是UVA1照射后,培养皿中的人类正常角质形成细胞IL-10mRNA及其蛋白表达增多,人体皮肤经UV辐射照射后,表皮角质形成细胞IL-10蛋白表达增多[10,11]。特应性皮炎的有效光疗(UVA-1或UVA/UVB)与其IFN-γ表达水平降低有关[9]。光疗诱导的IL-10表达和随后的IFN-γ产生的旁分泌抑制可能,至少部分解释了光疗的这种效应。

另一个例子是 UVB 和 UVA-1 辐射后诱导角质形成细胞产生可溶性因子，神经肽 α-促黑素细胞激素（α-MSH）来发挥抗炎或免疫抑制作用。UVB 辐射后的角质形成细胞的促黑素细胞激素的衍生肽包括 α-MSH 增加或合成增多[32]。α-MSH 具有多种抗炎（如抑制 IL-1 和肿瘤坏死因子（TNF）-α 介导的炎症反应）和免疫抑制（如抑制细胞介导的免疫应答）作用。因此可以推测 UV 辐射诱导 α-MSH 是的 UV 诱导的抗炎机制的一部分。

第三个例子是 UVB 和 UVA 辐射诱导表皮角质形成细胞产生前列腺素[8]。前列腺素（PG）E2 具有强烈的免疫抑制作用，它可以影响抗原递呈细胞表面协同共刺激因子的表达，从而抑制选择性 T 细胞亚群（尤其是 Th1 类细胞）的活化[12]。最新的研究表明除了角质形成细胞，UV 辐射的朗格汉斯细胞可以成为产生具有免疫抑制作用的前列腺素的重要细胞来源。UVB 和 UVA-1，尤其是 UVA-1，照射人类树突状细胞可诱导环氧合酶的活性，引起大量 PGE_2 和血栓素释放（J. Krutmann 等）。

UV 诱导细胞因子对水解蛋白酶的调控

UV 辐射诱导的可溶性细胞因子还包括 IL-1、IL-6，它们可以分泌促炎症因子，从而对治疗产生不利影响。然而，有趣的是 UVA-1 能够成功治疗局限性硬皮病，与光疗后改善皮损基质金属蛋白酶（MMP）-1 的表达上调 20 倍相关[47]。硬皮病患者的皮肤硬化是由于胶原的产生和沉积增加。光疗诱导皮损软化和硬皮皮损外观的恢复，这可能与其诱导 MMP-1 的产生有关。类似于 UVB，UVA-1 可能直接诱导 MMP-1 蛋白酶的表达，但是，在体外真皮成纤维细胞实验研究显示 UVA-1 诱导的 MMP-1 表达部分与 UVA-1 诱导的细胞因子 IL-1，IL-6 自分泌机制有关[52]。至少在治疗皮肤硬皮病中，高剂量 UVA-1 诱导产生的促炎症细胞因子是有利的而不是有害的。

影响细胞表面受体

越来越多的证据显示 UVB、UVA 和 PUVA 治疗能够直接影响细胞表面受体的表达和功能，这些受体包括黏附分子、细胞因子和生长因子受体。

调节黏附分子表达

银屑病、特应性皮炎和皮肤 T 淋巴细胞瘤等皮肤病对 UV 或 PUVA 治疗效果良好，与这些患者的表皮角质形成细胞表面的细胞间黏附分子（ICAM-1）的表达增多[31]有关。ICAM-1 是淋巴功能相关抗原（LFA）-1 的配体，存在于白细胞表面。体内外实验均证实 ICAM-1/LFA-1 调节细胞与细胞间的黏附，是皮肤各种炎症和免疫反应产生和维持的重要前提[21,25-28]。人类正常皮肤，角质形成细胞表面不表达或少表达 ICAM-1。而炎症皮肤显著不同，ICAM-1 表达明显上调，其原因是前炎症因子包括 IFN-γ, TNF-β 和 TNF-α 对角质形成细胞的刺激[31]。光疗让我们认识到亚致死量 UVB 或 UVA 照射人工培育的角质形成细胞可有效抑制细胞因子诱导的 ICAM-1 的表达。

UV 辐射的抗炎特性也可在体内研究中观察到[44,49]。亚致死剂量的 UVB 照射在人类皮肤，足以有效的抑制角质形成细胞 ICAM-1 表达上调，后者可通过皮内注射重组干扰素 γ 诱导。只有当 UVB 照射发生于细胞因子刺激之前，体内外才可观察到 ICAM-1 表达受到抑制。进一步的研究发现实际上 UVB 诱导的 ICAM-1 产生抑制是短暂的，因为研究者观察到 UVB 辐射后 24 小时，角质形成细胞 ICAM-1 大量表达[20,40]。如果在第一次 UVB 照射后 24 小时再照射一次，将再次诱导 ICAM-1 抑制，这说明持久的抗炎作用需要重复 UVB 辐射。

UV 抗炎作用的基因调控机制暂不清楚。细胞因子诱导 ICAM-1 表达抑制不依赖于 ICAM-1 诱导细胞因子的性质[20]。UVB 辐射不能通过干扰特殊细胞因子诱导的细胞内信号转导，而是通过更为常见的机制来抑制诱导基因转录。后者通过大量的研究得以证实，UVB 辐射也抑制其他细胞因子诱导的基因上调，包括 HLA-II 类细胞因子和 IL-7 的上调[15]。

PUVA 治疗使银屑病患者皮损处细胞因子 ICAM-1 表达明显减少[31]。然而目前并没有足够的证据表明 PUVA，如同 UVB 和 UVA 一样能够直接调节细胞因子诱导 ICAM-1 表达。PUVA 治疗诱导细胞因子 ICAM-1 表达下调可能通过间接机制，如细胞因子生成下调，炎症细胞浸润均可减少 ICAM-1 表达。

除了角质形成细胞，UVB 辐射能够显著抑制抗原递呈细胞如单核细胞或表皮朗格汉斯细胞细胞间分子的表达[19,45]。这些下调作用主要影响 ICAM-1 分子和 B7 家族成员。UVB 辐射诱导的细胞间黏附因子表达抑制作用与其功能相关，这是因为抗原递呈细胞共刺激的信号改变使效应性 Th1 细胞无能，优先激活调节 Th2 细胞。

以细胞因子和生长因子受体为靶点

角质形成细胞来源的 IL-1-α 是启动皮肤炎症最重要的细胞因子之一。因此，角质形成细胞 IL-1 受体表达在皮肤炎症反应过程中发挥重要的作用。人类表皮形成细胞表达两种不同的 IL-1 受体分子：IL-1 I 型受体（IL-1R I）和 IL-1 II 型受体（IL-1R II）。这些分子在功能上完全不同，IL-1R I 是信号受体，然而 IL-1R II 不介导 IL-1 诱导的信号的传递，IL-1R II 作为一个诱骗受体发挥限制和抑制 IL-1 介导的细胞应答的作用。由此光疗在于了解 UV 辐射对人类角质形成细胞 IL-R I 和 IL-R II 的调节作用的不同[13]。UVB 辐射后 IL-1R II 的表达快速急剧增多，然而，IL-1R I 的表达同时减少（虽然晚一些时候逐渐增多）。由此推测，UVB 可能通过以下 2 个途径限制炎症状态下 IL-1 激活角质形成细胞所产生的过度应答。

1. 上调诱导受体 IL-1RⅡ的表达
2. 下调信号分子 IL-1RⅠ的表达

UVB 辐射不仅下调 IL-1α 信号受体,也可以下调包括 TNFα 在内的其他细胞因子的受体。体外实验中将人类角质形成细胞暴露于亚致死剂量的 UVB 辐射中最初可以下调 TNFα 受体 55kDa mRNA 和蛋白的表达,随着 TNF 受体再表达,最终超过基线水平[50]。此外,在 TNF 受体表达减少时,UVB 辐射的角质形成细胞对 TNF 的反应性明显降低。UVB 辐射不影响人类角质形成细胞释放可溶性 TNF 受体。与之类似,UVB 或 UVA-1 辐射也不影响人类角质形成细胞产生可溶性 ICAM-1 分子[22]。除了细胞因子,生长因子受体如表皮生长因子受体(EGF)也是 UV 和 PUVA 治疗中的靶分子。EGF 受体表达和功能的调节在 UV 辐射诱导的基因表达有关的信号传导级联反应中居于核心地位。这些研究直接分析了哺乳动物细胞中的压力反应,运用的 UV 辐射剂量对治疗影响不大。然而相反,PUVA 治疗影响 EGF 受体功能。在哺乳动物和人类细胞中,PUVA 辐射抑制 EGF 与其受体的结合[30]。EGF 是促进角质形成细胞生长的因子,银屑病一种以角质形成细胞过度增殖为特征的皮肤病,我们推测 PUVA 可能通过抑制 EGF 结合在银屑病治疗中发挥作用。

诱发皮肤浸润细胞凋亡

相比其他细胞,如单核细胞或角质形成细胞而言,UV 辐射更易诱导 T 细胞凋亡。MoriTa 等人首次证实诱发皮肤浸润 T 细胞凋亡是 UVA 治疗特应性皮炎的机制[37]。特应性皮炎是 T 细胞介导的皮肤病,辅助 T 细胞被吸入性抗原(特异性抗原)激活,导致 T 细胞因子产生,随后发生湿疹样改变。此过程包括早期激活阶段,此阶段 Th-2 样细胞表达占有重要地位,随后进入第二个阶段[14]。第二个阶段的特点是 Th-1 样细胞因子 IFN-γ 占优势,产生和维持临床可见的湿疹样改变。UVA-1 辐射成功治疗特应性皮炎与皮肤浸润 T 细胞数量明显减少和随后在皮损处 IFN-γ 表达下调有关[9]。MoriTa 等人用双标技术鉴定 CD4$^+$T 细胞,凋亡 T 细胞,他的研究证明 UVA-1 诱导的辅助 T 细胞凋亡发生于特应性湿疹的真皮部分。仅仅将患者短暂的暴露于 130J/cm^2 UVA-1 辐射下,患者皮疹处可见 CD4$^+$,凋亡 T 细胞[37]。连续 UVA-1 辐射使辅助 T 细胞凋亡数量逐渐增多,随后炎症细胞浸润减少,临床症状改善。

诱发 T 细胞凋亡作用不是 UVA 光疗所特有的[6,17,33,55]。UVB 治疗的银屑病患者随着角质形成细胞形态学的正常化,浸润的 T 细胞数目减少。UVB 辐射体外诱导 T 细胞凋亡提示炎症浸润的减少是由于 UVB 辐射诱导 T 细胞凋亡引起的[17]。这种假说目前在对经过 UVB 光疗的银屑病患者皮损处凋亡 T 细胞的观察得到证实[41]。无论宽谱 UVB 或 311nm UVB 光疗均可诱导 T 细胞凋亡。然而值得注意的是,因其物理特性,311nm UVB 辐射可穿透皮肤真皮,故表皮和真皮中的 T 细胞均可发生凋亡。这种不同至少可以解释为何 311nm UVB 在治疗银屑病中的作用优于宽谱 UVB[42]。

诱导 T 细胞凋亡也是 PUVA 治疗的核心机制。有证据表明将 Sézary 综合征患者的外周血 T 细胞进行体外光化学免疫疗法,可见 PUVA 治疗后出现凋亡 T 细胞[55]。有趣的是诱导细胞凋亡不引起免疫失活,而是出现免疫抑制。吞噬凋亡细胞对单核巨噬细胞产生中间介质产生深远的影响[54]。凋亡 T 细胞被吞噬之后,巨噬细胞产生的抗炎/免疫抑制因子 IL-10 增多,而产生的促炎症因子如 TNF-α,IL-1 和 IL-12 减少[4,54]。进一步的研究显示自分泌产生 TGF-β 介导了对促炎细胞因子产生的抑制[34]。此外,选择性趋化因子生成增多,特别是 Mip-1-α 和 Mip-2。这些研究合理的解释了体外光化学免疫疗法的作用,通过诱导少部分外周血循环中的 T 细胞凋亡,产生免疫抑制作用,这个观点也在移植免疫中被证实。

UVA-1 和 UVB 诱导 T 细胞凋亡的机制有明显不同。在一般情况下,UVA-1 辐射能够引起预排程序的细胞死亡(早期凋亡),其蛋白独立合成,以及细胞程序性死亡(晚期凋亡),需要新的蛋白合成[5]。相反的,UVB 辐射(和 PUVA 治疗)只诱导晚期凋亡[6]。Morita 等人发现,对于 UVB 所致放射性皮炎的患者,UVA-1 辐射能够引起早期和晚期凋亡,UVA-1 辐射诱导的单线氧的产生是诱导 T 细胞凋亡的激发事件[37]。UVA 辐射诱导产生的单线态氧诱导 T 细胞 Fas 配体的表达。随后 Fas 配体与相同或邻近的 T 细胞表面的 Fas 结合诱发 T 细胞凋亡(图 2.2)。近期有关 Jurka T 细胞的独立研究证实了单线态氧在诱发人类 T 细胞早期凋亡中的重要作用。我们推测紫外线 A-1 辐射/单线态氧通过打开多通道和减少线粒体膜蛋白而作用于线粒体,诱导 Jurkat 细胞凋亡[6]。对 UVA-1 和单氧而言,其诱导哺乳动物细胞早期凋亡的能力是非常特殊和重要的。

以光疗的观点而言,这种性质上差异提示其在某些以炎症细胞增殖为其主要发病机制的皮肤病中可诱导细胞凋亡,因此,UVA-1 光疗优于 UVB 和 PUVA 治疗。研究显示,UVA-1 而非 PUVA 可诱导色素性荨麻疹患者皮肤浸润的肥大细胞凋亡,从而证实了以上假说(图 2.3)。结果,

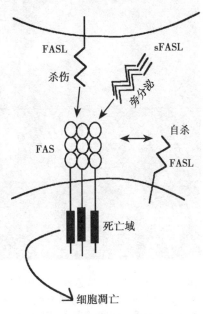

图 2.2 诱导 T 细胞凋亡机制示意图。sFASL,血清可溶性 Fas 配体

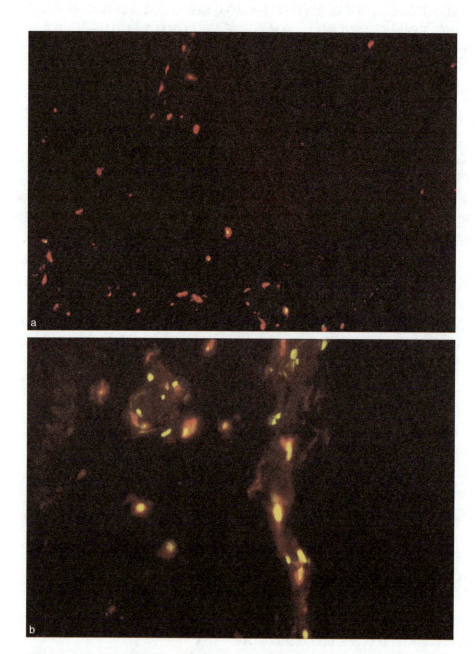

图 2.3 色素性荨麻疹患者皮损中的凋亡的肥大细胞在紫外线光疗前（a）和后（b）对照（3×130J/cm²）。红色是被抗肥大细胞胰蛋白酶抗体染色的肥大细胞,绿色是被末端脱氧核苷酸转移酶介导的 dUTP 缺口末端标记测定法（TUNEL）染色的凋亡细胞。橙色为细胞凋亡的肥大细胞

UVA-1 光疗,而非 PUVA,清除皮肤肥大细胞,使这些患者长期处于缓解期[46,48]。UVA-1 辐射的特性可用于治疗皮肤 T 细胞淋巴瘤[43]。体外实验研究发现恶性 T 细胞对 UVA-1 辐射诱导的凋亡非常敏感,UVA-1 治疗此疾病至少与 PUVA 相当[38]。

光(化学)疗法的光生物学作用

UVB 和 UVA-1 辐射发挥了几种光治疗相关的光调节作用,如诱导 IL-10 产生或抑制 ICAM-1 的产生。然而,不同的 UV 辐射类型,其免疫调节作用是不同的[24]。

和抗细胞增殖的作用类似,UVB 的免疫调节作用主要是由于 UVB 辐射诱导产生的 DNA 光产物诱导产生的,尤其是胸腺嘧啶。UVB 辐射可以抑制 IFN-γ 刺激角质形成细胞 ICAM-1 的表达,这与 UVB 照射人类皮肤诱导大量的胸腺嘧啶产生有关[49]。

局部使用 DNA 修复酶脂质体不仅能够使皮肤胸腺嘧啶二聚体阳性的角质形成细胞的数量减少 40%~50%,而且能够完全阻止 UVB 诱导的 ICAM-1 的抑制。在体外培养的小鼠角质形成细胞中,评估了胸腺嘧啶二聚体在 UVB 辐射诱导产生 IL-10 中的作用,得到了相同的结果[39]。鼠科动物的角质形成细胞(PAM212 细胞)胸腺嘧啶合成和 IL-10 表达与其 UVB 暴露呈剂量依赖关系,外源性 DNA 修复酶足以部分减少胸腺嘧啶的数量,同时可以完全抑制 UVB 辐射诱导的 IL-10 蛋白的合成。对胸腺嘧啶的部分逆转和对免疫调节作用的总体抑制,如 IL-10 蛋白合成或 ICAM-1 诱导抑制,这二者之间的矛盾目前还不清楚。因此可以推测基因特异性修复机制可解释这种现象。因此,胸腺嘧啶二聚物的产生是 UVB 辐射诱导治疗作用的核心。然而,UVB 辐射还有可能是独立于 DNA 损伤外的细胞膜作用[29]。

与 UVB 相比,UVA-1 诱导的免疫抑制作用的基础是氧化机制[22]。单线态氧的产生起重要作用。UVA 辐射诱导的基因调控事件,主要通过以下三点: UVA 辐射诱导的基因调节事件如 ICAM-1 的调控或胶原酶 I 表达能够:

1. 被单线态氧抑制
2. 通过增加单线态氧的半衰期而增强其作用
3. 用单线态氧产生系统刺激未经辐射的细胞可模拟此作用[7,53]

最近的研究发现 UVA 辐射和单线态氧诱导的基因表达均需通过转录因子 AP2 激活来介导,UVA 辐射诱导的基因表达通过 AP2 和其选择性片段产物 AP2B 来控制,这些研究有助于解释其机制[7]。单态氧不仅是 UVA 辐射诱导基因调控的重要机制,且在人类 T 辅助细胞中 UVA 辐射诱导凋亡起重要作用[37]。

PUVA 诱导免疫抑制作用还未被阐明。

展望

研究证实,光(生物)学治疗不简单是利用其抗增殖作用,更多的是与免疫调节作用有关,其中某些已在前文提到。然而,大量的光免疫学研究均基于离体或动物模型,直到最近原位技术才被用于监测 UV 辐射后患者皮肤的免疫改变。这些研究加强了我们对 UVA 和 UVB 光疗方法的认知,例如,确定识别凋亡细胞是光线疗法治疗 T 细胞介导的皮肤病的核心机制。这些成果将更迅速的运用于临床研究,即称为"光免疫治疗学"。

(周欣 译,张尔婷　孟珍　校,朱慧兰　审)

参考文献

1. Bevilaqua PM, Edelson RL, Gasparro FP (1991) High performance liquid chromatography analysis of 8-methoxypsoralen monoadducts and crosslinks in lymphocytes and keratinocytes. J Invest Dermatol 97:151–155
2. Epstein JH (1968) UVL-induced stimulation of DNA synthesis in hairless mouse epidermis. J Invest Dermatol 52:445–448
3. Everett M, Yeargers E, Sayre R, Olson R (1966) Penetration of epidermis by ultraviolet rays. Photochem Photobiol 5:533–542
4. Fadok VA, Bratton DL, Konowal A, Freed PW, Westcott JY, Henson PM (1998) Macrophages that have ingested apoptotic cells in vitro inhibit proinflammatory cytokine production through autocrine/paracrine mechanisms involving TGF-ß, PGE2, and PAF. J Clin Invest 101:890–896
5. Godar DE (1996) Preprogrammed and programmed cell death mechanisms of apoptosis: UV-induced immediate and delayed apoptosis. Photochem Photobiol 63:825–830
6. Godar DE (1999) UVA 1 radiation mediates singlet-oxygen and superoxide-anion production which trigger two different final apoptotic pathways: the S and P site of mitochondria. J Invest Dermatol 112:3–12
7. Grether-Beck S, Olaizola-Horn S, Schmitt H, Grewe M, Jahnke A, Johnson JP, Briviba K, Sies H, Krutmann J (1996) Activation of transcription factor AP-2 mediates UVA radiation- and singlet oxygen-induced expression of the human intercellular adhesion molecule-1 gene. Proc Natl Acad Sci USA 93:14586–14591
8. Grewe M, Trefzer U, Ballhorn A, Gyufko K, Henninger HP, Krutmann J (1993) Analysis of the mechanism of ultraviolet B radiation induced prostaglandin E2 synthesis by human epidermoid carcinoma cells. J Invest Dermatol 101:528–531
9. Grewe M, Gyufko K, Schöpf E, Krutmann J (1994) Lesional expression of interferon-γ in atopic eczema. Lancet 343:25–26
10. Grewe M, Gyufko K, Krutmann J (1995) Interleukin-10 production by cultured human keratinocytes: regulation by ultraviolet B and ultraviolet A1 radiation. J Invest Dermatol 104:3–6
11. Grewe M, Duvic M, Aragane Y, Schwarz T, Ullrich SE, Krutmann J (1996) Lack of induction of IL-10 expression in human keratinocytes. Reply. J Invest Dermatol 106:1330–1331
12. Grewe M, Klammer M, Stege H, Krutmann J (1996) Involvement of direct and indirect mechanisms in ultraviolet B radiation (UVBR)-induced inhibition of ICAM-1 expression in

human antigen presenting cells. Abstract. J Invest Dermatol 106:933
13. Grewe M, Gyufko K, Budnik A, Berneburg M, Ruzicka T, Krutmann J (1996) Interleukin-1 receptors type I and type II are differentially regulated in human keratinocytes by ultraviolet B radiation. J Invest Dermatol 107:865–871
14. Grewe M, Bruijnzeel-Koomen CAFM, Schöpf E, Thepen T, Langeveld-Wildschuh AG, Ruzicka T, Krutmann J (1998) A role for Th1 and Th2 cells in the immunopathogenesis of atopic dermatitis. Immunol Today 19:359–361
15. Khan IU, Boehm KD, Elmets CA (1993) Modulation of IFNγ-induced HLA-DR expression on the human keratinocyte cell line SCC-13 by ultraviolet radiation. Photochem Photobiol 57:103–106
16. Kripke ML (1981) Immunologic mechanisms in UV radiation carcinogenesis. Adv Cancer Res 34:69–106
17. Krueger JG, Wolfe JT, Nabeja RT, Vallat VP, Gilleaudeau P, Heftler NS, Austin LM, Gottlieb AB (1995) Successful ultraviolet B treatment of psoriasis is accompanied by a reversal of keratinocyte pathology and by selective depletion of intraepidermal T cells. J Exp Med 182:2057–2068
18. Krutmann J, Koeck A, Schauer E, Parlow F, Moeller A, Kapp A, Foerster E, Schoepf E, Luger TA (1990) Tumor necrosis factor β and ultraviolet radiation are potent regulators of human keratinocyte ICAM-1 expression. J Invest Dermatol 95:127–131
19. Krutmann J, Khan IU, Wallis RS, Zhang F, Koehler KA, Rich EA, Ellner JJ, Elmets CA (1990) The cell membrane is a major locus for ultraviolet-B-induced alterations in accessory cells. J Clin Invest 85:1529–1536
20. Krutmann J, Czech W, Parlow F, Trefzer U, Kapp A, Schoepf E, Luger TA (1992) Ultraviolet radiation effects on human keratinocyte ICAM-1 expression: UV-induced inhibition of cytokine induced ICAM-1 mRNA expression is transient, differentially restored for IFN-γ versus TNFα, and followed by ICAM-1 induction via a TNFα-like pathway. J Invest Dermatol 98:923–928
21. Krutmann J, Czech W, Diepgen T, Niedner R, Kapp A, Schöpf E (1992) High-dose UVA1 therapy in the treatment of patients with atopic dermatitis. J Am Acad Dermatol 26:225–230
22. Krutmann J (1994) Regulatory interactions between epidermal cell adhesion molecules and cytokines. In: Luger TA, Schwarz T (eds) Epidermal growth factors and cytokines. Dekker, New York, pp 415–432
23. Krutmann J, Elmets CA (eds) (1995) Photoimmunology. Blackwell Science, Oxford
24. Krutmann J, Grewe M (1995) Involvement of cytokines, DNA damage, and reactive oxygen species in ultraviolet radiation-induced modulation of intercellular adhesion molecule-1 expression. J Invest Dermatol 105:67S–70S
25. Krutmann J (1996) Phototherapy for atopic dermatitis. Dermatol Therapy 1:24–31
26. Krutmann J (1997) High-dose UVA-1 therapy for inflammatory skin diseases. Dermatol Ther 4:123–128
27. Krutmann J, Diepgen TL, Luger TA, Grabbe S, Meffert H, Sönnichsen N, Czech W, Kapp A, Stege H, Grewe M, Schöpf E (1998) High-dose UVA1 therapy for atopic dermatitis: results of a multicenter trial. J Am Acad Dermatol 38:589–593
28. Krutmann J (1999) Therapeutic photomedicine: phototherapy. In: Freedberg IM, Eisen AB, Wolff K, Austen KF, Goldsmith LA, Katz SI, Fitzpatrick TB (eds) Fitzpatrick's dermatology in general medicine, 5th edn. McGraw-Hill, New York, pp 2870–2879
29. Kulms D, Pöppelmann B, Yarosh D, Luger TA, Krutmann J, Schwarz T (1999) Nuclear and cell membrane effects contribute independently to the induction of apoptosis in human cells exposed to UVB radiation. Proc Natl Acad Sci USA 96:7974–7979
30. Laskin JD, Lee E, Yurkow EJ, Laskin DL, Gallo MA (1985) A possible mechanism of psoralen phototoxicity not involving direct interaction with DNA. Proc Natl Acad Sci USA 82:6158–6162
31. Lisby S, Ralfkier E, Rothlein R, Veijsgard GL (1989) Intercellular adhesion molecule-1

(ICAM-1) expression correlated to inflammation. Br J Dermatol 120:479–484
32. Luger TA, Schwarz T (1995) Effects of UV light on cytokines and neuroendocrine hormones. In: Krutmann J, Elmets CA (eds) Photoimmunology. Blackwell Science, Oxford, pp 55–76
33. Marks DI, Fox RM (1991) Mechanism of photochemotherapy induced apoptotic cell death in lymphoid cells. Biochem Cell Biol 69:754–760
34. McDonald PP, Fadok VA, Bratton D, Henson PM (1999) Transcriptional and translational regulation of inflammatory mediator production by endogenous TGF-β in macrophages that have ingested apoptotic cells. J Immunol 163:6164–6172
35. Morison WL (1993) Photochemotherapy. In: Lim HW, Soter NA (eds) Clinical photomedicine. Dekker, New York, pp 327–346
36. Morita A, Grewe M, Ahrens C, Grether-Beck S, Ruzicka T, Krutmann J (1997a) Ultraviolet A1 radiation effects on cytokine expression in human epidermoid carcinoma cells. Photochem Photobiol 65:630–635
37. Morita A, Werfel T, Stege H, Ahrens C, Karmann K, Grewe M, Grether-Beck S, Ruzicka T, Kapp A, Klotz O, Sies H, Krutmann J (1997b) Evidence that singlet oxygen-induced human T-helper cell apoptosis is the basic mechanism of ultraviolet-A radiation phototherapy. J Exp Med 186:1763–1768
38. Morita A, Yamauchi Y, Yasuda Y, Tsuji T, Krutmann J (2000) Malignant T-cells are exquisitely sensitive to ultraviolet A-1 (UVA-1) radiation-induced apoptosis. J Invest Dermatol (in press)
39. Nishigori C, Yarosh DB, Ullrich SE, Vink AA, Bucana CD, Roza L, Kripke ML (1996) Evidence that DNA damage triggers interleukin 10 cytokine production in UV-irradiated murine keratinocytes. Proc Natl Acad Sci USA 93:10354–10359
40. Norris DA, Lyons B, Middleton MH, Yohn JY, Kashihara-Sawami M (1990) Ultraviolet radiation can either suppress or induce expression of intercellular adhesion molecule-1 (ICAM-1) on the surface of cultured human keratinocytes. J Invest Dermatol 95:132–138
41. Ozawa M, Ferenci K, Kikuchi T, Cardinale I, Austin LM, Coven TR, Burack LH, Krueger JG (1999) 312-nanometer ultraviolet B light (narrow band UVB) induces apoptosis of T cells within psoriatic lesions. J Exp Med 189:711–718
42. Picot E, Meunier L, Picot-Deheze ML, Peyron JL, Meynadier J (1992) Treatment of psoriasis with a 311-nm UVB lamp. Br J Dermatol 127:509–512
43. Plettenberg H, Stege H, Megahed M, Ruzicka T, Hosokawa Y, Tsuji T, Morita A, Krutmann J (1999) Ultraviolet A1 (340–400nm) phototherapy for cutaneous T-cell lymphoma. J Am Acad Dermatol 41:47–50
44. Roza L, Stege H, Krutmann J (1996) Role of UV-induced DNA damage in phototherapy. In: Hönigsmann H, Jori G, Young AR (eds) The fundamental bases of phototherapy. OEMF spa, Milano, pp 145–152
45. Simon JC, Krutmann J, Elmets CA, Bergstresser PR, Cruz D (1992) Ultraviolet B irradiated antigen presenting cells display altered accessory signaling for T cell activation: relevance to immune responses initiated in the skin. J Invest Dermatol 98:66S–69S
46. Stege H, Schöpf E, Ruzicka T, Krutmann J (1996) High-dose-UVA1 for urticaria pigmentosa. Lancet 347:64
47. Stege H, Berneburg M, Humke S, Klammer M, Grewe M, Grether-Beck S, Dierks K, Goerz G, Ruzicka T, Krutmann J (1997) High-dose ultraviolet A1 (UVA1) radiation therapy for localized scleroderma. J Am Acad Dermatol 36:938–943
48. Stege H, Budde M, Kürten V, Ruzicka T, Krutmann J (1999) Induction of apoptosis in skin-infiltrating mast cells by high-dose ultraviolet A-1 radiation phototherapy in patients with urticaria pigmentosa. J Invest Dermatol 114:791
49. Stege H, Roza L, Vink AA, Grewe M, Ruzicka T, Grether-Beck S, Krutmann J (2000) Enzyme plus light therapy to repair DNA damage in ultraviolet-B-irradiated human skin. Proc Natl Acad Sci USA 97:1790–1795
50. Trefzer U, Brockhaus M, Lötscher H, Parlow F, Budnik A, Grewe M, Christoph H, Kapp A,

Schöpf E, Luger TA, Krutmann J (1993) The human 55-kd tumor necrosis factor receptor is regulated in human keratinocytes by TNFα and by ultraviolet B radiation. J Clin Invest 92:462–470
51. Volc-Platzer B, Hönigsmann H (1995) Photoimmunology of PUVA and UVB therapy. In: Krutmann J, Elmets CA (eds) Photoimmunology. Blackwell Science, Oxford, pp 265–273
52. Wlascheck M, Heinen G, Poswig A, Schwarz A, Krieg T, Scharfetter-Kochanek K (1994) UVA-induced autocrine stimulation of fibroblasts derived collagenase/MMP-1 by interrelated loops of interkeukin-1 and interleukin-6. Photochem Photobiol 59:550–556
53. Wlaschek M, Briviba K, Stricklin GP, Sies H, Scharfetter-Kochanek K (1995) Singlet oxygen may mediate the ultraviolet A-induced synthesis of interstitial collagenase. J Invest Dermatol 104:194–198
54. Voll RE, Herrmann M, Roth EA, Stach C, Kalden JR, Girkontaite I (1997) Immunosuppressive effects of apoptotic cells. Nature 390:330
55. Yoo EK, Rook AH, Elenitas R, Gasparro FP, Vowels BR (1996) Apoptosis induction by ultraviolet light A and photochemotherapy in cutaneous T-cell lymphoma: Relevance to mechanism of therapeutic action. J Invest Dermatol 107:235–242

第3章 银屑病的光(化学)疗法

H. Hönigsmann, A. Tanew, W. L. Morison

内容

引言 …………………………………………………… 66
光疗 …………………………………………………… 67
补骨脂光化学疗法 …………………………………… 70
临床总结 ……………………………………………… 79

要点

- 光疗和光化学疗法在银屑病的治疗中占有重要地位。
- 光疗可有效延长银屑病患者的缓解期。
- 尽管长时间 PUVA 治疗有一定致癌几率,但此疗法使患者缓解期延长,仍是一种较好的治疗方案。
- PUVA 或 UVB 联合维 A 酸治疗更安全有效,并可降低皮肤癌的发生。

引言

本章主要回顾紫外线(UV)和补骨脂光化学(PUVA)治疗银屑病。两种治疗方法均已被广泛接受,进一步的临床研究有助于完善治疗指南。同时可加深对 UV 照射的光生物学应答及补骨脂光敏作用机制的认识。最终,我们希望将通过优化治疗方案将潜在的长期副作用如诱发皮肤癌变降至最低。光疗方法是运用可控的 UVB 辐射多次照射皮肤,来改变皮肤生物学功能,进而治疗皮肤病。本章将讨论 UVB 疗法,而非光敏剂如补骨脂疗法(PUVA)。虽然 UVB 运用时间较 PUVA 更久,但后者已经被更详尽的研究和评价过。

光疗

历史

运用人工光源对银屑病进行光疗的传统要追溯到 75 年前,一个世纪以前主要是日光浴疗法。20 世纪早期,银屑病光疗主要用炭精电弧灯,这种灯由 Finsen 发明,最早用于治疗寻常狼疮。后来被中等压力的汞弧代替,后者更实用且能输出高能量的 UV。1925 年,Goeckerman 首先采用外涂粗煤焦油后接受 UV 照射的方法治疗银屑病。此后的半个世纪,尤其在美国,这一方法成为治疗银屑病的标准方法。20 世纪 70 年代开始,人们发现仅用宽谱 UVB 至轻度红斑反应的剂量,能够清除银屑病皮损,尤其是点滴型和脂溢性皮炎型。1984 年新设计出够发出窄波 312nm 的灯,使银屑病的治疗又向前迈进了重要的一步,这种灯被证实治疗效果优于宽波 UVB 灯。目前,这种灯仍是治疗银屑病最有效的方法。

日光浴疗法

人们在远古时代就认识到阳光照射对银屑病有益,20 世纪早期日光浴疗法治疗银屑病受到关注。目前,日光浴疗法,又称为气候疗法已经成功地在死海地区被运用。由于其位置在海平面 400M 以下且大气层中水蒸气的作用,这一地区 UVA 和 UVB 的比例非常高[1],日光浴既划算又有趣。然而,治疗后容易复发,可能是由于皮损清除后治疗突然中断,且未进行维持治疗,这种情况也常发生在运用人造 UV 治疗时。

光疗的原理和机制

传统的银屑病光疗是运用荧光灯发出的人造宽谱 UVB 照射,不采用其他外源性光敏剂。光线被内源性色基吸收,产生光化学反应,导致皮肤生物学改变从而起到治疗效果。UVB 最具特征性的色基是细胞核 DNA。核苷酸吸收紫外线,产生 DNA 光化学产物,主要嘧啶二聚体[2]。虽然二聚物在数量上占优势,但是嘧啶酮可能生物学上的作用更重要[3]。UV 照射产生许多特殊的 DNA 光产物[4,5]。人们对 DNA 光产物怎样干扰细胞周期,抑制细胞生长已经有较多的了解[6]。

UVB 照射抑制 DNA 合成[7,8],对银屑病的表皮细胞 DNA 合成亢进有抑制作用。UVB 和 UVB 诱导 DNA 损伤怎样干扰细胞分裂已有了更详尽的解释。

UVB 照射后肿瘤抑制因子 P53 上调。通过调控 WAF1/CIP1 基因而控制细胞周期[9]。以上机制可能与逆转银屑病患者表皮角质形成细胞增殖周期缩短相关。UVB 诱导细胞周期改变的调控机制对细胞凋亡亦很重要,后者见于 UVB 照射后的表皮(晒伤细胞)并影响皮肤细胞癌变[10]。

更多的证据显示 UV 照射除了影响 DNA 之外,还影响位于细胞质和细胞膜上的细胞核外靶分子,包括细胞表面受体,激酶,磷酸酯酶和转录因子。最近的研究显示细胞核内与细胞膜/质上受体的效应不是相互排斥的,而是相互协同,共同引起 UVB 的各种生物学效应[2,11,12]。

IL-6 和 IL-10 在 UV 光毒反应、免疫抑制反应引发全身症状中起重要作用[13-16]。这些机制在光疗产生疗效和副作用方面同等重要。另外,已证实 UV 诱导细胞分子效应与核 DNA 损伤无关,它们参与膜受体和分子信号途径以调节翻译活性[17,18]。因此,基因表达改变不依赖于 DNA 损伤,这种分子调控机制表明额外或类似的分子途径不能有助于识别光疗真实的靶细胞和效应机制。光疗机制另外一个重要方面是 UVB 改变皮肤的免疫应答。UV 诱导的系统免疫抑制作用也和嘧啶二聚体的形成有关[19]。UV 照射抑制接触过敏反应,迟发性超敏反应和免疫监视作用,后者使小鼠个体出现 UV 诱导的非黑素细胞瘤。朗格汉斯细胞对 UVB 非常敏感,UVB 可改变其表面抗原递呈作用。UV 照射影响角质形成细胞分泌可溶性介质,如 IL-1 和 IL-6,前列腺素 E2,肿瘤坏死因子 α 等。它们可直接作用于 T 细胞或通过影响表皮朗格汉斯细胞功能而改变表皮的免疫应答[2]。

各种光生物学通路之间的作用还未被阐明。银屑病中,表皮角质形成细胞和淋巴细胞均是 UVB 的靶细胞。免疫抑制,细胞因子表达的改变以及细胞周期停滞都是 UVB 治疗银屑病的机制[20]。

作用光谱和光源

作用光谱是指在 UV 诱导过程相对有效的特定的波长,在光疗中,此过程表示治疗效果。诱发红斑的作用光谱可被测量,银屑病光疗的有效剂量和诱发红斑剂量相等。然而,超过红斑剂量其光疗作用反而有限。

所以,Fisher 比较了各种光谱发现治疗银屑病最有效的光谱在 313nm 左右[21]。Parrish 和 Jaenicke[22] 的研究发现波长小于 296nm 的紫外线治疗银屑病无效,即使可使不同个体产生最小红斑量(MEDS)。相反,304nm 和 313nm 乃是最佳作用波长,即使在亚红斑剂量。标准 UVB 荧光灯发射的波长在 295nm 和 350nm 之间,峰值为 305nm,符合这一作用光谱。产生红斑剂量的 UVA 在理论上也有效,但需要超过 1000 倍的辐射剂量,实际操作难以实现。照射 UVB 同时增加 UVA 照射并不能提高银屑病的疗效[23]。

设计出优于传统光源的新型灯具来满足治疗的作用光谱。金属卤化物灯增加了295nm和330nm的辐射,被认为是选择性紫外光治疗(SUP)[25],SUP比宽谱治疗仪更有效,但无法和PUVA相比[25]。312nm窄谱UVB灯(飞利浦TL-10灯发出的波长位于311~313nm之间)治疗银屑病的效果最佳[26]。

光疗方法

光疗之前需评估每个患者对紫外线的敏感性。UVB照射较小的范围(如直径1cm的圆形)从较低能量逐渐递增,以10mJ/cm²的梯度递增或以$\sqrt{2}$倍的剂量递增,导致出现境界清楚的粉红色斑片反应的剂量称为最小红斑量(MED)。目前,将最小可见红斑反应作为评估临界值的可靠方法[27]。虽然对是否靠视觉评估MED做为放射量测定的最佳方法仍有争议,但它不需要任何特殊仪器,简单易行。

UVB最初的治疗剂量为MED的75%~100%,每周治疗2~5次。UVB红斑出现的高峰期在照射后24小时内,每次连续治疗UVB剂量均会递增,增加的比例取决于治疗频率和前一次治疗后的效果。照射剂量增加的目的是维持最小可见红斑,临床评估最佳放射量测定。如果一周治疗三次,如果未出现红斑则每次增加40%照射量,如出现轻度红斑则增加20%照射量,如果红斑持续存在,则不增加照射剂量。如果每天都照射,增加量分别不能超过30%、15%和0%。如果红斑严重且疼痛,则要停止照射直到症状消失。一直治疗至达到总体缓解或在病情未进一步发展后继续光疗维持。英国皮肤光疗小组颁布了UVB治疗指南,他们为同时患有多种疾病的患者提供以实例为基础的治疗指南以及在准备治疗时的鉴别诊断[28]。

银屑病光疗

点滴型和脂溢性皮炎型银屑病对宽谱UVB反应良好,但慢性斑块型银屑病则效果欠佳。虽然宽谱UVB治疗银屑病有效,但在临床清除皮疹和缓解时间方面不及PUVA[20]。除了上文提到的治疗方案,其他方案也被采用。某些方案以皮肤类型确定起始剂量和固定增量,无论皮肤反应如何,患者四肢照射增加剂量大于躯干。患者头部若未被累及,光疗时需佩戴防护头盔以最大限度减少光损伤。有时,患者四肢UV照射增量高于躯干。

皮疹清除后,对治疗终止或继续维持治疗各国看法不一,且其有效性和必要性也受到争议。一般认为,维持治疗可使患者患者长期缓解。英国的一些皮肤病学者不主张维持治疗,而在美国,皮疹清除后维持治疗数年。

UVB维持治疗存在一些问题,浪费时间或影响患者的生活质量,随着维持治疗的延长,UVB积累剂量迅速增多,提前光老化和及光致癌性风险增加。需要更多的多中心研究来判定长期治疗的危险性和维持治疗的必要性。

维持治疗已经形成一定的规范,一般而言,患者的皮疹清除,就应减少 UVB 照射的频率,同时采用皮疹清除时最后一次的剂量来维持。辅助用药和联合治疗的目的是提高疗效,降低 UVB 治疗的积累剂量以减轻其长期副作用。照光之前用疏水性药膏减少痂皮,以增加紫外线照射的作用[29]。UVB 可联合局部使用煤焦油[30]或蒽林[31]。不推荐联合局部运用糖皮质激素,因为可能导致缓解时间缩短[32]。系统用药,如维 A 酸类药物,可增加疗效,尤其对慢性和增生肥厚性斑块型银屑病[33,34],除此之外,维 A 酸类药物还可以降低 UVB 光疗的潜在致癌性。

窄谱紫外线(312nm)光疗在皮疹清除和延长缓解时间方面均优于传统宽谱 UVB[26,35,36]。这是由于提高了照射强度以达到最佳治疗效果。在欧洲,窄谱 UVB 在很多地方已经取代了传统光疗。在美国,飞利浦 TL01 灯由于部分技术不匹配近期才投入使用。根据研究和其他报道,我们认为窄谱 UVB 的疗效和 PUVA 类似[37,38]。窄谱 UVB 的唯一缺点是对于手掌和足底皮损无效。窄谱 UVB 已经成功用于联合治疗,如与维 A 酸类(RePUVA)[39]、蒽林[31,40]和钙泊三醇[41]。亚红斑量窄谱 UVB 辐射治疗银屑病的作用有待更进一步的开发和改进。

副作用

短期副作用包括红斑(晒伤),皮肤干燥伴瘙痒,光毒性水疱少见,复发性单纯疱疹发作频率增加。过度暴露引起的中度疼痛性红斑可局部运用皮质类固醇缓解。严重病例可系统运用非甾体类抗炎药物和皮质类固醇。温水浴后外用温和的润滑剂可缓解瘙痒、皮肤干燥等亚急性症状。长期副作用包括光老化和致癌性。

众所周知 UVB 具有致癌性,尽管其潜在的致癌性低于 PUVA。Stern 和 Laird 对 16 个中心的研究未发现 UVB 治疗和非黑素细胞瘤之间存在相关性。然而,他们肯定的认为更多的研究可能会发现 UVB 治疗会增加皮肤非黑素细胞瘤的发生。英国的一项研究显示观察了 1908 个经窄谱 UVB 治疗的患者,发现基底细胞癌的发病率小量增加,而非鳞状细胞癌。作者认为,调查偏倚可能是部分原因,窄谱 UVB 光疗的致癌性仍然需要进一步确定[43]。

补骨脂光化学疗法

补骨脂光化学疗法(PUVA)是补骨脂(P)联合长波紫外线(UVA)。药物联合照射用于单独治疗效果欠佳的患者。可控的光毒反应可用来治疗皮肤病[44]。

补骨脂可以口服,可以制成溶液、软膏外用,也可以用来沐浴。

历史

古埃及及古印度的医师用含有补骨脂的植物的汁、种子等涂抹白癜风患者皮疹并将其暴露于太阳下来进行治疗已经有几千年历史。西方国家最早用暴露于阳光下或紫外线照射治疗白癜风开始于20世纪。El Mofty[45,46]最先提出口服或局部外用补骨脂。

1974年,研究者发现口服8-甲氧补骨脂,然后再进行人工UVA照射治疗银屑病效果显著。这个新的治疗方法被定义为光化学疗法,简称PUVA(补骨脂和紫外线治疗)[47]。新型高强度UVA辐射光源的出现使得口服补骨脂的PUVA治疗得以发展。波士顿的哈佛大学是第一个用其治疗银屑病的机构。同时,越南,澳大利亚的大样本队列研究证实其疗效显著[48]。几年后,PUVA的显著疗效得到全世界的认可。

然而,在发现高强度UVA光源之前局部使用补骨脂加低强度UVA(黑光)就能够清除银屑病皮损[49,50]。口服补骨脂光化学疗法的有效性已经被广泛证实,它对皮肤病的治疗产生了深远的影响,因为它为除了银屑病以外的其他皮肤病提供了治疗方法[51]。

原理和机制

PUVA是在照射UVA前连续间断性注射一定剂量的补骨脂。保持不变的参数有利于维持补骨脂的血浆浓度。根据UVA变化决定初始计量和对计量进行调整。

通过不断的可控的光毒反应银屑病得以缓解。这些反应只发生在通过UVA照射补骨脂具有活性时。根据UVA的穿透特性,能量的吸收仅限于皮肤。药量过大,PUVA诱导的光毒反应类似迟发性晒伤,如红斑和炎症反应,可发展为炎性水疱甚至浅表皮肤溃疡。因此,UVA放射量测定对PUVA治疗的安全性和有效性十分重要[47,48]。为了光化学疗法最大程度的安全有效,需遵循以下准则:

1. 熟悉光生物学原理,临床反应和光毒反应的过程
2. 了解UVA的放射量测定和补骨脂动力学
3. 精确定义UVA的照射计量
4. 患者摄入补骨脂后计算个体的光敏性

补骨脂是线性呋喃豆香素,最初来源于植物成分,它结合日光照射用于治疗白癜风[52]。8-甲氧补骨脂(甲氧沙林)是目前运用最多的药物,5-甲氧补骨脂(佛手内酯)也有运用。欧洲主要将人工合成的线性呋喃香豆素,4,5′,8-三甲基

补骨脂素放入洗澡水中进行 PUVA 治疗。目前,8-MOP 和 5-MOP 都可以作为口服制剂,它们可以是结晶体,微粉化结晶体,或者溶于胶体基质中。液体补骨脂较固体补骨脂更早、更快达到血药峰值,代谢也更容易。口服补骨脂在肝脏中代谢,12~24h 才能经尿液中排出。由于首过效应补骨脂浓度的微小改变都会影响药物血浆浓度,这可能是个体之间血浆浓度显著不同的原因[53-55]。尽可能地保证各个参数一致是非常重要的,包括每天吃饭的时间,和摄入食物的品种、数量。

补骨脂是线性呋喃豆香素,最初来源于植物成分,它结合日光照射用于治疗白癜风[52]。8-甲氧补骨脂(甲氧沙林)是目前运用最多的药物,5-甲氧补骨脂(佛手内酯)也有运用。欧洲主要将人工合成的线性呋喃香豆素,4,5′,8-三甲基补骨脂素放入洗澡水中进行 PUVA 治疗。目前,8-MOP 和 5-MOP 都可以作为口服制剂,它们可以是结晶体,微粉化结晶体,或者溶于胶体基质中。液体补骨脂较固体补骨脂更早、更快达到血药峰值,代谢也更容易。口服补骨脂在肝脏中代谢,12~24 小时才能经尿液中排出。由于首过效应补骨脂浓度的微小改变都会影响药物血浆浓度,这可能是个体之间血浆浓度显著不同的原因[53-55]。尽可能地保证各个参数一致是非常重要的,包括每天吃饭的时间,和摄入食物的品种、数量。

补骨脂在被 UV 辐射激活后才发生反应,其活性局限于 UVA 穿透的皮肤层。辐射可以穿透表皮,真皮乳头到达真皮浅层血管丛。激发补骨脂产生改变生物分子学的光化学反应,从而改变皮肤的生物学。

细胞核 DNA 光化学反应与其生物学高度相关,已经被完全阐明[56]。2 种不同功能的补骨脂与 DNA 反应分三步。第一步,在 UV 照射前,补骨脂整合到双链 DNA 中。经过辐射后,活性双键之一增加一个嘧啶碱形成环丁烷状,根据补骨脂成为双键的一部分被称为 3,4-单加合物或 4′,5′-单加合物。只有 4′,5′-单加合物在吸收二光子之后能够形成补骨脂-DNA 交联物。在临床上,单加合物是更加突出的加合物,但是不同的补骨脂-DNA 光化合物的关系取决于补骨脂的种类和照射波长[57]。虽然关于补骨脂-DNA 光化学产物已知很多,但是其他 8-MOP 光化学反应可能与治疗作用相关[58]。激活的补骨脂能够与分子氧起化学反应,导致活性氧分子如单氧分子形成。活性氧分子通过脂质过氧化作用引起细胞膜损伤,并且激活环氧合酶和花生四烯酸的代谢途径[59]。

DNA-补骨脂交联抑制 DNA 复制导致细胞周期终止。所涉及的细胞分子路径已经阐明,进一步增加了我们对其作用机制的了解。补骨脂光化学作用影响细胞因子和细胞因子受体表达以及细胞因子分泌[60]。PUVA 能够逆转角质细胞分化标志的病理改变,减少表皮细胞增殖数量。PUVA 能够明显抑制淋巴细胞浸润,前者对 T 细胞不同亚群作用不一[61]。已经证实 PUVA 在对淋巴细胞和角质形成细胞抗增殖活性相似的情况下,更易使淋巴细胞凋亡[62]。这说明 PUVA 更易诱导淋巴细胞凋亡。这种特殊的反应模式可用于解释为何 PUVA 治疗 T 细胞淋巴瘤和炎症性皮肤病效果显著。虽然这些研究已经证实补骨脂光化学路径和机制,但是与 PUVA 治疗其他特殊疾病的相互关系仍不清楚。

光谱

曾经认为 8-MOP 诱导的迟发性红斑的光谱峰值为 365nm,近期的研究显示最大活性为在 330nm 范围[63,64]。就光疗而言,只有在银屑病的治疗中需要评估与治疗相关的引起红斑的光谱。由于补骨脂浓度在不同个体的血浆和皮肤中的差异,这些数据难以收集。然而目前认为 8-MOP 治疗银屑的光谱与产生红斑的光谱相似[65,66]。已经获得体内与 8-MOP DNA 交联反应相匹配的光谱[67]。这表明补骨酯-DNA 交联在治疗银屑病中产生作用。

补骨脂光谱恰好与传统的荧光灯发出产生治疗作用的 UVA 重叠。金属卤化物灯,用于不产光敏反应的 UVA 光疗,发射出的光谱波长在 UVB 和 UVC 范围。由于其光谱较长,治疗效果相对较差,但仍可用于光化学疗法。但是 UVA 的高输出率大大降低了治疗时间。

光敏作用

PUVA 治疗产生炎症反应表现为迟发性光毒性红斑。此反应取决于药物剂量,UVA 剂量以及个体敏感性(皮肤类型)。研究发现改变 8-MOP 剂量并未影响 PUVA 红斑剂量-反应曲线的最大斜率。因此,个体 8-MOP 剂量改变,幅度较大但在临床范围内,出现对 PUVA 照射受红斑反应阈值的显著性改变,但红斑的发生率并未随着 UVA 剂量的增加而增加[68]。PUVA 照射后红斑与晒斑及 UVB 照射后红斑显著不同,后者发生于照射后 4~6 小时,12~24 小时达到高峰。PUVA 照射后红斑发生于照射后 24~36 小时,72~96 小时达到高峰。其剂量-反应曲线较 UVB 照射后红斑低平,这种差异一直持续到最大红斑量[69]。PUVA 照射后红斑持续时间较长(超过 1 周),可呈暗红色甚至紫罗兰色。反应剧烈可出现水疱及浅表坏死。超量的 PUVA 常引起照射区水肿、剧烈瘙痒,有时出现异常刺痛感。此时,红斑是评估 PUVA 反应严重程度的有效参数,因此它在调整 UVA 剂量中发挥重要作用[20]。

PUVA 第二个重要影响是不出现临床上可见的红斑,而为色素沉着。正常皮肤,PUVA 照射后色素沉着发生的高峰为照射后 7 天,一般持续数周到数月。和日光引起的晒黑相似,个体晒黑耐受力需要评估,但是剂量-反应曲线较陡峭。小剂量 PUVA 暴露导致的晒黑较多重日光照射引起的晒黑更明显。

PUVA 治疗炎症和肿瘤性疾病的目标是在诱发严重的色素沉着之前产生临床反应。

PUVA 治疗方案

最初临床研究补骨脂治疗银屑病是局部外用 8-MOP[49,50]。局部补骨脂联合 UVA 光疗在清除银屑病皮损中有效,但也有部分副作用。光毒性红斑反应不可预知且可能引起水疱,所以 UVA 放射量测定标准难以制定。如果皮损较多,补骨脂的应用费时费力,常会出现色素沉着。而且,若在银屑病的进展期,新的损害会出现在先前未累及和治疗的部位。根据笔者经验,局部外用 PUVA 联合口服用于治疗较顽固的斑块,尤其是掌跖银屑病。另一方面,PUVA 浴治疗,将全身浸入 TMP 或 8-MOP 后进行全身 UVA 照射,可产生满意的治疗效果。尤其对于不容易晒黑的患者,PUVA 浴是有效的治疗方法。

PUVA 治疗银屑病

事实上,PUVA 对各种类型的银屑病均有效,虽然红皮病型银屑病和泛发型脓疱型银屑病相比其他类型银屑病治疗困难[20]。两种方法效果均较好且一直沿用。它们常在美国和欧洲指南中被提及。表 3.1 显示了两种口服 8-MOP 进行 PUVA 治疗的方法[70,71]。

表 3.1　欧洲 PUVA(EPS) 和 US16 中心试验(UST) 的治疗方案和结果

	EPS	UST
起始剂量	1MPD	依赖皮肤的类型
每周治疗的次数	4	2~3
UVA 剂量的增加量	个体化	固定
清除率	88.8%	88%
暴露次数	20	25
清除时间	5.7 周	12.7 周
累积 UVA 剂量	96J/cm^2	245J/cm^2

常规治疗包括分别口服 0.6~0.8mg/kg 8-MOP 溶液或 1.2mg/kg 5-MOP 溶液 1~2 小时后进行 UVA 照射。对于斑块型银屑病,每周 4 次,周三作为间歇期休息,直到皮疹清除。欧洲指南推荐持续治疗,用皮疹清除时的 UVA 剂量照射每周 2 次,连续四周,然后每周 1 次。英国光线性皮肤病学组认为只需对皮疹清除后很快复发的患者进行持续治疗[72]。运用左右比较研究法对慢性复发性斑

块型患者运用短期持续疗法,发现约 8.8% 的患者缓解期明显延长,其他 91.2% 的患者对其缓解期无影响。本研究显示维持治疗对预防银屑病的早期复发无明显作用,应该避免。需要更多的研究来阐明维持治疗的作用[73]。

新方法或改进已存在的旧方法以增加 PUVA 的疗效而降低其副作用。而 5-MOP 可用安全计量较宽,即使服用超过 1.8mg/kg 的剂量,也只产生较少的胃肠道副作用。口服之后,5-MOP 较 8-MOP 临床光毒反应小,因此在超剂量 UVA 照射引起的副作用方面较安全[74]。

在治疗过程中通过重复测定光毒阈值来优化 UVA 照射。治疗每周 2 次,间隔 72 小时,目的是优化放射量,从而增加疗效,降低总体 UVA 影响[75,76]。近期,非皮损区使用 UVA 保护剂二羟基丙酮再联合 PUVA 可增加银屑病的清除率[77]。

PUVA 治疗局限性皮损,可外用补骨脂溶液。将浓度为 0.15% 的 8-MOP 溶液涂抹于皮损处,20 分钟后进行照射。通过洗澡水局部使用 TMP 在北欧半岛非常流行[78],但直到最近才受到世界范围内的关注。8-MOP 加入洗澡水中能够避免胃肠道和口腔的副反应,因为不会产生系统性光敏感。和口服药物相比,外涂药物皮肤补骨脂可重复性强且光敏感持续时间更短。降低初始治疗剂量(30%~50% 最小红斑量)和治疗初期细致的辐射量测定能够降低不可预知的光毒性的发生几率[79]。浓度为每公升洗澡水 0.5~5.0mg 8-MOP。洗浴 15~20 分钟,然后将皮肤轻柔的拍干,立即进行 UVA 照射,否则光敏性将迅速减低。局部外用 TMP 的光毒性更大,因此使用浓度较 8-MOP 的小,为 0.125~0.5mg/L。

研究人员为了减少副作用而不断探索新的补骨脂素,他们合成了角呋喃香豆素 4,6,4-三补骨脂素和功能型 7-甲基吡啶补骨脂素。这两种化合物均显示出良好的光合参数,在局部治疗银屑病时均有较好的疗效[80,81]。目前为止,这些呋喃香豆类补骨脂素仍在研究阶段。

联合治疗

PUVA 可联合其他治疗方式以提高疗效降低副作用[82]。局部联合皮质类固醇,地蒽酚和煤焦油制剂取得了部分成功,最近联合局部使用钙泊三醇取得了较好的效果。然而,局部治疗并非被所有患者接受,因为有人它较常规治疗落后。联合 PUVA 和甲氨蝶呤可缩短治疗时间,照射次数和 UVA 总剂量,且对单独 PUVA 和 UVB 治疗反应不佳的患者有效[83]。

环孢素 A 联合 PUVA 治疗和 RePUVA 可清除泛发性斑块型银屑病患者皮损。然而,严重和早期复发患者需要积累 UVA 剂量以清除皮疹,RePUVA 在治疗这类患者中具有明显优势。此外,环孢素联合 PUVA 可明显增加皮肤肿瘤的罹患率,故不推荐两者合用[85-87]。

PUVA 联合系统使用维 A 酸是治疗银屑病最有潜力的方法之一[88]。PUVA 开始前 5~10 天,开始联合每日口服维 A 酸类药物(阿维 A 酯,阿维 A,异维 A 酸;1mg/kg),能够显著提高 PUVA 的治疗效果[89,90]。此治疗方案称为 RePUVA,可降低 1/3 的照射剂量及超过一半的 UVA 累积剂量。RePUVA 对 PUVA 单独治疗不能完全缓解的"PUVA 反应不佳"的患者亦有效。

维 A 酸和 PUVA 联合的相互作用机制暂不清楚,可能是加速银屑病斑块的脱屑从而改善皮肤情况和减轻炎症细胞浸润。作为额外的效能,阿维 A 酯和阿维 A 在理论上通过减少 PUVA 的照射次数和其潜在的抗癌作用来降低 PUVA 长期使用的致癌性。维 A 酸类药物的短期副作用停药后可逆,由于一般只在皮疹清除期用药,其长期副作用不确定。维 A 酸类药物的致畸性应受到重视。在欧洲,阿维 A 酯已被其活性代谢物阿维 A 代替,这是由于后者的半衰期较前者短,且在 RePUVA 治疗中同样有效[91,92]。同时有证据表明,部分由阿维 A 酯代谢的阿维 A 可在体内继续累积[93,94],因此认为阿维 A 并不优于阿维 A 酯。异维 A 酸可用于育龄期妇女,因其在结束治疗后只需避孕 2 个月,而阿维 A 和阿维 A 酯则要避孕 2 年。

HIV 感染患者的光疗和 PUVA 治疗

皮肤病亦常发生于 HIV 感染患者[95]。银屑病和其他对光疗有效的皮肤病如 CTCL 和白癜风也可发生于 HIV 感染患者[96,97]。1985 年,报道了第一例 AIDs 合并银屑病的患者[98]。有报道显示两种疾病有一定的相关性,但是是否 HIV 感染者较正常人更易患银屑病目前尚不清楚。这两种疾病有一定的矛盾性,因为 HIV 感染导致免疫抑制,而银屑病常采用免疫抑制疗法[99]。

HIV 影响机体的免疫系统,能够触发银屑病的发生和加重。HIV 感染耗尽 $CD4^+$ 辅助 T 细胞和表皮朗格汉斯细胞[100,101]。病毒感染并不一定杀死细胞。它可以改变细胞基因的表达模式,导致细胞生长和功能的异常[100]。HIV 引起机体细胞和体液免疫失调,打乱细胞因子之间微妙的平衡。细胞因子模式的紊乱被认为是银屑病的触发因素[102]。偶然的,CD4 细胞计数较低的银屑病患者能够自然缓解,可能因 AID 患者不能够产生表皮过度增殖所需的细胞因子。这种现象也见于其他疾病末期的患者。

HIV 感染的银屑患者通常对例如局部使用皮质类固醇等治疗抵抗。UVB 光疗或 PUVA 治疗对此类患者有效。此种治疗的安全性存在争议。首先,UVB 和 PUVA 均能引起系统免疫抑制,改变患者的免疫状态,导致 HIV 恶化[103]。其次,UV 和补骨脂的光敏性可能会激活 HIV 促发因子,后者可促进病毒基因转录,最终产生病毒[104]。第三,病毒诱导的免疫抑制作用可能会加速 UVB 或

PUVA 治疗的患者的皮肤癌变[105]。这种治疗不会导致 HIV 恶化或增加并发症的几率[106]。

若 UVB 光疗失败,可选择 PUVA 治疗。此外,运用 PUVA 治疗银屑病不会导致 HIV 感染的进展且不会增加其副作用[107,108]。一些研究发现 UVB 光疗或 PUVA 治疗对 HIV 阳性的银屑病患者是安全的。UVB 或 PUVA 诱导人类皮肤 HIV 激活的模型显示在体内 UVB 较 PUVA 更易激活病毒[109]。由于不会导致 HIV 加重使得最初的临床研究得以进行,长期观察的资料目前还在整理之中。因此,目前广泛推荐使用 PUVA 和 UVB 光疗治疗 HIV 免疫抑制的个体,但其主要的危险暂不清楚。已获得的资料和理论显示在治疗 HIV 感染患者中 UVB 的安全性较 PUVA 差[109,110]。需要长期的研究来评估 UVB 光疗和 PUVA 治疗 HIV 感染患者的远期利弊。

副作用和长期治疗的危险性

UVB 和 PUVA 过量的短期副作用相似,包括红斑、肿胀、偶见水疱,类似过度晒伤。主要区别在于出现时间不同:UVB 诱发的红斑高峰期出现在 24 小时之前,而 PUVA 最明显的反应出现在 72 小时之后。泛发的瘙痒和刺痛感是警示信号,提示光毒性反应。如果累及范围较大,将发生如发热、全身不适等光毒性反应的系统症状,这是由于释放了大量的细胞因子。除了调节放射量剂量,其他处理手段取决于光毒反应的深度和广度。冷敷、非甾体抗炎药、局部甚至系统皮质类固醇的使用均可减轻症状。PUVA 诱导的与光毒晒伤无关的皮肤疼痛罕见,一旦发生需中断治疗。使用 5-MOP 进行 PUVA 治疗的最初阶段,少数病人出现无临床症状的暂时性斑丘疹,与光毒反应无关[74]。日光性甲脱离和甲下出血是甲床对急性光毒性的迟发反应。

除了光毒性反应外,无光照的情况下补骨脂能够诱发系统副作用。口服 8-MOP 最常见不良反应的是恶心、呕吐。8-MOP 溶液最常发生此不良反应。口服 5-MOP 可以明显减少这些不良反应的发生,这也是两者混合物的使用增加的主要原因。

UVA 照射时的眼部防护是必需的,此外不透 UVA 的防护镜需要保护非照射区直至治疗当晚。通过这些预防来避免眼部副作用的发生。眼部意外暴露于 UVB 下,由于眼结膜和角膜吸收 UVB 可引起光性角膜炎。UVA 可穿通晶状体发生白内障。系统补骨脂过敏者可能是产生了补骨脂蛋白光产物。年纪越小的患者,晶状体更易被穿透,故 12 岁以下儿童禁忌口服 PUVA。虽然有实验数据有过早发生白内障的风险,但是临床观察发现那些忽略眼部防护的患者也并未出现晶状体浑浊[111,112]。然而这些患者发生如眼球结膜改变等其他眼部副作用[112]。

UVB 和 PUVA 的长期副作用相似,如光老化,即皮肤长期暴露于阳光下,高积累剂量导致皮肤过度损害。损害常出现在过度曝光部位,如面部、颈部、前臂。高积累剂量的 UVB 和 PUVA 全身照射引起色素沉着、皮肤干燥、缺乏弹性、皱纹形成和发生光线性角化病。此外,PUVA 还可以导致多毛症,大面积黑色雀斑形成,称为 PUVA 着色斑病[70]。

长期重复光化学疗法可诱发或促进皮肤肿瘤的发生和发展(综述,见[113])。日光照射在黑素瘤和非黑素瘤的发生中起重要作用。因此,进行 PUVA 治疗的患者在治疗初期就应仔细监测其发生恶性黑素瘤的征兆。所有的信息均来自银屑病患者,因为银屑病患者接受 PUVA 治疗的占大部分。

PUVA 最大的副作用是发生 DNA 损伤,但是其诱导的免疫应答下调亦发挥重要作用。PUVA 治疗的患者与对照组相比,发生鳞状细胞癌的风险显著增高且具有剂量依赖性[114-117],而发生基底细胞癌的风险并未升高。然而,并不确定 PUVA 在起癌变中所起多大作用,报道的部分患者先前已经过度暴露于日光下或者接受过具有致癌性物质的治疗,包括砷、UVB 和抗代谢物[115,118]。高剂量的 UVB 暴露增加接受 PUVA 治疗患者的皮肤非黑素细胞癌的发生[119]。先前用煤焦油和 UVB 治疗过的男性患者经 PUVA 治疗后外阴容易发生癌变[120],但单纯用 PUVA 治疗的患者无此风险[121]。

5-MOP-UVA 治疗在接受 PUVA 治疗的患者中的致癌性暂不清楚,但是体外小鼠研究中发现 5-MOP 和 8-MOP 的致突变和致癌活性相似[122]。只有散在个别长期接受 PUVA 治疗的银屑病患者发生恶性黑素瘤[123]报道,迄今为止,大范围研究中并未发现恶性黑素瘤的风险增高。然而,Stern[124]最近报道一项始于 1975 年的有 1380 名患者参加的 PUVA 随访研究(16 个研究中心),发现 23 名患者发生了 26 种侵袭性或原位黑素瘤。暴露于 PUVA 后最初 15 年,PUVA 治疗组发生黑素瘤的风险增加。作者推断可能和 PUVA 治疗不平衡有关。对于严重的银屑病患者,相比运用其他方法,如甲氨蝶呤和免疫抑制治疗如环孢素 A,PUVA 长期治疗的副作用更需要严密监视。

除了患者详细信息的数据缺乏,此报告强调 PUVA 治疗指南需严格遵守。长期 PUVA 治疗的患者需进行终生随访[125]。不管怎样,累积照射剂量保持低水平可降低癌变风险,因此,UVA 节制且积极的治疗方案不延长维持治疗可能比维持治疗更安全,非积极的方案可能改变了 PUVA 的致癌时间[113]。在该方面,最近的研究表明运用 PUVA 和系统维 A 酸联合治疗的银屑病患者鳞状细胞癌的罹患率降低,但基底细胞的罹患率无明显改变[126]。

基于对 944 例瑞典和芬兰的患者和以前的动物试验研究发现,用 TMP 进行 PUVA 浴并未增加致癌性。另外,158 名银屑病患者中并未发现皮肤癌和 8-MOPPUVA 浴之间的相关性[129]。这些信息提示 PUVA 浴远期是安全的,但是不能得出任何过早的结论。

对比 PUVA 和 UVB 光疗的副作用是必需的。动物实验显示 UVB 具有致癌性,但是模型研究显示接受 PUVA 治疗发生鳞状细胞癌的几率高于接受 UVB 辐射者[130,131]。目前的趋势是运用窄谱 UVB(飞利浦 TL-01)。此光源与 PUVA 相比,其致癌性大小暂不清楚,这将成为长期接受治疗的银屑病患者的监测重点。

重度银屑病需要长期治疗计划。经验丰富的医师能够严格筛选病人,采用个体化治疗方案或联合疗法。对于可能致残的银屑病患者,治疗方案的选择不考虑安全与风险的大小,而是在甲氨蝶呤、环孢素 A,或维 A 酸和 UVB 之间选择,以上没有一种药物均是绝对安全的。PUVA 治疗的利与弊仍有争议[132],目前,或许除了窄谱 UVB,没有其他治疗被认为是安全而有效的。

临床总结

光(化学)疗法需要由训练有素的人员进行操作。最初的照射剂量取决于皮肤类型或光实验(MED 或 MPD 计算)。所有患者均需被告知副作用和慢性危害,需要建立详尽的个体治疗记录。治疗过程需要有经过培训的人员进行和陪同,医师需根据患者对治疗反应进行合理的调整,以降低其副作用。

窄谱 UVB 治疗

窄谱 UVB 是荧光灯发射波长为 311 到 313nm 的辐射。窄波 UVB 较宽谱 UVB 清除银屑病皮疹更快且缓解期更长,其治疗效果和 PUVA 相当,且引起皮肤癌的几率低。但窄波 UVB 不及 PUVA 治疗后缓解期长。联合系统治疗,包括甲氨蝶呤和维 A 酸类药可提高疗效。常规每周治疗 3 次,平均治疗 30 次可到达最大缓解。

PUVA 治疗

PUVA 治疗是补骨脂联合 UVA 照射。运用于临床的有三种补骨脂:运用于 PUVA 浴的甲氧沙林(8-甲氧补骨脂),佛手内酯(5-甲氧补骨脂),以及三甲补骨脂内酯(三甲基补骨脂素;TMP)。

治疗开始前 1~2 小时先口服补骨脂或用进行局部补骨脂溶液浴。口服 8-MOP 的患者中 10% 可发生不适和恶心。将总剂量分两次口服,中间间隔 15 分钟可进食,这样可以减轻恶心症状。另外,对于有严重恶心反应的患者可进行

PUVA 浴。UVA 照射应在 PUVA 浴后 15 分钟内。1 小时后光敏性明显降低。

UVA 剂量大小根据亚红斑量来选择，但是由于个体对补骨脂的吸收不同，部分患者仍会出现不可避免的红斑反应。和 UVB 治疗类似，PUVA 联合口服如阿维 A 等维 A 酸类药物或甲氨蝶呤能够增加其治疗效果。除此之外，联合疗法能够降低辐射剂量，使其长期副作用减至最小。维 A 酸类药物也可以预防皮肤癌的发生。已经明确联合环孢素能够增加光疗或 PUVA 的致癌性，尽量避免使用。仔细的放射量测定能够减少包括瘙痒、晒伤、水疱等皮肤反应的发生。

每周治疗 3～4 次，皮疹清除平均需要治疗 25 次，严重银屑病患者治疗次数需更多。PUVA 对重症银屑病患者仍然是最有效的治疗，但是同时使用环孢素或生物制剂会增加其副作用，并且价格昂贵。PUVA 维持疗法有诱发鳞状细胞癌的风险，故常规不推荐，但对于知情的患者，在没有更安全的方法可以选择的前提下可以尝试这种疗法。

（周欣 译，田歆　孟珍 校，朱慧兰 审）

参考文献

1. Abels DJ, Kattan-Byron J (1985) Psoriasis treatment at the Dead Sea: a natural selective ultraviolet phototherapy. J Am Acad Dermatol 12:639–643
2. Weichenthal M, Schwarz T (2005) Phototherapy: how does UV work? Photodermatol Photoimmunol Photomed 21:260–266
3. Petit Frere C, Clingen PH, Arlett CF, Green MH (1996) Inhibition of RNA and DNA synthesis in UV-irradiated normal human fibroblasts is correlated with pyrimidine (6–4) pyrimidone photoproduct formation. Mutat Res 354:87–94
4. Ronai ZA, Lambert ME, Weinstein IB (1992) Inducible cellular responses to ultraviolet light irradiation and other mediators of DNA damage in mammalian cells. Cell Biol Toxicol 6:105–126
5. Moan J, Peak MJ (1989) Effects of UV radiation of cells. J Photochem Photobiol B Biol 4:21–34
6. Liu M, Pellingo JC (1995) UV-B/A irradiation of mouse keratinocytes results in p53-mediated WAF-1/CIP-1 expression. Oncogene 10:1955–1960
7. Kramer DM, Pathak MA, Kornhauser A, Wiskemann A (1974) Effects of ultraviolet radiation on biosynthesis of DNA in guinea pig skin. J Invest Dermatol 62:388–393
8. Epstein WL, Fukuyama K, Epstein JH (1969) Early effects of ultraviolet light on DNA synthesis in human skin in vivo. Arch Dermatol 100:84–89
9. Liu M, Pellingo JC (1995) UV-B/A irradiation of mouse keratinocytes results in p53-mediated WAF1/CIP1 expression. Oncogene 10:1955–1960
10. Brash DE, Rudolph JA, Simon JA, Lim A, McKenna GJ, Baden HP, Halperin AJ, Ponten J (1991) A role for sunlight in skin cancer: UV-induced p53 mutations in squamous cell carcinoma. Proc Natl Acad Sci USA 88:10124–10128
11. Hruza LL, Pentland AP (1993) Mechanisms of UV-induced inflammation. J Invest Dermatol 100:35S–41S

12. Greaves MW (1986) Ultraviolet erythema: causes and consequences. In: Hönigsmann H, Stingl G (eds) Therapeutic photomedicine. Current problems in dermatology, vol 15. Karger, Basel, pp 18–24
13. Schwarz T, Luger TA (1989) Effect of UV irradiation on epidermal cell cytokine production. J Photochem Photobiol B Biol 4:1–13
14. Beissert S, Hosoi J, Grabbe S, Asahina A, Granstein RD (1995) IL-10 inhibits tumor antigen presentation by epidermal antigen-presenting cells. J Immunol 154:1280–1286
15. Urbanski A, Schwarz T, Neuner P, Krutmann J, Kirnbauer R, Köck A, Luger TA (1990) Ultraviolet light induces increased circulating interleukin-6 in humans. J Invest Dermatol 94:808–811
16. Ullrich SE (1995) Modulation of immunity by ultraviolet radiation: key effects on antigen presentation. J Invest Dermatol 105:30S–36S
17. Warmuth I, Harth Y, Matsui MS, Wang N, DeLeo VA (1994) Ultraviolet radiation induces phosphorylation of the epidermal growth factor receptor. Cancer Res 54:374–376
18. Devary Y, Rosette C, DiDonato JA, Karin N (1993) NF-kB activation by ultraviolet light not dependent on a nuclear signal. Science 261:1442–1445
19. Kripke ML, Cox PA, Alas LG, Yarosh DB (1992) Pyrimidine dimers in DNA initiate systemic immunosuppression in UVB-irradiated mice. Proc Natl Acad Sci USA 89:7516–7520
20. Hönigsmann H (2001) Phototherapy for psoriasis. Clin Exp Dermatol 6:343–350
21. Fisher T (1976) UV-light treatment of psoriasis. Acta Derm Venereol 56:473–479
22. Parrish JA, Jaenicke KF (1981) Action spectrum for phototherapy of psoriasis. J Invest Dermatol 76:359–362
23. Diette KM, Momtaz K, Stern RS, Arndt KA, Parrish JA (1984) Role of ultraviolet A in phototherapy for psoriasis. J Am Acad Dermatol 11:441–447
24. Schröpl F (1977) Zum heutigen Stand der technischen Entwicklung der selektiven Phototherapie. Dtsch Dermatol 25:499–504
25. Hönigsmann H, Fritsch P, Jaschke E (1977) UV-Therapie der Psoriasis. Halbseitenvergleich zwischen oraler Photochemotherapie (PUVA) und selektiver UV-Phototherapie (SUP). Z Hautkr 52:1078–1082
26. Van Weelden H, De La Faille HB, Young E, Van der Leun IC (1988) A new development in UVB phototherapy of psoriasis. Br J Dermatol 119:11–19
27. Quinn AG, Diffey BL, Craig PS, Farr PM et al (1994) Definition of the minimal erythema dose used for diagnostic phototesting (abstract). Br J Dermatol 131:56
28. Ibbotson SH, Bilsland D, Cox NH et al (2004) An update and guidance on narrowband ultraviolet B phototherapy: a British Photodermatology Group Workshop Report. Br J Dermatol 151:283–97
29. Lebwohl M, Martinez J, Weber P, De Luca R (1995) Effects of topical preparations on the erythemogenicity of UVB: implications for psoriasis phototherapy. J Am Acad Dermatol 32:469–471
30. Tanenbaum L, Parrish JA, Pathak MA, Anderson RR, Fitzpatrick TB (1975) Tar phototoxicity and phototherapy for psoriasis. Arch Dermatol 111:467–470
31. Storbeck K, Hölzle E, Schurer N, Lehmann P, Plewig G (1993) Narrow-band UVB (311nm) versus conventional broad-band UVB with and without dithranol in phototherapy for psoriasis. J Am Acad Dermatol 28:227–231
32. Meola T Jr, Soter NA, Lim HW (1991) Are topical corticosteroids useful adjunctive therapy for the treatment of psoriasis with ultraviolet radiation? A review of the literature. Arch Dermatol 127:1708–1713
33. Steigleder GK, Orfanos CE, Pullmann H (1979) Retinoid-SUP-Therapie der Psoriasis. Z Hautkr 54:19–23
34. Iest J, Boer J (1989) Combined treatment of psoriasis with acitretin and UVB phototherapy compared with acitretin alone and UVB alone. Br J Dermatol 120:665–670
35. Green C, Ferguson J, Lakshmipathi T, Johnson BE (1988) 311nm UVB phototherapy—an

effective treatment for psoriasis. Br J Dermatol 119:691–696
36. Picot E, Meunier L, Picot-Debeze MC, Peyron JL, Meynadier J (1992) Treatment of psoriasis with a 311-nm UVB lamp. Br J Dermatol 127:509–512
37. Van Weelden H, Baart de la Faille H, Young E, Van der Leun JC (1990) Comparison of narrow-band UV-B phototherapy and PUVA photochemotherapy in the treatment of psoriasis. Acta Derm Venereol 70:212–215
38. Tanew A, Radakovic-Fijan S, Schemper M, Hönigsmann H (1999) Paired comparison study on narrow-band (TL-01) UVB phototherapy versus photochemotherapy (PUVA) in the treatment of chronic plaque type psoriasis. Arch Dermatol 135:519–524
39. Green C, Lakshmipathi T, Johnson BE, Ferguson J (1992) A comparison of the efficacy and relapse rates of narrowband UVB (TL-01) monotherapy vs. etretinate (re-TL-01) vs. etretinate-PUVA (re-PUVA) in the treatment of psoriasis patients. Br J Dermatol 127:5–9
40. Karvonen J, Kokkonen EL, Ruotsalainen E (1989) 311 nm UVB lamps in the treatment of psoriasis with the Ingram regimen. Acta Derm Venereol 69:82–85
41. Kerscher M, Volkenandt M, Plewig G, Lehmann P (1993) Combination phototherapy of psoriasis with calcipotriol and narrow-band UVB. Lancet 342:9
42. Stern RS, Laird N (1994) The carcinogenic risk of treatments for severe psoriasis. Cancer 73:2759–2764
43. Man I, Crombie IK, Dawe RS, Ibbotson SH, Ferguson J (2005) The photocarcinogenic risk of narrowband UVB (TL-01) phototherapy: early follow-up data. Br J Dermatol 152:755–57
44. Hönigsmann H, Szeimies RF, Knobler R et al (1999) Photochemotherapy and photodynamic therapy. In: Freedberg IM, Eisen AZ, Wolff K, Austen KF, Goldsmith LA, Katz SI (eds) Fitzpatrick's dermatology in general medicine, 5th edn. McGraw-Hill, New York, pp 2880–2900
45. El Mofty AM (1948) A preliminary report on the treatment of leukoderma with *Ammi majus* Linn. J R Egypt Med Assoc 31:651–655
46. Lerner AB, Denton CR, Fitzpatrick TB (1953) Clinical and experimental studies with 8-methoxypsoralen in vitiligo. J Invest Dermatol 20:299–314
47. Parrish JA, Fitzpatrick TB, Tanenbaum L, Pathak MA (1974) Photochemotherapy of psoriasis with oral methoxsalen and long wave ultraviolet light. N Engl J Med 291:1207–1211
48. Wolff K, Hönigsmann H, Gschnait F, Konrad K (1975) Photochemotherapie bei Psoriasis. Klinische Erfahrungen bei 152 Patienten. Dtsch Med Wochenschr 100:2471–2477
49. Mortazawi SAM (1972) Meladinine mit UVA bei Vitiligo, Psoriasis, Parapsoriasis und Akne vulgaris. Dermatol Wochenschr 158:908–911
50. Walter JF, Voorhees JJ (1973) Psoriasis improved by psoralen plus light. Acta Derm Venereol 53:469–472
51. Honig B, Morison WL, Karp D (1994) Photochemotherapy beyond psoriasis. J Am Acad Dermatol 31:775–790
52. Pathak MA, Fitzpatrick TB (1992) The evolution of photochemotherapy with psoralens and UVA (PUVA): 2000 BC to 1992 AD. J Photochem Photobiol B Biol 14:3–22
53. Hönigsmann H, Jaschke E, Nitsche V, Brenner W, Rauschmeier W, Wolff K (1982) Serum levels of 8-methoxypsoralen in two different drug preparations. Correlation with photosensitivity and UVA dose requirements for photochemotherapy. J Invest Dermatol 79:233–236
54. Herfst MJ, De Wolff FA (1983) Intraindividual and interindividual variability in 8-methoxypsoralen kinetics and effect in psoriatic patients. Clin Pharmacol Ther 34:117–125
55. Brickl R, Schmid J, Koss FW (1984) Pharmacokinetics and pharmacodynamics of psoralens after oral administration: considerations and conclusions. Natl Cancer Inst Monogr 66:63–67
56. Dall'Acqua F (1986) Furocoumarin photochemistry and its main biological implications. In: Hönigsmann H, Stingl G (eds) Therapeutic photomedicine. Current problems in dermatology, vol 15. Karger, Basel, pp 137–163
57. Tessman JW, Isaacs ST, Hearst JE (1985) Photochemistry of the furan-side 8-methoxypso-

ralen-thymidine monoadduct inside the DNA helix. Conversion to diadduct and to pyroneside monoadduct. Biochemistry 24:1669–1676
58. Schmitt I, Chimenti S, Gasparro F (1995) Psoralen-protein photochemistry—the forgotten field. J Photochem Photobiol B Biol 27:101–105
59. Averbeck D (1989) Recent advances in psoralen phototoxicity mechanism. Photochem Photobiol 50:859–882
60. Neuner P, Charvat B, Knobler R, Kirnbauer R, Schwarz A, Luger TA, Schwarz T (1994) Cytokine release by peripheral blood mononuclear cells is affected by 8-methoxypsoralen plus UV-A. Photochem Photobiol 59:182–188
61. Vallat V, Gilleaudeau P, Battat L, Wolfe J, Nabeya R, Heftler N, Hodak E, Gottlieb AB, Krueger JG (1994) PUVA bath therapy strongly suppresses immunological and epidermal activation in psoriasis: a possible cellular basis for remittive therapy. J Exp Med 180:283–296
62. Johnson R, Staiano-Coico L, Austin L, Cardinale I, Nabeya-Tsukifuji R, Krueger JG (1996) PUVA treatment selectively induces a cell cycle block and subsequent apoptosis in human T-lymphocytes. Photochem Photobiol 63:566–571
63. Cripps DJ, Lowe NJ, Lerner AB (1982) Action spectra of topical psoralens: a re-evaluation. Br J Dermatol 107:77–82
64. Kaidbey KH (1985) An action spectrum for 8-methoxypsoralen-sensitized inhibition of DNA synthesis in vivo. J Invest Dermatol 85:98–101
65. Brücke J, Tanew A, Ortel B, Hönigsmann H (1991) Relative efficacy of 335 and 365 nm radiation in photochemotherapy of psoriasis. Br J Dermatol 124:372–374
66. Farr PM, Diffey BL, Higgins EM, Matthews JSN (1991) The action spectrum between 320 and 400 nm for clearance of psoriasis by psoralen photochemotherapy. Br J Dermatol 124:443–448
67. Ortel B, Gange RW (1990) An action spectrum for the elicitation of erythema in skin persistently sensitized by photobound 8-methoxypsoralen. J Invest Dermatol 94:781–785
68. Ibbotson SH, Dawe RS, Farr PM (2001) The effect of methoxsalen dose on ultraviolet-A-induced erythema. J Invest Dermatol 116:813–815
69. Ibbotson SH, Farr PM (1999) The time-course of psoralen ultraviolet A (PUVA) erythema. J Invest Dermatol 113:346–350
70. Henseler T, Wolff K, Hönigsmann H, Christophers E (1981) The European PUVA study (EPS) on oral 8-methoxypsoralen photochemotherapy of psoriasis. A cooperative study among 18 European centres. Lancet 1:853–857
71. Melski JW, Tanenbaum L, Fitzpatrick TB, Bleich HL, Parrish JA (1977) Oral methoxsalen photochemotherapy for the treatment of psoriasis: a cooperative clinical trial. J Invest Dermatol 68:328–335
72. British Photodermatology Group (1994) British Photodermatology Group guidelines for PUVA. Br J Dermatol 130:246–255
73. Tanew A, Radakovic-Fijan S, Seeber A, Hönigsmann H (2008) PUVA maintenance treatment for psoriasis. J Am Acad Derm, in press
74. Tanew A, Ortel B, Rappersberger K, Hönigsmann H (1988) 5-methoxypsoralen (Bergapten) for photochemotherapy. J Am Acad Dermatol 18:333–338
75. Green C, George S, Lakshmipathi T, Ferguson J (1993) A trial of accelerated PUVA in psoriasis. Clin Exp Dermatol 18:297–299
76. Tanew A, Ortel B, Hönigsmann H (1999) Halfside comparison of erythemogenic versus suberythemogenic UVA doses in oral photochemotherapy of psoriasis. J Am Acad Dermatol 41:408–413
77. Taylor CR, Kwangsukstith C, Wimberly J, Kollias N, Anderson RR (1999) Turbo-PUVA: dihydroxyacetone-enhanced photochemotherapy for psoriasis: a pilot study. Arch Dermatol 135:540–544
78. Fischer T, Alsins J (1976) Treatment of psoriasis with trioxsalen baths and dysprosium lamps. Acta Derm Venereol 56:383–390

79. Calzavara-Pinton PG, Ortel B, Carlino AM, Hönigsmann H, De Panfilis G (1993) Phototesting and phototoxic side effects in bath-PUVA. J Am Acad Dermatol 28:657–659
80. Cristofolini M, Recchia G, Boi S, Piscioli F, Bordin F, Baccichetti F, Carlassare F, Tamaro M, Pani B, Babudri N, Guiotto A, Rodighiero P, Vedaldi D, Dall'Acqua F (1990) 6-Methylangelicins: new monofunctional photochemotherapeutic agents for psoriasis. Br J Dermatol 122:513–524
81. Dubertret L, Averbeck D, Bisagni E, Moron J, Moustacchi E, Billardon C, Papadopoulo D, Nocentini S, Vigny P, Blais J, Bensasson RV, Ronfard-Haret JC, Land EJ, Zajdela F, Latarjet R (1985) Photochemotherapy using pyridopsoralens. Biochimie 67:417–422
82. Morison WL (1985) PUVA combination therapy. Photodermatol 2:229–236
83. Morison WL (1992) Phototherapy and photochemotherapy. Adv Dermatol 7:255–270
84. Petzelbauer P, Hönigsmann H, Langer K, Anegg B, Strohal R, Tanew A, Wolff K (1990) Cyclosporin A in combination with photochemotherapy (PUVA) in the treatment of psoriasis. Br J Dermatol 123:641–647
85. Molin L, Larkö O (1997) Cancer induction by immunosuppression in psoriasis after heavy PUVA treatment (letter). Acta Derm Venereol 77(5):402
86. Van-de-Kerkhof PC, De-Rooij MJ (1997) Multiple squamous cell carcinomas in a psoriatic patient following high-dose photochemotherapy and cyclosporin treatment: response to long-term acitretin maintenance. Br J Dermatol 136(2):275–278
87. Marcil I, Stern RS (2001) Squamous-cell cancer of the skin in patients given PUVA and ciclosporin: nested cohort crossover study. Lancet 358:1042–1045
88. Fritsch PO, Hönigsmann H, Jaschke E, Wolff K (1978) Augmentation of oral methoxsalen-photochemotherapy with an oral retinoic acid derivative. J Invest Dermatol 70:178–182
89. Hönigsmann H, Wolff K (1989) Results of therapy for psoriasis using retinoid and photo-chemotherapy (RePUVA). Pharmacol Ther 40:67–73
90. Hönigsmann H, Wolff K (1983) Isotretinoin-PUVA for psoriasis. Lancet 1:236
91. Saurat JH, Geiger JM, Amblard P, Beani JC, Boulanger A, Claudy A, Frenk E, Guilhou JJ, Grosshans E, Merot Y, Meynadier J, Tapernoux B (1988) Randomized double-blind multicenter study comparing acitretin-PUVA, etretinate-PUVA and placebo-PUVA in the treatment of severe psoriasis. Dermatologica 177:218–224
92. Tanew A, Guggenbichler A, Hönigsmann H, Geiger JM, Fritsch P (1991) Photochemotherapy for severe psoriasis without or in combination with acitretin: a randomized double-blind comparison study. J Am Acad Dermatol 25:682–684
93. Chou RC, Wyss R, Huselton CA, Wiegand UW (1992) A potentially new metabolic pathway: ethyl esterification of acitretin. Xenobiotica 22:993–1002
94. Maier H, Hönigsmann H (1996) Concentration of etretinate in plasma and subcutaneous fat after long-term acitretin. Lancet 348:1107
95. Stern RS (1994) Epidemiology of skin disease in HIV infection: a cohort study of health maintenance organization members. J Invest Dermatol 102:34S–37S
96. Duvic M, Rapini R, Hoots WK, Mansell PW (1987) Human immunodeficiency virus-associated vitiligo: expression of autoimmunity with immunodeficiency? J Am Acad Dermatol 17:656–662
97. Crane GA, Variakojis D, Rosen ST, Sands AM, Roenigk HH Jr (1991) Cutaneous T-cell lymphoma in patients with human immune deficiency virus infection. Arch Dermatol 127:989–994
98. Johnson TM, Duvic M, Rapini RP, Rios A (1985) Acquired immunodeficiency syndrome exacerbates psoriasis (letter). N Engl J Med 313:1415
99. Duvic M, Crane MM, Conant M, Mahoney SE, Reveille JD, Lehrman SN (1994) Zidovudine improves psoriasis in human immunodeficiency virus positive males. Arch Dermatol 130:447–451
100. Stingl G, Rappersberger K, Tschachler E, Garner S, Groh V, Mann DL, Wolff K, Popovic M (1990) Langerhans cells in HIV-1 infections. J Am Acad Dermatol 22:1210–1217

101. Mahoney SE, Duvic M, Nickoloff BJ, Minshall M, Smith LC, Griffiths CE, Paddock SW, Lewis DE (1991) Human immunodeficiency virus transcripts identified in human immunodeficiency virus related psoriasis and Kaposi's sarcoma lesions. J Clin Invest 88:174–185
102. Kadunce DP, Krueger GG (1995) Pathogenesis of psoriasis, current concepts. Dermatol Clin 13:723–737
103. Ullrich SE (1996) Does exposure to UV radiation induce a shift to a Th-2-like immune reaction? Photochem Photobiol 64:254–258
104. Morrey JD, Bourn SM, Bunch TD, Jackson MK, Sidwell RW, Barrows LR, Daynes RA, Rosen CA (1991) In vivo activation of human immunodeficiency virus type I long terminal repeat by UV type A (UV-A) light plus psoralen and UV-B light in the skin of transgenic mice. J Virol 65:5045–5051
105. Wang CY, Brodland DG, Su WP (1995) Skin cancers associated with acquired immunodeficiency syndrome. Mayo Clin Proc 70:766–772
106. Meola T, Soter NA, Ostreicher R, Sanchez M, Moy JA (1993) The safety of UVB phototherapy in patients with HIV infection. J Am Acad Dermatol 29:216–220
107. Ranki A, Puska P, Mattinen S, Lagerstedt A, Krohn K (1991) Effect of PUVA on immunologic and virologic findings in HIV-infected patients. J Am Acad Dermatol 24:404–410
108. Horn TD, Morison WL, Farzadegan H, Zmudzka BZ, Beer JZ (1994) Effects of psoralen plus UVA radiation (PUVA) on HIV-1 in human beings: a pilot study. J Am Acad Dermatol 31:735–740
109. Zmudzka BZ, Miller SA, Jacobs ME, Beer JZ (1996) Medical UV exposures and HIV activation. Photochem Photobiol 64:246–253
110. Morison WL (1996) PUVA therapy is preferable to UVB phototherapy in the management of HIV-associated dermatoses. Photochem Photobiol 64:267–268
111. Cox NH, Jones SK, Downey DJ, Tuyp EJ, Jay JL, Moseley H, MacKie RM (1987) Cutaneous and ocular side-effects of oral photochemotherapy: results of an 8-year follow-up study. Br J Dermatol 116:145–152
112. Calzavara-Pinton PG, Carlino A, Manfredi E, Semerano F, Zane C, De Panfilis G (1994) Ocular side effects of PUVA-treated patients refusing eye sun protection. Acta Derm Venereol [Suppl] 186:164–165
113. Young AR (1996) Photochemotherapy and skin carcinogesis: a critical review. In: Hönigsmann H, Jori G, Young AR (eds) The fundamental bases of phototherapy. OEMF, Milano, pp 77–87
114. Stern RS, Laird N for the Photochemotherapy Follow-up Study (1994) The carcinogenic risks of treatments for severe psoriasis. Cancer 73:2759–2764
115. Maier H, Schemper M, Ortel B, Binder M, Tanew A, Hönigsmann H (1996) Skin tumours in photochemotherapy for psoriasis. A single centre follow-up of 496 patients. Dermatology 193:185–191
116. Stern RS, Lunder EJ (1998) Risk of squamous cell carcinoma and methoxsalen (psoralen) and UV-A radiation (PUVA). A meta-analysis. Arch Dermatol 134(12):1582–1585
117. Stern RS, Liebman EJ, Vakeva L (1998) Oral psoralen and ultraviolet-A light (PUVA) treatment of psoriasis and persistent risk of nonmelanoma skin cancer. PUVA follow-up study. J Natl Cancer Inst 90:1278–1284
118. Henseler T, Christophers E, Hönigsmann H, Wolff K (1987) Skin tumors in the European PUVA study: eight year follow-up of 1643 patients treated with PUVA for psoriasis. J Am Acad Dermatol 16:108–116
119. Lim JL, Stern RS (2005) High levels of ultraviolet B exposure increase the risk of nonmelanoma skin cancer in psoralen and ultraviolet A-treated patients. J Invest Dermatol 124:505–513
120. Stern RS, Members of the photochemotherapy follow-up study (1990) Genital tumors among men with psoriasis exposed to psoralens and ultraviolet A (PUVA) radiation and ultraviolet B radiation. N Engl Med J 322:1093–1097

121. Wolff K, Hönigsmann H (1991) Genital carcinomas in psoriasis patients treated with photochemotherapy. Lancet 1:439
122. Young AR, Magnus IA, Davies AC, Smith NP (1983) A comparison of the phototumorigenic potential of 8-MOP and 5-MOP in hairless albino mice exposed to solar simulated irradiation. Br J Dermatol 108:507–518
123. Gupta AK, Stern RS, Swanson NA, Anderson TF, the PUVA follow-up study (1988) Cutaneous melanomas in patients treated with psoralen plus ultraviolet A. J Am Acad Dermatol 19:67–76
124. Stern RS (2001) The PUVA Follow up Study. The risk of melanoma in association with long-term exposure to PUVA. J Am Acad Dermatol 44:755–761.
125. Wolff K (1997) Should PUVA be abandoned? Editorial. N Engl J Med 336:1090–1091
126. Nijsten TEC, Stern RS (2003) Oral retinoid use reduces cutaneous squamous cell carcinoma risk in patients with psoriasis treated with psoralen-UVA: a nested cohort study. J Am Acad Dermatol 49:644–50
127. Hannuksela-Svahn A, Sigurgeirsson B, Pukkala E, Lindelöf B, Berne B, Hannuksela M, Poikolainen K, Karvonen J (1999) Trioxsalen bath PUVA did not increase the risk of squamous cell skin carcinoma and cutaneous malignant melanoma in a joint analysis of 944 Swedish and Finnish patients with psoriasis. Br J Dermatol 141:497–501
128. Hannuksela M, Stenbäck F, Lahti A (1986) The carcinogenic properties of topical PUVA. A lifelong study in mice. Arch Dermatol Res 278:347–351
129. Hannuksela-Svahn A, Pukkala E, Koulu L, Jansén CT, Karvonen J (1999) Cancer incidence among Finnish psoriasis patients treated with 8-methoxypsoralen bath PUVA. J Am Acad Dermatol 40:694–696
130. Slaper H, Schothorst AA, Van der Leun JC (1986) Risk evaluation of UVB therapy for psoriasis: comparison of calculated risk for UVB therapy and observed risk in PUVA-treated patients. Photodermatol 3:271–283
131. Young AR (1995) Carcinogenicity of UVB phototherapy assessed. Lancet 345:1431–1432
132. Morison WL, Baughman RD, Day RM, Forbes PD, Hönigsmann H, Krueger GG, Lebwohl M, Lew R, Naldi L, Parrish JA, Piepkorn M, Stern RS, Weinstein GD, Whitmore SE (1998) Consensus workshop on the toxic effects of long-term PUVA therapy. Arch Dermatol 134:595–598

第4章 特应性皮炎的光治疗

J. Krutmann, A. Morita

内容

特应性皮炎:从日光浴到现代光疗 ········· 87
特应性皮炎的发病机制 ················· 88
特应性皮炎概念相关的光疗 ············· 89
展望 ································· 97

要点

> 现代光疗作为特应性皮炎的日常治疗手段,是一种对症光治疗。
> UVA-1 治疗代表了一种针对急性和重症进展期特应性皮炎患者的新颖的单一治疗方法。
> PUVA 在特应性皮炎患者的治疗中有限制。
> 体外光化学免疫疗法可能对治疗重度特应性皮炎患者有益。
> 311nm UVB 治疗可能代表了诱导特应性皮炎患者长期改善的光疗模式。

特应性皮炎:从日光浴到现代光疗

几十年来普遍认为紫外线(UV)的照射对特应性皮炎患者有益[29]。1929年,德国皮肤学专家 Buschke 声明海洋气候对特应性皮炎的效果让人"惊喜"。1940年,Lomhold 和 Norrlind 认为大多数特应性皮炎患者的症状在夏季得到改善[42]。1948年,Nexman 首先系统性地评价了光疗在特应性皮炎患者的有益作用,在他的研究中,特应性皮炎患者使用炭精电弧灯照射治疗[48]。20世纪70年代末期,特应性皮炎的光疗一直是使用现代荧光灯作为发射光源。在过去的5年中,一些新的光疗形式开始出现,包括 UVA-1 治疗[35,36]和 311nm UVB 治疗[15]。这使得现在的皮肤科专家可以从不同光疗模式的多样化光谱中为其患者做出特定的光疗选择。

同时,在对特应性皮炎发病机制的了解上取得了突破性的进展。光疗作为特应性皮炎现代治疗的方法是由当前它的发病机制的观点所决定的[38]。下面的章节将简要地概述特应性皮炎发病机制的最新认识。

特应性皮炎的发病机制

现在普遍认为特应性皮炎是针对吸入性变应原诱导的 T 细胞介导的免疫反应[26]。特应性皮炎的主要临床、组织学、免疫组织化学特征显著类似变应性接触性皮炎这一事实支持了这一观点。在特应性皮炎患者皮损中,包括了以 Th 淋巴细胞为主的炎性浸润和由这些细胞原位产生的细胞因子,导致了特应性皮炎患者皮损的产生和迁延。目前已知表达于特应性皮炎患者皮损的细胞因子的类型主要取决于疾病的阶段[22]。来自急性特应性皮炎或湿疹样皮炎的皮损的活检显示 Th2 样细胞因子白介素(IL-4)的表达占优。特应性皮炎患者的表皮在接触标准化的吸入性变应原后激发产生皮损,然后对皮损发展的早期阶段进行研究(变应原接触24小时后)。同时活检也发现 Th1 样细胞因子干扰素-γ 的表达低于正常水平。在晚一些阶段的时候,即在特应性皮炎的慢性苔藓样皮损或在48小时吸入性变应原斑贴试验诱发的皮损中,这一细胞因子的模式发生了逆转。在后期阶段,Th1 样细胞因子干扰素-γ 的表达显著增加,而 IL-4 表达降低[18-20,23]。干扰素-γ 表达的增加导致了特应性皮炎患者临床上明显皮损的产生和迁延,即观察到在特应性皮炎的临床进程和特应性皮炎患者皮损中干扰素-γ 表达有密切相关性。这些发现可能更好地阐释了特应性皮炎发病机制的双相模式,初始激发阶段以 Th2 样的炎症反应为主,临床上没有明显的皮损,之后转换为2期湿疹样模式,此阶段以 Th1 样细胞因子干扰素-γ 表达占优,临床上表现为湿疹样[25]。最近研究显示细胞因子 IL-12 的表达增加可能使 Th2 细胞因子模式向 Th1 细胞因子模式的转化(图4.1)。

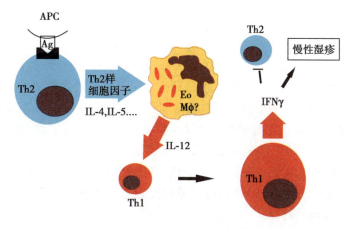

图 4.1 特应性皮炎的发病机制

特应性皮炎概念相关的光疗

基于这种双相模式,目前可以认为光疗策略是针对特应性皮炎的初始阶段,光疗可以直接作用于疾病的湿疹样阶段,通过下调特应性皮炎皮损处 IFN-r 的表达而达到症状的缓解,因此,从广义上来说,光疗被认为是预防性的措施[38]。特应性皮炎的光疗进一步分为两种,一种是可以短期有效治疗特应性皮炎急性加重期的有效单一光疗模式,另一种是低效的光疗模式,可以成功的长期联合治疗特应性皮炎患者慢性形式(表4.1)。现代光疗作为特应性皮炎的日常治疗手段,是对症的光治疗。

表 4.1 特应性皮炎的光疗

指征	模式	备注	行为模式
急性,严重性的	高剂量 UVA-1,PUVA,体外光化学免疫疗法	单一治疗,糖皮质激素的替代治疗	症状学的,抗湿疹样作用
慢性,温和的	311nm, UVB, UVA/UVB,低剂量 UVA-1,宽谱 UVB,宽谱 UVA	联合治疗,为了节省糖皮质激素	症状学的,抗湿疹样作用,维持治疗

急性严重特应性皮炎的光(化学)治疗

一般情况下,急性、严重特应性皮炎可使用 UVA-1 光疗,系统性运用补骨脂素联合 UVA(PUVA)和体外光化学免疫疗法,而传统的 UVA/UVB 和窄谱 UVB

治疗的光疗模式主要用于该种疾病的慢性期(表4.1)。

UVA-1 光疗

应用 UVA-1 照射,即波长(340~400nm)UVA 照射,治疗特应性皮炎患者的理论依据是以免疫学研究为基础的,该研究显示人体皮肤暴露于 130J/cm² 单一剂量的 UVA-1 照射与表皮朗汉细胞激活同种反应性 T 细胞的功能消失有关[3]。同时,有越来越多的证据显示表皮朗汉细胞凭借其与 IgE 分子结合的能力,可能在吸入变应原介导的 T 细胞活化中发挥重要作用,也因此在特应性皮炎的发病机制中起到关键作用[6]。另外,对比宽谱 UVB、UVA/UVB 治疗特应性皮炎功效的临床研究显示,传统的 UVB 治疗功效可能通过增加光谱中 UVA 比例(UVA/UVB 治疗)得以显著提高[27]。

针对特应性皮炎患者使用 UVA-1 照射治疗功效的首次研究中,运用单一剂量 130J/cm² 的 UVA-1(大剂量 UVA-1 治疗)照射急性、重症特应性皮炎患者,每天一次,连续 15 天[36]。运用单一疗法模式对比 UVA-1 与传统 UVA/UVB 的治疗功效,即两组均禁止使用润肤霜。从两个方面对治疗功效进行评估:由 Costa 等[11]初始完善和建立的临床评分系统,其由严重度和基线评分组成,以及嗜酸粒细胞阳离子蛋白的血清水平检测。既往认为,嗜酸粒细胞阳离子蛋白的血清水平是反应特应性皮炎疾病活动性的敏感性参数,因此被用于评估 UVA-1 照射的治疗功效的客观参数[12]。临床评分的评估显示 UVA-1 治疗可以快速有效的诱导特应性皮炎患者临床症状的改善,与传统的 UVA/UVB 治疗相比,UVA-1 照射 6 和 15 次后临床症状更显著地改善(图 4.2a,b)。类似地,特应性皮炎患者升高的嗜酸粒细胞阳离子蛋白的血清水平在 UVA-1 治疗后显著降低,而在 UVA/UVB 治疗后基本维持不变。

这些初步但令人鼓舞的结论显示 UVA-1 治疗能代表一种崭新的光疗模式,用于治疗急性、严重加重的特应性皮炎。在随后的数年里,这些初步的观察结果被大量的研究所确认,这些研究主要代表了非标准的,开放性的,有些甚至是无对照的研究[1,33,34,43,68]。Krutmann 等的首次研究并未成功地提供 UVA-1 治疗与局部使用糖皮质激素的直接对比,而后者是用于治疗急性、严重进展的特应性皮炎的金标准。在随后的多中心试验中,53 例患者随机地被分配使用 UVA-1 治疗(一天一次,130J/cm²,共 10 天),传统的 UVA/UVB 治疗(一天一次,最小红斑量决定,共 10 天),或局部使用氟考龙(一天一次,共 10 天)[39]。至今,这项研究也是唯一运用可控的、随机方式对 UVA-1 治疗的功效提供多中心评估的研究。在 10 次治疗后发现,三个治疗组患者病情均改善,总的临床评分的降低,与 UVA/UVB 治疗组对比,接受糖皮质激素治疗和 UVA-1 治疗的患者的临床改善更为显著。而与糖皮质激素治疗组相比,UVA-1 治疗可以更好的下调临床评分。

第4章　特应性皮炎的光治疗

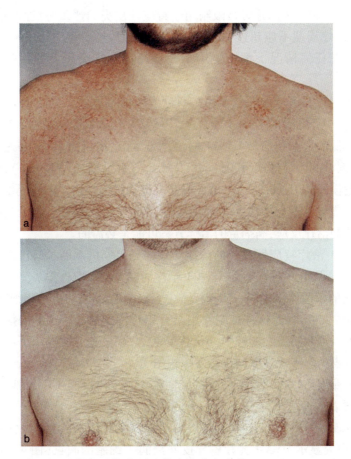

图4.2　急性加重期的严重特应性皮炎患者 UVA1（10×130J/cm^2）光疗前（a）、后（b）

这些临床观察在实验室研究中通过对比三组治疗组治疗前后嗜酸粒细胞阳离子蛋白的血清水平和外周血的嗜酸粒细胞数量得到证实。汇总多中心试验研究结果显示，UVA-1 和糖皮质激素在治疗急性、严重加重的特应性皮炎疗效显著优于传统的 UVA/UVB。因此 UVA-1 治疗可替代糖皮质激素用于治疗严重的特应性皮炎。

UVA-1 治疗不可用于 UVA-1 敏感的特应性皮炎或多形性日光疹等光敏性皮肤病的治疗[38]。因此在 UVA-1 治疗前必须排除这些疾病。这能通过简单的光激发试验来完成。除了疱疹样湿疹，在 UVA-1 治疗特应性皮炎过程中未发现其他急性副作用，尽管其潜在的致癌风险在理论上是存在的[40]。将无毛的白化病 skh-hr1 鼠暴露于 UVA-1 照射时，能诱导鳞状细胞癌，因此 UVA-1 照射是否诱发人类形成恶性肿瘤，现在仍存着争议，但尚不能被排除。在对 UVA-1 治疗有更多认识之前,UVA-1 治疗常被限制用于特应性皮炎的严重、急性加重期,一般来说,一个治疗周期不应超过 10~15 次连续照射,且一年中运用不超过一次。UVA-1 光疗在任何情况下都不能用于儿童特应性皮炎患者的治疗(小于 18 岁)[40]。

UVA-1 照射的治疗功效是否存在剂量依赖仍有争议。类似于 $130J/cm^2$ 的高剂量照射,中等剂量的 UVA-1 也优于 UVA/UVB 治疗[33]。最近 J. C. Simon 等直接对比了低剂量和高剂量 UVA-1 的治疗方案(手稿待出版)。在这项开放性研究中,高剂量的治疗模式($130J/cm^2$)优于中等剂量模式($50J/cm^2$),后者明显优于低剂量模式($20J/cm^2$)[28]。因此看起来低剂量治疗模式不能提供任何超过传统光疗的优势。这与中等和高剂量 UVA-1 光疗形成对比。为了获得最佳的和长期持续的治疗反应,高剂量的治疗方案可能是必需的[1]。

对 UVA-1 治疗特应性皮炎的治疗功效的光免疫机制的了解已经取得了重大的进展[37]。从这些研究来看,UVA-1 治疗能够下调特应性皮炎患者原位皮损中 γ-干扰素的表达。由于同一病理标本中管家基因 β-肌动蛋白和细胞因子 IL-4 的表达都减少了,因此这种抑制作用具有相对特异性。UVA-1 治疗和糖皮质激素应用可以抑制特应性湿疹中 γ-干扰素表达,这很有可能提示了不同治疗方案在特应性皮炎患者通过共同机制发挥作用[19]。

UVA-1 照射治疗可以直接影响特应性湿疹真皮内浸润 Th1 细胞,因此下调了 γ-干扰素表达[16,17]。

研究发现体外的 UVA-1 照射高效的诱导人 T 细胞凋亡(程序性的细胞死亡)。在体研究显示 UVA-1 光疗诱导皮肤浸润 T 细胞的凋亡(图 4.3a~d),因此使炎性浸润逐步减少,患者皮肤疾患的改善[47]。这些发现也引起了使用 UVA-1 光疗治疗其他 T 细胞介导的皮肤疾病的兴趣[49]。

除了直接作用于表皮和真皮的 T 细胞,UVA-1 照射可能通过间接机制,例如诱导产生抗炎性细胞因子如由表皮角质形成细胞产生的 IL-10 改变了 Th1 细胞 γ-干扰素的表达,这也依次可能以旁泌方式作用于 T 细胞。为了证实这一观点,体内试验显示,UVA-1 照射后,培养的人角质形成细胞的 IL-10 mRNA 和分泌的 IL-10 蛋白表达增加[21]。

免疫组织化学研究发现接受 UVA-1 治疗的特应性皮炎患者的病理活检标本显示,除了 T 细胞和角质形成细胞,上皮朗汉细胞和真皮的肥大细胞也是 UVA-1 照射的靶细胞[19]. 与 UVA/UVB 治疗相比,UVA-1 治疗不仅降低了表皮中 IgE 耐受的朗汉细胞的相对数量,也降低了真皮 CD1a+朗汉细胞和肥大细胞的数量。近期的观察结果使得 UVA-1 治疗在色素性荨麻疹的处理中得到使用,皮肤和系统的症状在治疗中获得了立即的和长期持续的缓解[62]。

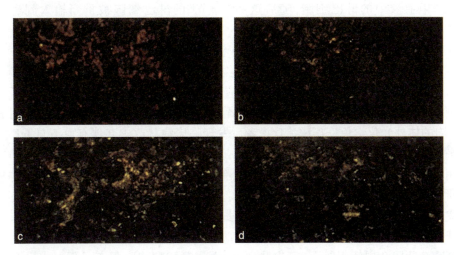

图4.3 在之前(a)、之后一次(b)、两次(c)、三次(d)UVA-1照射(单一剂量130J/cm²)特应性湿疹患者皮损中T细胞的凋亡。红色的CD4+T细胞(辅助性T细胞);绿色凋亡TUNEL试验细胞;橙色T细胞

PUVA 治疗

系统性光化学治疗(PUVA)是联合了口服的补骨脂素和 UVA 照射的治疗方法[31]。自从 30 年前 PUVA 引入皮肤病学光疗以来,它对一系列皮肤病的治疗都具有高效性(见[45]),包括特应性皮炎。尽管 PUVA 可以成功治疗中度、重度甚至红皮病性的特应性皮炎,但必须认识到 PUVA 治疗具有较大的不良反应[2,4,42,45,46,58,59,61,66]。与 PUVA 治疗银屑病相比,治疗特应性皮炎缓解的实际数目相对较高。更重要的是,如果光化学治疗不与系统性糖皮质激素联合使用,不能继续维持治疗更长的时间而间隔超过数年,那么 PUVA 治疗的终止与高比例患者出现反弹现象有关[53]。相对低龄的特应性皮炎患儿长期应用 PUVA 应得到特别关注,近期报道显示,PUVA 的长期应用可能与发生皮肤癌的风险增加有关,包括恶性黑素瘤[64,65]。进一步的不利结论来自光敏感性延长,这需要太阳镜保护来防止白内障的出现,和系统性副作用的出现,如在相对高比例患者中出现的恶心(高达百分之二十)。特应性皮炎患者 PUVA 治疗的使用受到限制,同时 PUVA 不能作为替代糖皮质激素或 UVA-1 治疗严重的特应性皮炎的手段。

体外光化学治疗

证据证明体外光化学免疫疗法对治疗重度特应性皮炎患者有效。体外光化学免疫疗法是包含光激活补骨脂素(8-甲氧补骨脂素)的新鲜提取血液经过体外UVA暴露[14]。普遍认为 UVA 照射活化了药理学上失活的 8-甲氧补骨脂素,后者影响血液中的淋巴细胞,随后这些"调节"的淋巴细胞被重新输入到患者体内。

体外光化学免疫疗法较成功地用于治疗 Sézary 综合征的患者。也有推荐其可以用于一些免疫基础的皮肤疾病如移植物抗宿主病的治疗[67]。Prinz 等最早将体外光化学免疫疗法成功的用于特应性皮炎患者的治疗[51]。他们报道了三例终身伴有症状的重症特应性皮炎患者。由于他们病情对传统治疗抵抗,间隔 4 周的体外光化学免疫疗法治疗患者后发现临床症状改善并伴有血清总 IgE 水平的降低,但体外光化学免疫疗法并不是作为单一的治疗方法而是联合局部外用泼尼卡酯,然而后者单独使用并不能有效地控制这类病人病情的活动。这些研究结果已在一项非相关研究中被证实,在此项研究中,三例早前难治性特应性皮炎患者使用单一体外光化学免疫疗法后得到了控制[56]。所有的患者临床症状得到巨大的改善,这也取决于治疗周期的频率(图 4.4a,b)。当体外光化学免疫疗法间隔 2 周使用时,全身皮肤评分、血清嗜酸粒细胞阳离子蛋白水平和总 IgE 均快速降低。然而治疗间隔期在从 2 周调整至 4 周时,这些疗效快速消失了,但是恢复间隔 2 周治疗后这些疗效重新开始。总的来说这些研究提示体外光化学免疫疗法对特应性皮炎患者的治疗有效,但是需要更大病人样本量的随机对照研究来确证这些早期的观察。同时这一模式昂贵又费时,因此它的使用被限制于其他治疗方式无效的特应性皮炎患者的治疗。

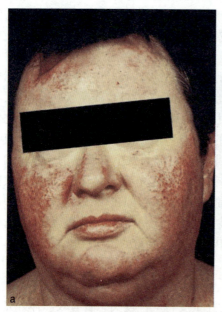 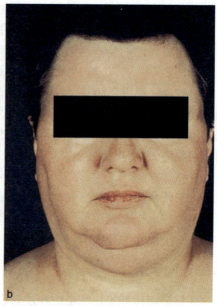

图 4.4 难治性特应性皮炎的患者运用体外光化学免疫疗法前(a)、后(b)(4 个周期)

慢性中度特应性皮炎的光(化学)治疗

宽谱 UVB 治疗,联合 UVA/UVB 治疗、311nm UVB 治疗、宽谱 UVA 治疗,或低剂量 UVA-1 治疗是有效的治疗轻度和中度特应性湿疹的方法,但是对治疗急性重症的特应性湿疹无效[1,10,13,15,24-29,34,35,44,50,52,58]。这些 UV 光疗的形式通常不会作为单独的治疗方法而通常是为了减少糖皮质激素的使用而与局部糖皮质激素联合应用。

UVA/UVB 光疗

近期研究显示联合 UVB 照射与 UVA 照射(UVA/UVB 治疗)相对于传统的宽谱 UVB 治疗,传统的 UVA 治疗和低剂量的 UVA-1 治疗在处理慢性、中度特应性皮炎上更有效。在两项配对对比研究中,Jekler 和 Larko 发现 UVB 治疗比安慰剂有效。有趣的是,高剂量 UVB(0.8MED)与中等剂量 UVB(0.4MED)等效[28]。相同的作者通过应用临床评分系统,在一项配对对比研究中发现 UVA/UVB 治疗与宽谱 UVB 治疗效果上存在统计学上的显著差异[27]。在这项试验中,患者可连续局部使用糖皮质激素,另外以 UVB-MED 方式,每周 3 次,最多 8 周进行照射光疗。这些仔细的观察进一步证实了 UVA/UVB 治疗在治疗特应性皮炎上是优于 UVB 治疗[38]。

窄谱 UVB 光疗

特应性皮炎患者对光疗抱怨最多的是瘙痒加剧,受热后汗液分泌减少,这也与 UV 治疗,尤其 UVA 治疗有关。在近期的研究中,George 等在 311nm UVB 照射单元中安装了空调[15]。通过应用 50 台装有反射镜的 TL-01(100W)台灯获得了 5mw/cm^2 的 UVB 输出,这使得最大治疗时间少于 10 分钟。在这项设计好的研究中,监测慢性、中度特应性皮炎患者在光疗前使用类固醇 12 周,光疗 12 周,在光疗停止后跟踪了 24 周。311nm UVB 治疗的开始不仅降低了总体的临床评分,还大幅度上降低了强效皮质类固醇的使用。这些有利的作用仍旧存在于中断光疗 6 周后的大部分的病人。

这些研究显示选择 311nm UVB 光疗模式治疗可诱导特应性皮炎患者病情获得长期改善。一项独立研究最近证实了他们的结果,这项研究提示获得 George 等人报道的良好治疗效果并不需要特别的制冷系统[25]。

我们认为 311nm UVB 治疗是仅次于 UVA-1 治疗的理想治疗模式,而后者是用于急性、严重进展期特应性皮炎的初始阶段的治疗。UVA-1 是有效和较安全的治疗模式,而 311nm UVB 治疗可作为维持治疗代替 UVA-1 治疗[70]。311nm UVB 治疗也被推荐用于儿童[10],但是对其长期副反应的担忧仍存在[9,30,41]。

慢性水疱性手足湿疹的光(化学)治疗

手足的水疱性湿疹是特应性皮炎慢性病程中普遍存在的临床症状。由于临床表现仅限于皮肤的某些区域,全身 UV 治疗似乎并不合适。近期发展的霜剂-PUVA 治疗为治疗单个、病变范围明确如手足部,而避免非皮损处皮肤暴露于 UV 照射的治疗提供了可能[63]。另外,某些报道认为这样的情况可使用局部皮肤的 UVA-1 照射[60]。

霜剂-PUVA 光化学治疗

对于霜剂-PUVA,将包含 0.0006% 8-甲氧补骨脂的油包水在 UVA 照射前一小时应用于照射部位。理想的光毒反应在霜剂使用 1~3 小时后,然后迅速消退。最早期的报道显示霜剂-PUVA 治疗慢性手部湿疹特别有效[63]。在平均 40 次治疗后,10 个病人中有 7 人获得完全的缓解(图 4.5a,b)。最近一项非独立研究证实了这些发现,这项研究中发现霜剂-PUVA 比 PUVA 浴有效[32]。这可能是因为与淋浴-PUVA 相比,霜剂-PUVA 的重复使用不会导致湿疹样皮肤的干燥。另外,与淋浴-PUVA 相比,霜剂-PUVA 更简便,更便宜,可以更安全的使用。

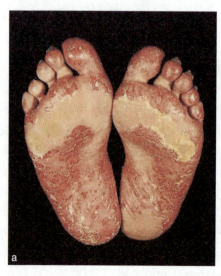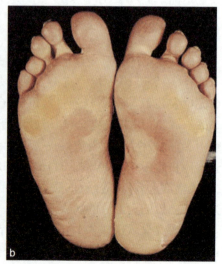

图 4.5　PUVA 霜剂治疗慢性足部湿疹前(a)、后(b)(34 次治疗)

局部皮肤的 UVA-1 光疗

在最近的研究中,12 例慢性汗疱疹患者的手掌和背部暴露于单一剂量

40J/cm² 的局部 UVA-1 光疗[60]。局部 UVA-1 光疗是作为单一疗法使用。在 15 次治疗后,12 例患者中有 10 例患者病情获得逐步的改善。在超过 3 个月的随访期内病情无复发。与局部 PUVA 光疗相比,局部 UVA-1 光疗具有更大的优势。至今尚无标准化的对比研究证明此观点。

展望

与银屑病不同的,绝大多数情况下,银屑病的光化学治疗常常作为一种单一的治疗模式而被评估。由于特应性皮炎类似于银屑病,是一种无治愈手段的慢性疾病,治疗的安全性是重要的关注点。在这种情况下,由于联合治疗可同时提高治疗的有效性和安全性,因此得到广泛关注。标准化的,随机的,对照研究局部类固醇治疗联合新的光疗模式如 311nm UVB 或 UVA-1 光疗模式具有重要的实用意义。近期将局部免疫抑制剂运用于特应性皮炎患者为这种疾病的系统治疗提供了一种完全崭新的视野。在这点上,联合治疗提出了优先关注安全的考虑,因为免疫抑制剂如他克莫司有可能增加皮肤肿瘤罹患的风险,尤其是当与 UV 照射联合使用时。为了公平的判断这一问题,安全性研究是不可缺少的。

使用光疗对是否预防特应性湿疹的可能性仍几乎未知。预防性的光疗方法可能基于紫外线照射可干预此疾病初始阶段。在这点上尤其有意识的反复暴露于高剂量 UVA-1 照射能够抑制特应性皮炎患者吸入性变应原斑贴试验阳性的皮肤反应的形成[69]。

将变应原试验敏感的吸入性变应原,如屋尘螨变应原,应用于特应性皮炎患者皮肤非皮损区,发现接触变应原 48 小时内可诱导了大约 45% ~ 50% 受试患者的产生湿疹样皮损[54,55,57]。关于诱发出的皮损主要是由接触到皮肤的吸入性变应原引起的免疫组织化学和尤其免疫学的大量研究已经清晰的建立,它们不仅仅是非特异性的刺激反应。作为后果,吸入性变应原斑贴试验因此被认为是特应性皮炎初始阶段的一种模型,它包含了由皮肤对空气中变应原接触并发展到湿疹样皮损形成的时间。在同一患者,诱导吸入性变应原斑贴试验反应阳性已经是高度可复制的事件,这一观察使我们询问究竟 UV 照射对这一系统是否存在作用[69]。

我们发现人的皮肤暴露于 UVA-1 照射可高效的完全抑制吸入性变应原斑贴试验的阳性反应。这种抑制作用是相对特异性的,因为在同一患者,皮肤照射等量 UVA-1 并不能成功的抑制由之前表皮接触刺激性十二烷基硫酸钠激起的斑贴试验的阳性反应。这些初步的观察提示重复 UVA-1 照射可能对由吸入性变应原导致的特应性皮炎皮损的激发提供保护作用。这一观点与高剂量 UVA-1 治疗的中断和特应性皮炎患者湿疹的反弹或快速复发无关的临床观察一致。进一步的研究需要评估 UVA-1 照射抑制吸入性变应原斑贴试验反应的潜在机制。同 e 样让人感兴趣的是其他波长紫外线照射是否具有相同的效果，如 311nm UVB 治疗。这些研究将最大程度的让光疗策略得到发展，让特应性皮炎患者间隔照射后获得缓解，在抑制病情重新加重的同时，提供最大的安全保护。

（杨艳 译，罗育武　孟珍 校，朱慧兰 审）

参考文献

1. Abeck D, Schmidt T, Fesq H (2000) Long-term efficacy of medium dose UVA-1 phototherapy in atopic dermatitis. J Am Acad Dermatol 42:254–257
2. Atherton DJ, Carabott F, Glover MT, Hawk JM (1988) The role of psoralen photochemotherapy (PUVA) in the treatment of severe atopic eczema in adolescents. Br J Dermatol 118:791–795
3. Baadsgard O, Lisby S, Lange-Wantzin G, Wulf HC, Cooper KD (1989) Rapid recovery of Langerhans cell alloreactivity, without induction of autoreactivity, after in vivo ultraviolet A, but not ultraviolet B exposure of human skin. J Immunol 142:4213–4217
4. Binet O, Aron-Brunetiere C, Cuneo M, Cesaro M-J (1982) Photochimiotherapie par voie orale et dermatite atopique. Ann Dermatol Venereol 109:589–590
5. Bos JD, Wierenga EA, Smitt JHS, van der Heijden FL, Kapsenberg ML (1992) Immune dysregulation in atopic eczema. Arch Dermatol Res 128:1509–1514
6. Bruijnzeel-Koomen C (1986) IgE on Langerhans cells: new insights into the pathogenesis of atopic dermatitis. Dermatologica 172:181–184
7. Bruijnzeel-Koomen CAFM, van Wichen DF, Spry CJF, Venge P, Bruynzeel PLB (1988) Active participation of eosinophils in patch test reactions to inhalant allergens in patients with atopic dermatitis. Br J Dermatol 118:222–233
8. Buckely CC, Ivison C, Poulter LW, Rustin MHA (1992) FceR11/CD23 receptor distribution in patch test reactions to aeroallergens in atopic dermatitis. J Invest Dermatol 99:184–188
9. Clayton TH, Clark SM, Turner D, Goulden V (2006) The treatment of severe atopic dermatitis in childhood with narrowband ultraviolet B phototherapy. Clin Exp Dermatol 32:28–33
10. Collins P, Ferguson J (1995) Narrowband (TLO1) UVB airconditioned phototherapy for atopic eczema in children. Br J Dermatol 133:653–654
11. Costa C, Rillet A, Nicolet M, Saurat JH (1989) Scoring atopic dermatitis: the simpler the better. Acta Derm Venereol (Stockh) 69:41–47
12. Czech W, Krutmann J, Schöpf E, Kapp A (1992) Serum eosinophil cationic protein is a sensitive measure for disease activity in atopic dermatitis. Br J Dermatol 126:351–355
13. Falk ES (1985) UV-light therapies in atopic dermatitis. Photodermatol Photoimmunol Photomed 2:241–246
14. Gasparro F, Edelson RL (1995) Extracorporeal photochemotherapy. In: Krutmann J, Elmets CA (eds) Photoimmunology. Blackwell Scientific, Oxford, pp 231–245
15. George SA, Bilsland DJ, Johnson BE, Fergusson J (1993) Narrow-band (TL01) UVB air-conditioned phototherapy for chronic severe adult atopic dermatitis. Br J Dermatol 128:49–56
16. Godar DE (1996) Preprogrammed and programmed cell death mechanisms of apoptosis: UV-induced immediate and delayed apoptosis. Photochem Photobiol 63:825–830
17. Godar DE (1999) UVA 1 radiation mediates singlet-oxygen and superoxide-anion production which trigger two different final apoptotic pathways: the S and P site of mitochondria. J Invest Dermatol 112:3–12
18. Grabbe J, Welker P, Humke S, Grewe M, Schöpf E, Henz BM, Krutmann J (1996) High-dose UVA-1 therapy, but not UVA/UVB therapy, decreases IgE binding cells in lesional skin of

第 4 章 特应性皮炎的光治疗

patients with atopic eczema. J Invest Dermatol 107:419–423
19. Grewe M, Gyufko K, Schöpf E, Krutmann J (1994) Lesional expression of interferon-γ in atopic eczema. Lancet 343:25–26
20. Grewe M, Walther S, Gyufko K, Czech W, Schöpf E, Krutmann J (1995) Analysis of the cytokine pattern expressed in situ in inhalant allergen patch test reactions of atopic dermatitis patients. J Invest Dermatol 105:407–410
21. Grewe M, Gyufko K, Krutmann J (1995) Interleukin-10 production by cultured human keratinocytes: regulation by ultraviolet B and A1 radiation. J Invest Dermatol 104:3–6
22. Grewe M, Bruijnzeel-Koomen CAFM, Schöpf E, Thepen T, Langeveld-Wildschuh AG, Ruzicka T, Krutmann J (1998) A role for Th1 and Th2 cells in the immunopathogenesis of atopic dermatitis. Immunol Today 19:359–361
23. Hamid Q, Boguniewicz M, Leung DYM (1994) Differential in situ cytokine gene expression in acute versus chronic atopic dermatitis. J Clin Invest 94:870–876
24. Hannuksela M, Karvonen J, Husa M, Jokela R, Katajamäki L, Leppisaari M (1985) Ultraviolet light therapy in atopic dermatitis. Acta Derm Venereol (Stockh) 114:137–139
25. Hudson-Peacock MJ, Diffey BL, Farr PM (1996) Narrow-band UVB phototherapy for severe atopic dermatitis. Br J Dermatol 135:332
26. Jekler J, Larkö O (1988) UVB phototherapy of atopic eczema. Br J Dermatol 119:697–705
27. Jekler J, Larkö O (1990) Combined UV-A-UV-B versus UVB phototherapy for atopic dermatitis. J Am Acad Dermatol 22:49–53
28. Jekler J, Larkö O (1991) Phototherapy for atopic dermatitis with ultraviolet A (UVA), low-dose UVB and combined UVA and UVB: two paired comparison studies. Photodermatol Photoimmunol Photomed 8:151–156
29. Jekler J (1992) Phototherapy of atopic dermatitis with ultraviolet radiation (dissertation). Graphics Systems AB, University of Göteborg, Göteborg, 1992, 10
30. Jury CS, McHenry P, Burden AD, Lever R, Bilsland D (2006) Narrowband ultraviolet B (UVB) phototherapy in children. Clin Exp Dermatol 31:196–199
31. Kavli G (1978) Fotokjemoterapi med psoralen og langbolget ultrafiolett lys. 1 1/2 ars erfaring fra hudavdelingen in Tromso. Tidsskr Nor Lageforen 98:269–271
32. Kerscher M (1998) Creme-PUVA und Bade-PUVA. In: Plewig G, Wolff H (eds) Fortschritte der Dermatologie und Venerologie. Springer, Heidelberg, pp 135–139
33. Kobyletzki G, Pieck C, Hoffmann K, Freitag M, Altmeyer P (1999) Medium-dose UVA-1 cold-light phototherapy in the treatment of severe atopic dermatitis. J Am Acad Dermatol 41:931–937
34. Kowalzick L, Kleinhenz A, Weichenthal M, Ring J (1995) Low dose versus medium dose UVA-1 treatment in severe atopic dermatitis. Acta Derm Venereol (Stockh) 75:43–45
35. Krutmann J, Schöpf E (1992) High-dose UVA1 therapy: a novel and highly effective approach for the treatment of patients with acute exacerbation of atopic dermatitis. Acta Derm Venereol (Stockh) 176:120–122
36. Krutmann J, Czech W, Diepgen T, Niedner R, Kapp A, Schöpf E (1992) High-dose UVA1 therapy in the treatment of patients with atopic dermatitis. J Am Acad Dermatol 26:225–230
37. Krutmann J (1995) UVA1-induced immunomodulation. In: Krutmann J, Elmets CA (eds) Photoimmunology. Blackwell Scientific, Oxford, pp 246–256
38. Krutmann J (1996) Phototherapy for atopic dermatitis. Dermatol Ther 1:24–31
39. Krutmann J, Diepgen TL, Luger TA, Grabbe S, Meffert H, Sönnichsne N, Czech W, Kapp A, Stege H, Grewe M, Schöpf E (1998) High-dose UVA1 therapy for atopic dermatitis: results of a multicenter trial. J Am Acad Dermatol 38:589–593
40. Krutmann J (2007) Therapeutic photomedicine: phototherapy. In: Freedberg IM, Eisen AZ, Wolff K, Austen KF, Goldsmith LA, Katz SI, Fitzpatrick TB (eds) Fitzpatrick's dermatology in general medicine, 5th edn. McGraw-Hill, New York, pp 2870–2879
41 Kunisada M, Kumimoto H, Ishizaki K, Sakumi K, Nakabeppu Y, Nishigori C (2007) Narrowband UVB induces more carcinogenic skin tumors than broad-band UVB through the forma-

tion of cyclobutane pyrimidine dimers. J Invest Dermatol 127:2865–2871
42. Lomhold S (1974) Hudsygdommene og deres behandling, 2nd edn. Copenhagen 97:425
43. Meffert H, Sönnichsen N, Herzog M, Hutschenreuther A (1992) UVA-1 cold light therapy of severe atopic dermatitis. Dermatol Monatsschr 78:291–296
44. Midelfart K, Stenvold S-E, Volden G (1985) Combined UVB and UVA phototherapy of atopic eczema. Dermatologica 171:95–98
45. Morison WL, Parrish JA, Fitzpatrick TB (1978) Oral psoralen photochemotherapy of atopic eczema. Br J Dermatol 98:25–30
46. Morison WL (1985) Phototherapy and photochemotherapy of skin disease, 2nd edn. Raven, New York, pp 148–152
47. Morita A, Werfel T, Stege H, Ahrens C, Karmann K, Grewe M, Grether-Beck S, Ruzicka T, Kapp A, Klotz O, Sies H, Krutmann J (1997) Evidence that singlet oxygen-induced human T-helper cell apoptosis is the basic mechanism of ultraviolet-A radiation phototherapy. J Exp Med 186:1763–1768
48. Nexman P-H (1948) Clinical studies of Besnier's prurigo (dissertation). Rosenkilde and Bagger, Copenhagen
49. Plettenberg H, Stege H, Megahed M, Ruzicka T, Hosokawa Y, Tsuji T, Morita A, Krutmann J (1999) Ultraviolet A1 (340–400 nm) phototherapy for cutaneous T-cell lymphoma. J Am Acad Dermatol 41:47–50
50. Potekaev NS, Sevidova LY, Vladimirov VV, Kochergin NG, Shinaev NN (1987) Selective phototherapy and dimociphon immunocorrective therapy in atopic dermatitis. Vestn Dermatol Venereol 9:39–42
51. Prinz B, Nachbar F, Plewig G (1994) Treatment of severe atopic dermatitis with extracorporeal photopheresis. Arch Dermatol Res 287:48–52
52. Pullmann H, Möres E, Reinbach S (1985) Wirkungen von Infrarot- und UVA-Strahlen auf die menschliche Haut und ihre Wirksamkeit bei der Behandlung des endogenen Ekzems. Z Hautkr 60:171–177
53. Rajka G (1980) Recent therapeutic events: cimetidine and PUVA. Acta Derm Venereol (Stockh) [Suppl] 92:117–118
54. Ramb-Lindhauer CH, Feldmann A, Rotte M, Neumann CH (1991) Characterization of grass pollen reactive T-cell lines derived from lesional atopic skin. Arch Dermatol Res 283:71–76
55. Reitamo S, Visa K, Kähönen K, Stubb S, Salo OP (1986) Eczematous reactions in atopic patients caused by epicutaneous testing with inhalant allergens. Br J Dermatol 114:303–308
56. Richter H, Billmann-Eberwein C, Grewe M, Stege H, Berneburg M, Ruzicka T, Krutmann J (1998) Successful monotherapy of severe and intractable atopic dermatitis by photopheresis. J Am Acad Dermatol 38:585–588
57. Sager N, Feldmann A, Schilling G, Kreitsch P, Neumann C (1992) House dust-mite specific T cells in the skin of subjects with atopic dermatitis: frequency and lymphokine profile in the allergen patch test. J Allergy Clin Immunol 89:801–807
58. Salo O, Lassus A, Juvaksoski T, Kanerva L, Lauharanta J (1983) Behandlung der Dermatitis atopica und der Dermatitis seborrhoica mit selektiver UV-Phototherapie und PUVA. Dermatol Monatsschr 169:371–375
59. Sannwald C, Ortonne JP, Thivolet J (1979) La photochimiotherapie orale de l'eczema atopique. Dermatologica 159:71–77
60. Schmidt T, Abeck D, Boeck K, Mempel M, Ring J (1998) UVA1 irradiation is effective in treatment of chronic vesicular dyshidrotic hand eczema. Acta Derm Venereol (Stockh) 78:318–319
61. Soppi E, Viander M, Soppi A-M, Jansen CT (1982) Cell-mediated immunity in untreated and PUVA-treated atopic dermatitis. J Invest Dermatol 79:213–217
62. Stege H, Schöpf E, Krutmann J (1995) High-dose UVA1 therapy in the treatment of patients with urticaria pigmentosa. J Invest Dermatol 105:499A
63. Stege H, Berneburg M, Ruzicka T, Krutmann J (1997) Cream-PUVA-Photochemotherapy.

Hautarzt 48:89–93
64. Stern RS and members of the Photochemotherapy Follow-Up Study (1990) Genital tumors among men with psoriasis exposed to psoralen and ultraviolet A radiation (PUVA) and ultraviolet B radiation. N Engl J Med 322:1093–1096
65. Stern RS, Nichols KT, Vakeva LH (1997) Malignant melanoma in patients treated for psoriasis with methoxsalen (psoralen) and ultraviolet A radiation (PUVA). N Engl J Med 336:1041–1045
66. Vaatainen N, Hannuksela M, Karvonen J (1979) Local photochemotherapy in nodular prurigo. Acta Dermatol 59:544–547
67. Volcz-Platzer B, Hönigsmann H (1995) Photoimmunology of PUVA and UVB therapy. In: Krutmann J, Elmets CA (eds) Photoimmunology. Blackwell Scientific, Oxford, pp 265–273
68. von Bohlen F, Kallusky J, Woll R (1994) The UVA1 cold light treatment of atopic dermatitis. Allergologie 17:382–384
69. Walter S, Grewe M, Gyufko K, Czech W, Kapp A, Stege H, Schöpf E, Krutmann J (1994) Inhalant allergen patch tests as a model for the induction of atopic dermatitis: analysis of the in situ cytokine pattern and modulation by UVA1. Abstract. Arch Dermatol Res 286:220
70. Young AR (1995) Carcinogenicity of UVB phototherapy assessed. Lancet 345:1431–1432

5 第5章 特发性光线性皮肤病的光疗和光化学疗法

A. Tanew, J. Ferguson

内容

概要	103
引言	103
多形性日光疹	103
种痘样水疱病	107
光化性痒疹	108
日光性荨麻疹	109
慢性光化性皮炎	111
总结	112

要点

- 特发性光线性皮肤病是一类具有免疫异常背景的日光诱发的皮肤疾病。
- 患者存在明显的个体差异,作用光谱包括从 UVB 到可见光。
- 光治疗手段可以对患者进行成功脱敏,纠正异常的光敏感性。
- 窄谱 UVB 和 PUVA 对于多形性日光疹(polymorphic light eruption, PLE)的光预防有相当好的效果。
- 总的来说,对 PLE 以外的光线性皮肤病进行光脱敏更困难,但有助于持续性的提高患者对日光的耐受。

概要

特发性光线性皮肤病是一类日光诱发的不同类型的皮肤疾病,包括多形性日光疹、种痘样水疱病、光化性痒疹、日光性荨麻疹和慢性光化性皮炎。在这些疾病中,多形性日光疹是最常见的,其他疾病相对少见。疾病的主要作用光谱包括从 UVB 到可见光的范围,因此防晒剂往往不能提供足够的保护。因此对这些患者,通过进行可控制的 UVB 暴露和光化学疗法可以对患者进行有效的光脱敏,从而治疗这种异常的光敏感性。

引言

"特发性光线性皮肤病"这个名词是指一类发生在相对健康的患者身上,在没有外源性光敏剂的情况下,接受自然或者人工光线暴露后出现的皮肤疾病。这一类疾病包括多形性日光疹、种痘样水疱病、光化性痒疹、日光性荨麻疹和慢性光化性皮炎。所有这类疾病有两个共同点:①它们可以因为紫外线或者可见光范围的电磁辐射诱发;②这类疾病临床表现的具体病理机制尚待阐明,但可能和免疫相关。特别需要指出的是,开始是具体哪种色基导致光化学反应,以及最终导致皮肤的炎症反应仍然是未解之谜。诊断光线性皮肤病主要基于临床特点和光试验,组织病理学改变和实验室检查为次要的诊断手段。

基本上所有的光线性皮肤病都是 UVB 光疗和光化学疗法[补骨脂素结合 UVA 光疗(psoralen plus UVA,PUVA)]的明确适应证。治疗的目标是提高患者对日光的耐受,预防疾病发作。在后面的章节中,会对每种光线性皮肤病的光疗和光化学疗法应用进行介绍。介绍包括简单描述疾病,概括光疗的方案和治疗注意事项,以及概述可预期的结果。

多形性日光疹

和其他的光线性皮肤病相反,多形性日光疹(polymorphic light eruption,PLE)非常常见。报道称 PLE 的发病率大概为 3%～21%,好发于女性,和纬度相关。PLE 的患者可能有家族史。可能是常染色体显性遗传,有不完全外显性;但目前没有发现特定的 HLA 型和发病有关。

PLE 具有季节性发作的特点,常与晚春或者夏季假期中开始出现。开始日光暴露到皮疹发作的时间间隔可以从小于一小时到数天不等。主要症状是剧烈瘙痒,之后在日光暴露的部位常出现丘疹、水疱或斑块样的皮疹[25]。其他少见的皮疹形态包括多形红斑样或出血性皮疹。也有报道只有瘙痒而没有临床体征。

最重要的诊断方法是光试验。当明确 UVA 和 UVB 的最小红斑量(minimal erythema dose,MED)后,应该在之前受累部位的皮肤重复进行红斑量的光线照射,以诱导出特异的皮损。PLE 的确诊需要进行光激发试验,虽然大多数诊断仅仅基于临床病史。光激发试验同时可以明确患者发生 PLE 的作用光谱,这点对于预防是有用的。对大量患者的光试验表明,50%~75% 的 PLE 是 UVA 诱发,10%~15% 为 UVB 诱发,15%~35% 为 UVA 和 UVB 共同诱发[24,43]。本病可以自愈[21],临床严重程度差异很大,大多数患者的治疗仅需避光和使用高强度的广谱防晒剂。但对少数患者这种方法效果不佳,需要进行 UVB 或者 PUVA 的光脱敏。

多形性日光疹的光疗

虽然刚开始看起来,使用光疗预防光线引起的疾病似乎是个悖论。但是大多数患者都可以体会到在夏季皮疹发作减少或者完全缓解。这种逐渐增加的日光耐受被称为"硬化效应"(hardening effect)。

这种效应的可能机制为皮肤黑色素形成增加,角质层增厚和皮肤免疫反应改变,导致皮肤滤过作用增强。

PLE 的光疗预防或者光化学疗法预防可能是通过类似机制发挥作用。通常短期的照射足够引发硬化效应。为了避免在这一过程中激发 PLE 的发作,可以采取两种策略:一是采用不能诱发 PLE 的 UV 光谱进行光脱敏;另一是采用致病波长的光线,但使用低于诱发阈值的剂量进行治疗。

基于这些考虑,对于 UVA 诱发的 PLE 患者更加适合使用 UVB 进行脱敏。多项研究发现,每周进行 3~5 次的照射,在 12~15 次疗程后可以增加患者对日光的耐受,有效预防和减少 PLE 的发作[41,42]。尽管缺乏临床证据,一般认为没有必要使用红斑量的 UVB 治疗。治疗导致的色素沉着不是治疗效果的可靠指标,因为 I 型和 II 型皮肤的患者很少晒黑,但仍然对 PLE 有较好的预防效果。

尽管光疗已经广泛应用,但不同的治疗中心之间治疗方案差异很大[9](表 5.1)。在一些治疗中心,窄谱 UVB(TL-01)已经逐渐取代了宽谱 UVB 和 PUVA,是 PLE 脱敏的首选治疗。这些治疗中心中,PUVA 是对那些不能获得满意防护效果的患者的保留选择。在一项最近进行的观察者盲性随机对照试验中,对 25 名患者比较了窄谱 UVB 和 PUVA 的效果,发现两种治疗不但对预防 PLE 是等效的,同时在治疗过程中诱发 PLE 发作也是有类似的效果[5]。在这个独立研究中,使用窄谱 UVB 治疗 PLE 效果优于宽谱 UVB,而不及 PUVA。

表5.1　UVB和PUVA用于PLE脱敏治疗的方案示例

	治 疗 方 案
UVB脱敏（窄谱或者宽谱）	24h时判读最小红斑量（minimal erythema dose，MED） 起始照射量：70% MED 没有红斑[a]或者PLE发作[b]的情况下，每次治疗增量20% 门诊病人：每周三次治疗持续五周（共15次） 住院病人：每日治疗持续两周（共10次）
PUVA脱敏	使用8-MOP或者5-MOP 72~96小时判读最小光毒性剂量（minimal phototoxic dose，MPD） 起始剂量：70% MPD 没有红斑[a]或者PLE发作[b]的情况下，每次治疗增量20% 治疗每周三次持续四周（共12次治疗）
如果产生红斑	1度：重复前次剂量 2度：推迟下一次治疗，重复前次剂量，后续采用20%增量 3/4度：红斑消退之前不进行治疗，剂量减半后续采用10%增量
如果PLE发作	瘙痒或者轻度PLE：必要时外用皮质类固醇激素 中度：维持同等剂量，外用中效/强效皮质类固醇激素，后续采用10%增量 重度：推迟1~2次治疗，外用强效皮质类固醇激素，重新开始采用倒数第二次治疗剂量，后续采用10%增量

[a]若相反，参考"如果产生红斑"部分。
[b]若相反，参考"如果PLE发作"部分。

相较于PUVA，窄谱UVB的优点有：

1. 无需补骨脂素致敏，没有相关的消化道不适；
2. 治疗后不需要眼保护；
3. 儿童和孕妇可以进行治疗；
4. 应用更为方便廉价，特别适用于那些需要每年进行脱敏疗程的患者；
5. 在诱发非黑素瘤的皮肤癌风险方面，宽谱和TL-01UVB均比PUVA安全[11,33,58]。

多形性日光疹的光化学疗法

因为对PLE进行光化学疗法需要使用光敏剂，所以只需要使用小剂量的UVA。一般来说这些剂量远远低于诱发PLE发作的剂量，但仍然可以诱导色素沉着，调节皮肤免疫反应。最早的使用PUVA预防PLE的报道诞生于1970年代晚期。在一项研究报道中，在全部5名患者中使用PUVA硬化治疗，都获得完全的防护效果[19]；另一项研究报道在10名PLE患者中,9名患者的发作显著减少[45]。所有研究中,患者的PLE病史很长,严重发作,并且使用防晒剂不能成功缓解。另外四项研究也证实了光化学疗法对于预防PLE发作有相当好的效果[2,36,42,43]。此外,已经证实光化学疗法较宽谱UVB明显有效。对于90%~100%的患者,PUVA可以近乎完全或者完全预防PLE症状,而宽谱UVB的治疗反应率在60%~80%之间。

PUVA硬化治疗适用于使用防晒剂或者UVB光疗效果不佳的严重PLE患者。一般每周进行三次治疗,持续四周。在最近一次患者间对照研究中,6到12次PUVA治疗效果没有显著性差异,特别是对于程度较轻的患者[44]。8-甲氧补骨脂素(methoxypsoralen,MOP)和5-MOP都可以作为光敏剂使用,但是一般更倾向使用5-MOP,它有两大优点：一是胃肠道和中枢神经系统副作用常见于8-MOP,使用5-MOP几乎不发生；二是5-MOP产生色素沉着的效果优于8-MOP。

亚红斑量的UVA剂量通常已经足够产生治疗效果。较低的累积UVA量就可以产生光保护效果,而超过保护阈值剂量的治疗效果并不见得获益更多[36]。

虽然使用的是低剂量的UVA照射,少部分患者在PUVA硬化治疗的初期仍然可能发生短暂的PLE发作。这表明PUVA可能通过特定机制诱发PLE。通常仅需要对症处理,外用皮质类固醇激素即可。

预防性光化学疗法对于预防PLE的治疗价值应该与长期应用的副作用权衡。对银屑病患者进行PUVA治疗的随访研究发现累积超过200次治疗,发生鳞状细胞癌的风险显著增高[55,56]。因为光保护需要的治疗疗程少,累积UVA剂量低(根据皮肤类型和光致敏剂的不同,每次疗程的剂量从15到40J/cm^2),以及PLE可以严重影响患者的户外活动,当其他预防方法失败时权衡利弊值得采用PUVA来治疗PLE。

总而言之,对于70%~90%的严重PLE患者,2~4周的短期窄谱UVB光疗或者光化学疗法可以预防发作。

脱敏治疗的操作

当和患者讨论脱敏疗程时(表5.2),很重要的一点是对患者强调自然的"硬化"过程不是产生治疗效用的必须过程,每名患者的反应不同,因此治疗必须个体化。在PLE的治疗中,研究发现已脱敏患者的一半人数可能出现至少一次轻度的PLE发作。第一次发作是探索性的。应该提前提醒患者可能诱发皮疹,无需停止继续治疗。对那些发作严重或者反复的患者,治疗时应该注意增加剂量的步骤,同时光(化学)疗法后使用强效皮质类固醇激素,使治疗继续得以完成。

表5.2 脱敏治疗：需要注意的操作要点

病史是否存在自然"硬化"不是必需的前提条件
每名患者的反应可能不同
第一次疗程是试验性的
只需要对光暴露部位（即手臂、腿和面部）进行治疗
对于严重病例，治疗后外用皮质类固醇激素可以缓解症状
每次治疗时，患者应该穿着厚的棉质衣物或者在同一部位覆盖不透过紫外线的敷料
脱敏治疗后，鼓励患者在夏季谨慎地进行日光暴露，以维持硬化效应。给患者提供一份脱敏后注意事项的手册
已经进行三次脱敏疗程，并且疗效好的患者应该鼓励其停止治疗一年。因为确实存在自愈的可能

对于那些在夏季只希望暴露手臂、腿部和面部的患者，治疗可以局限在这些部位，可以建议患者在每次治疗过程中穿着同样厚度的棉质短袖衫和短裤。每次治疗时衣料应该严格覆盖在相同位置，避免未治疗部位出现晒伤反应。完成脱敏治疗后，应该鼓励患者谨慎地进行一些日光暴露，从而不断补充这种人工的光保护效果。不这样做的风险是保护效果可能会在4~6周内消失[43]。一些效果不好的患者可能是因为春天的治疗进行太早，而初夏的日晒不够，导致光保护效果消失。无论是PUVA还是窄谱UVB的光脱敏的效果都是暂时的，治疗应该以年为单位重复进行。遵循以上疗程，不会出现效果消失，对于已经成功脱敏3~4年的患者可以尝试停止治疗一年[38]。

异常光敏感的儿童或者成人患者，每年重复进行光疗，存在长期风险如光损伤和非黑素瘤皮肤癌，这是一个严重的问题。如有必要，临床医生是否应该建议患者在长达二三十年的时间里进行重复光疗？答案可能是肯定的，对于PLE患者，终生累积的日光暴露量可能不会高于，甚至低于正常人，考虑到明显有益的治疗效果，还是值得承担轻度增加的风险[32]。

种痘样水疱病

种痘样水疱病是非常罕见的光线性皮肤病，典型表现为光照诱发的丘疹水疱，主要累及面部、胸部、前臂和手。皮损进展为浆液性-出血性水疱，坏死的表皮愈合伴有结痂，导致痘疮样瘢痕。累及到眼部表现为结膜炎，同时伴有畏光或角膜溃疡。本报始于儿童时期，表现为慢性反复的病程。自发缓解多发生在成年早期。男性患病高于女性。

数个研究发现种痘样水疱病的作用光谱在UVA范围内[13,17,20,30,34]。使用30~60J/cm^{2}的UVA照射可以诱发皮损重现。

种痘样水疱病的治疗比 PLE 困难。常规防晒剂对 UVA 的过滤作用有限,大多时候不能提供足够的防护。倍他胡萝卜素和抗疟药物的作用同样效果不佳。因此光疗和光化学疗法对于种痘样水疱病的治疗十分重要。

种痘样水疱病的光疗

因为种痘样水疱病的患病率很低,关于本病的光预防治疗也仅有个例报道[20]。Sonnex 和 Hawk[54] 总结了 10 名接受了不同治疗的患者,两名使用了 UVB 光疗的患者在夏季保持无皮疹发作的状态。

应用窄谱 UVB 治疗的资料同样稀有。Collins 和 Ferguson[6] 在一项研究窄谱 UVB 对光线性皮肤病预防效果的报道中,治疗了四例种痘样水疱病。其中两名患者对治疗反应较好,在夏季保持很好的光保护效果。

种痘样水疱病的光化学疗法

最早的通过 PUVA 治疗种痘样水疱病的病例是 Jaschke 和 Hönigsmann[30] 于 1981 年报道出版的。12 次治疗之后,患者在整个夏季没有症状发作。另一个患者连续两年分别接受了 12 次和 8 次 PUVA 治疗,虽然未能完全防止疾病发作,但是有效减轻症状[17]。

在维也纳,我们数年内成功地对四名患者进行了光化学疗法。治疗后,患者正常皮肤从未出现皮损,瘢痕部位仅有散在皮损出现。治疗方案和 PLE 类似,包括每周三次 PUVA,持续 4~6 周。

总而言之,种痘样水疱病是一种罕见的 UVA 诱导的光线性皮肤病。已有的个案报道证实,光化学疗法和窄谱 UVB 对于减轻种痘样水疱病的症状以及预防复发均有效。

光化性痒疹

光化性痒疹是另一种罕见,很多患者可能未得到正确诊断的光线性皮肤病[1,15,26]。这种慢性疾病常始发于儿童,主要为女性罹患。患者通常有特应性体质或者光敏感的家族史。HLA 的 DR4 等位基因和本病呈强相关联,特别是最近报道的罕见的 DRB1*0407 亚型[18]。本病的临床表现独特,包括以光暴露部位为主分布的痒疹样皮损,但可以不局限于光暴露部位。面部常常受累,鼻远端是典型部位。另一个常见的表现是下唇的剥脱性唇炎。日光诱发的急性反应是水肿性红斑,后期进展为痒疹样的皮损。本病始发时发作为季节性,后期全年都可以发病,夏季显著加重。到成年后,患者有症状缓解甚至自发消退。

光试验的结果可以是正常的,或者 UVB 和 UVA 的红斑阈值降低。通过光

第5章 特发性光线性皮肤病的光疗和光化学疗法

激发试验可以诱发特异性皮损。作用光谱包括全部紫外线范围,但主要集中在UVA部分[26]。

光化性痒疹的光疗

在一项开放性研究中,对六名光化性痒疹的患者评估了窄谱UVB的光疗效果,发现其非常有效,在随后的夏季提高了他们日常活动的紫外线耐受性,不低于6小时[6]。其中的两名患者之前接受了宽谱的UVB治疗也是有效的,其他四名患者接受了PUVA治疗,效果类似。后来使用的窄谱UVB为每周进行3次治疗,持续5周,住院患者采用每周5次治疗,持续2周。根据记录,五名患者出现瘙痒,四名患者有诱发皮损出现。如果症状较重,可以外用强效皮质类固醇激素,后续的光疗增量限制在10%。

光化性痒疹的光化学疗法

Farr和Diffey[14]利用PUVA治疗了五名患者,每周进行两次,持续15周。第四周后观察到患者光敏感性下降。治疗结束时的平均累积UVA剂量是58J/cm^2,所有的患者在夏季即使暴露于日光下达数小时都未发作。光化学疗法的总体耐受性好,除个别有红斑反应。

总的来说,光化性痒疹是一种慢性光线性皮肤病,有非常特殊的临床特点,但临床上可能很多患者未得到正确诊断。光疗和光化学疗法可以实质性的改善患者对日光的耐受性。

日光性荨麻疹

日光性荨麻疹是罕见的,典型表现为日光暴露或者人工辐射,例如美黑设备,后出现的风团反应。这种荨麻疹样的皮损在几分钟内出现,局限在日光暴露的部位,伴有严重瘙痒。一些严重光敏患者或者大量光暴露后,患者可能发生弥漫性的荨麻疹以及过敏性休克。较轻的亚型是固定型日光性荨麻疹,荨麻疹反应局限于皮肤局部[50]。和其他特发性光线性皮肤病一样,本病也可能发生自发缓解,但并不是普遍规律。

每个人的作用光谱不同,从短波紫外线到可见光都有可能诱发本病。因为几乎所有的患者都对UVA和可见光有反应,防晒剂基本上是无效的。报道称一些患者存在光抑制(photoinhibition)现象,光诱发的荨麻疹可以被后续更长波长(罕见的病例报道也可以为较短的波长)的光暴露所抑制[29]。

光试验是诊断治疗日光性荨麻疹的重要依据[53]。通过照射逐渐增加剂量的UVB、UVA和可见光来判断最小荨麻疹量(minimal urticarial dose,MUD)。这可以指导患者开始光疗或者光化学疗法时可耐受的治疗剂量。日光性荨麻疹患者还需要检查血浆中的光反应因子[27]。因此，需要抽取患者血浆，在体外用作用光谱进行照射。照射后的血浆再注射进入患者真皮内，以未照射的血浆作为对照。如果光激活的血浆导致了风团反应，治疗可以考虑通过血浆置换清除循环的光反应因子[12]。

总而言之，日光性荨麻疹患者必须在进行光（化学）疗法之前进行最小荨麻疹量的判断，以避免在治疗开始时发生严重反应。

日光性荨麻疹的光疗

荨麻疹发作之后，皮肤可以抵抗后续光照不发生皮疹达数小时，这就是脱敏治疗的概念基础。脱敏的目的是通过重复给予可以诱发日光性荨麻疹的波长的光照，帮助患者保持在一个慢性抵抗的状态[49]。这种治疗通常采用 UVA，这是大部分患者的作用光谱。但是通过 UVB 诱导耐受也有文献报道[31]。在脱敏治疗的起始阶段，每天可以使用小于 MUD 剂量进行一到多次照射。随后，治疗的间隔时间和照射剂量都应随之增加，直到达到个体可耐受的最大程度。人们提出假说认为，照射导致光变应原阻滞了肥大细胞结合的 IgE 抗体上的结合位点，进一步阻止了肥大细胞脱颗粒[35]。

Bernhard 等人[4]报道了单用 UVA 治疗，使用低于 MUD 剂量，每周 3~5 次，持续 6 周。五名患者中的三名在后续的夏季里症状持续改善。另一项报道在两名严重的日光性荨麻疹患者中，使用 UVA 光疗后，症状得到类似持续性的改善。这项研究的治疗方案为每天两次持续 2~3 周。单色光的光试验证实光疗后 3 个月，仍然有持续性效果[8]。对于特别敏感的患者，可以使用 UVA 皮疹硬化方案（UVA rush hardening regimen），间隔一个小时照射多次 UVA，可以在三天之内获得保护效果[3]。

针对 UVA 或者可见光诱发的日光性荨麻疹使用 UVB 照射，是一种完全不同的理论[37]。这里的理论是避免作用光谱，而不是利用其抵抗效应。治疗的目的是为了通过色素沉着和表皮增生，提高患者皮肤的光滤过作用。

窄谱 UVB 用于日光性荨麻疹的资料极少。一项研究治疗了少数高度 UVA/可见光敏感的患者，但是治疗效果仅持续了 3~4 周[6]。

日光性荨麻疹的光化学疗法

1980 年代报道了几项使用光化学疗法治疗日光性荨麻疹的研究[1,46,47]。PUVA 的效果优于光疗，前者诱导的保护作用总体持续时间明显更长久[52]。

PUVA 使用剂量为 0.6mg/kg 的 8-MOP，每周进行三次治疗。使用 5-MOP 时，药物和照射剂量均更高，但不可以应用于 UVA 明显光敏的患者。起始 UVA

剂量应该刚刚低于诱发红斑和荨麻疹的阈值剂量。对于 UVA 高度敏感的患者，PUVA 之前可以辅助使用短程的 UVA 光疗[48,51]。Hudson-Peacock 等人[28] 报道了一例患者，血浆中可检测到光变应原，因为患者的 MUDUVA 低至 $0.05J/cm^2$ 而不能使用 PUVA。进行了 5 次血浆置换后，MUDUVA 提高至 $1.3J/cm^2$，才可以开始 PUVA 治疗。

在治疗的第一阶段，患者的日光耐受性逐渐增强，直到他们可以在户外活动，而不出现日光性荨麻疹发作。在这一阶段，照射频率保持在一周三次，UVA 剂量持续增加。一旦达到适当的脱敏效果，可以进行维持阶段。这一阶段，每 1~2 周照射一次通常已足够。报道一例对其他治疗无反应的严重患者，联合 PUVA 和静脉使用免疫球蛋白的治疗获得成功[7]，另一例治疗抵抗的患者使用体外光化学免疫疗法也取得成功[39]。

PUVA 治疗日光性荨麻疹的作用尚未完全明确。除了 PUVA 导致的色素沉着，治疗效应可能还包括对肥大细胞脱颗粒的作用，抗原-IgE 相互作用以及下调 IgE 产生。

脱敏治疗的操作

进行光（化学）疗法期间，存在诱发荨麻疹，甚至危重的过敏性休克的可能性。因此脱敏治疗前必须判断 MUD，即使患者的日光性荨麻疹仅对抗组胺药物有部分反应，也必须使用抗组胺药罩。开始可以只治疗少数部位，例如手臂和面部，因为这些可以诱发弥漫性荨麻疹，从而最小化休克的风险。

慢性光化性皮炎

本病并不如既往认为的那样少见，它多见于男性，在一项 370 人的病例研究中，90% 为男性[16]。本病偶发于 50 岁以下的人群，90% 的患者发病在 50 岁到 70 岁中间。大多数患者的临床表现为曝光部位的非特异皮炎，但皮疹可以播散至光遮蔽的部位。慢性光化性皮炎的一种严重假性淋巴瘤亚型，称为"光化性类网状细胞增多症"，典型表现为结节聚合形成斑块。经典的检查表现为 UVA 和 UVB 的高度光敏感性，超过一半的患者还存在对可见光的敏感[10]。此外，很多患者伴有接触性或者光接触性变态反应。本病的防治包括行为上避光，穿着厚织的棉质衣物，以及使用不含已知接触性变应原的防晒剂。

对于老年男性，出现光暴露部位分布的湿疹样皮疹时，都必须考虑慢性光化性皮炎的诊断，光试验可以帮助鉴别诊断。

慢性光化性皮炎的光（化学）疗法

1979 年，Morison 等人[40] 报道了使用 8-MOP 成功治疗慢性光化性皮炎的经验,起始阶段加用系统性的泼尼松龙,后期单用光化学疗法作为维持治疗。Hölzle 等人[23]治疗了两名严重 UV 敏感的患者,诱导了长期缓解。在治疗的起始阶段,只使用非常低剂量的 UVA,并且只照射患者的部分身体。进一步的研究中,对四名患者进行 PUVA 照射,光照后立刻给予外用强效皮质类固醇激素,所有患者均有良好效果[22]。虽然缺乏进一步的资料,但人们认为轻中度患者效果较好,因为病情严重者无法耐受最低剂量的 PUVA 增量。最近,Toonstra 等人[57]报道了使用高压汞弧灯发射 UVB,采用小增量治疗了 13 例光化性类网状细胞增生症,取得较好的效果。但仍需要进一步工作来评判这种治疗的效果,特别是考虑到这类患者表现出来对 UVB 的高度敏感性。

总结

尽管特发性光线性皮肤病的人工硬化的机制尚不明确,正在进行多项研究来探索这个领域,当机制更加明确时,可能影响未来的治疗方法。毫无疑问,目前的这些治疗方法还是令人满意的,但对于部分患者,也是耗时的治疗。

(陈荃 译,杨艳 孟珍 校,朱慧兰 审)

参考文献

1. Addo HA, Frain-Bell W (1984) Actinic prurigo—a specific photodermatosis? Photodermatology 1:119–128
2. Addo HA, Sharma SC (1987) UVB phototherapy and photochemotherapy (PUVA) in the treatment of polymorphic light eruption and solar urticaria. Br J Dermatol 116:539–547
3. Beissert S, Ständer H, Schwarz T (2000) UVA rush hardening for the treatment of solar urticaria. J Am Acad Dermatol 42:1030–1032
4. Bernhard JD, Jaenicke K, Momtaz-T K, Parrish JA (1984) Ultraviolet A phototherapy in the prophylaxis of solar urticaria. J Am Acad Dermatol 10:29–33
5. Bilsland D, George SA, Gibbs NK, Aitchison T, Johnson BE, Ferguson J (1993) A comparison of narrow band phototherapy (TL-01) and photochemotherapy (PUVA) in the management of polymorphic light eruption. Br J Dermatol 129:708–712
6. Collins P, Ferguson J (1995) Narrow-band UVB (TL-01) phototherapy: an effective preventive treatment for the photodermatoses. Br J Dermatol 132:956–963
7. Darras S, Segard M, Mortier L, Bonnevalle A, Thomas P (2004) Treatment of solar urticaria by intravenous immunoglobulins and PUVA therapy. Ann Dermatol Venereol 131:65–69
8. Dawe RS, Ferguson J (1997) Prolonged benefit following ultraviolet A phototherapy for solar urticaria. Br J Dermatol 137:144–148
9. Dawe RS, MacKie RM, Ferguson J (1998) The Scottish phototherapy audit: the need for evidence based guidelines? Br J Dermatol 139[Suppl 51]:17
10. Dawe RS, Ferguson J (2003) Diagnosis and treatment of chronic actinic dermatitis. Dermatol Ther 16:45–51
11. de Gruijl FR (1998) What do we know about skin cancer risk? PUVA vs UVB vs TL01. In: Hönigsmann H, Knobler RM, Trautinger F, Jori G (eds) Landmarks in photobiology. OEMF spa, Milano, pp 448–450

12. Duschet P, Leyen P, Schwarz T, Höcker P, Greiter J, Gschnait F (1987) Solar urticaria—effective treatment by plasmapheresis. Clin Exp Dermatol 12:185–188
13. Eramo LR, Garden JM, Esterly NB (1986) Hydroa vacciniforme. Diagnosis by repetitive ultraviolet-A phototesting. Arch Dermatol 122:1310–1313
14. Farr PM, Diffey BL (1989) Treatment of actinic prurigo with PUVA: mechanism of action. Br J Dermatol 120:411–418
15. Ferguson J (1990a) Polymorphic light eruption and actinic prurigo. Curr Probl Dermatol 19:130–147
16. Ferguson J (1990b) Photosensitivity dermatitis and actinic reticuloid syndrome (chronic actinic dermatitis). Semin Dermatol 9:47–54
17. Galosi A, Plewig G, Ring J, Meurer M, Schmoeckel C, Schurig V, Dorn M (1985) Experimentelle Auslösung von Hauterscheinungen bei Hydroa vacciniformia. Hautarzt 36:566–572
18. Grabczynska SA, McGregor JM, Kondeatis E, Vaughan RW, Hawk JLM (1999) Actinic prurigo and polymorphic light eruption: common pathogenesis and the importance of HLA-DR4/DRB1 × 0407. Br J Dermatol 140:232–236
19. Gschnait F, Hönigsmann H, Brenner W, Fritsch P, Wolff K (1978) Induction of UV light tolerance by PUVA in patients with polymorphous light eruption. Br J Dermatol 99:293–295
20. Halasz CLG, Leach EE, Walther RR, Poh-Fitzpatrick MB (1983) Hydroa vacciniforme: induction of lesions with ultraviolet A. J Am Acad Dermatol 8:171–176
21. Hasan T, Ranki A, Jansen CT, Karvonen J (1998) Disease associations in polymorphous light eruption: a long-term follow up study of 94 patients. Arch Dermatol 134:1081–1085
22. Hindson C, Spiro J, Downey A (1985) PUVA therapy of chronic actinic dermatitis. Br J Dermatol 113:157–160
23. Hölzle E, Hofmann C, Plewig G (1980) PUVA-treatment for solar urticaria and persistent light reaction. Arch Dermatol Res 269:87–91
24. Hölzle E, Plewig G, Hofmann C, Roser-Maass E (1982) Polymorphous light eruption. Experimental reproduction of skin lesions. J Am Acad Dermatol 7:111–125
25. Hölzle E, Plewig G, von Kries R, Lehmann P (1987) Polymorphous light eruption. J Invest Dermatol 88:32s–38s
26. Hölzle E, Rowold J, Plewig G (1992) Aktinische Prurigo. Hautarzt 43:278–282
27. Horio T, Minami K (1977) Solar urticaria: photoallergen in a patient's serum. Arch Dermatol 113:157–160
28. Hudson-Peacock MJ, Farr PM, Diffey BL, Goodship THJ (1993) Combined treatment of solar urticaria with plasmapheresis and PUVA. Br J Dermatol 128:440–442
29. Ichihashi M, Hasei K, Hayashibe K (1985) Solar Urticaria. Further studies on the role of inhibition spectra. Arch Dermatol 121:503–507
30. Jaschke E, Hönigsmann H (1981) Hydroa vacciniforme—Aktionsspektrum. UV-Toleranz nach Photochemotherapie. Hautarzt 32:350–353
31. Kalimo K, Jansen C (1986) Severe solar urticaria: active and passive action spectra and hyposensitizing effect of different UV modalities. Photodermatology 3:194–195
32. Larkö O, Diffey BL (1983) Natural UV-B radiation received by people with outdoor, indoor, and mixed occupations and UV-B treatment of psoriasis. Clin Exp Dermatol 8:279–285
33. Lee E, Koo J, Berger T (2005) UVB phototherapy and skin cancer risk: a review of the literature. Int J Dermatol 44:355–360
34. Leenutaphong V (1991) Hydroa vacciniforme: an unusual clinical manifestation. J Am Acad Dermatol 25:892–895
35. Leenutaphong V, Hölzle E, Plewig G (1990) Solar urticaria: studies on mechanisms of tolerance. Br J Dermatol 122:601–606
36. Leonard F, Morel M, Kalis B, Amblard P, Avenel-Audran M, Beani JC, Bonnetblanc JM, Leroy D, Marguery MC, Peyron JL, Rouchouze B, Thomas P (1991) Psoralen plus ultraviolet A in the prophylactic treatment of benign summer light eruption. Photodermatol Photoimmunol Photomed 8:95–98

37. Machet L, Vaillant L, Muller C, Henin P, Brive D, Lorette G (1991) Traitement par UVB therapie d'une urticaire solaire induite par les UVA. Ann Dermatol Venereol 118:535–537
38. Man I, Dawe RS, Ferguson J (1999) Artificial hardening for polymorphic light eruption: practical points from ten years' experience. Photodermatol Photoimmunol Photomed 15:96–99
39. Mang R, Stege H, Budde MA, Ruzicka T, Krutmann J (2002) Successful treatment of solar urticaria by extracorporeal photochemotherapy (photopheresis)—a case report. Photodermatol Photoimmunol Photomed 18:196–198
40. Morison WL, White HAD, Gonzalez E, Parrish JA, Fitzpatrick TB (1979) Oral methoxsalen photochemotherapy of uncommon photodermatoses. Acta Derm Venereol (Stockh) 59:366–368
41. Morison WL, Momtaz K, Mosher DB, Parrish JA (1982) UV-B phototherapy in the prophylaxis of polymorphous light eruption. Br J Dermatol 106:231–233
42. Murphy GM, Logan RA, Lovell CR, Morris RW, Hawk JLM, Magnus IA (1987) Prophylactic PUVA and UVB therapy in polymorphic light eruption—a controlled trial. Br J Dermatol 116:531–538
43. Ortel B, Tanew A, Wolff K, Hönigsmann H (1986) Polymorphous light eruption: action spectrum and photoprotection. J Am Acad Dermatol 14:748–753
44. Palmer RA, Friedmann PS (2004) A comparison of six and 12 PUVA treatments in the prophylaxis of polymorphic light eruption. Clin Exp Dermatol 29:141–143
45. Parrish JA, Le Vine MJ, Morison WL, Gonzalez E, Fitzpatrick TB (1979) Comparison of PUVA and beta-carotene in the treatment of polymorphous light eruption. Br J Dermatol 100:187–191
46. Parrish JA, Jaenicke KF, Morison WL, Momtaz K, Shea C (1982) Solar urticaria: treatment with PUVA and mediator inhibitors. Br J Dermatol 106:575–580
47. Plewig G, Hölzle E, Lehmann P (1986) Phototherapy for photodermatoses. Curr Probl Dermatol 15:254–264
48. Pont M, Deleporte E, Bennevalle A, Thomas P (2000) Solar urticaria: pre-PUVA UVA desensitization. Ann Dermatol Venereol 127:296–299
49. Ramsay CA (1977) Solar urticaria treatment by inducing tolerance to artificial radiation and natural light. Arch Dermatol 113:1222–1225
50. Reinauer S, Leenutaphong V, Hölzle E (1993) Fixed solar urticaria. J Am Acad Dermatol 29:161–165
51. Roelandts R (1985) Pre-PUVA UVA desensitization for solar urticaria. Photodermatology 2:174–176
52. Roelandts R, Ryckaert S (1999) Solar urticaria: the annoying photodermatosis. Int J Dermatol 38:411–418
53. Ryckaert S, Roelandts R (1998) Solar urticaria. A report of 25 cases and difficulties in phototesting. Arch Dermatol 134:71–74
54. Sonnex TS, Hawk JLM (1988) Hydroa vacciniforme: a review of ten cases. Br J Dermatol 118:101–108
55. Stern RS, Laird N (1994) The carcinogenic risk of treatments for severe psoriasis. Cancer 73:2759–2764
56. Studniberg HM, Weller P (1993) PUVA, UVB, psoriasis, and nonmelanoma skin cancer. J Am Acad Dermatol 29:1013–1022
57. Toonstra J, Henquet CJM, van Weelden H, van der Putten SCJ, van Vloten WA (1989) Actinic reticuloid: a clinical, photobiologic, histopathologic, and follow-up study of 16 patients. J Am Acad Dermatol 21:205–214
58. Young AR (1995) Carcinogenicity of UVB assessed. Lancet 345:1431–1432

第6章 皮肤T细胞淋巴瘤的光（化学）疗法

H. Hönigsmann, A. Tanew

内容

引言 ································· 116
UVB 光疗 ····························· 117
光化学疗法（PUVA）···················· 118
展望 ································· 124
临床总结 ····························· 124

要点

> 皮肤T细胞淋巴瘤（CTCL）指一组原发于皮肤的，包含不同非霍奇金淋巴瘤的大群体。
> 由于临床的病情（分期）不同，CTCL 的治疗方案各异，一般采取联合治疗的方式。
> 许多 CTCL 患者疾病仅局限于皮肤，这为采用光疗提供了理想的条件，需或不需要额外的治疗。
> 有三种光疗的方法在治疗 CTCL 上取得了相当大的成功：①传统宽光谱 UVB 照射；②系统口服光敏药物结合 UVA 照射，如 8-甲氧补骨脂素；③局部给与光敏药物结合 UVA 照射。
> 成功的光疗法会使 CTCL 患者获得长期缓解，甚至治愈。

引言

皮肤T细胞淋巴瘤(CTCL)指一组原发于皮肤的非霍奇金淋巴瘤。由于皮肤暴露在外,光疗及光化学疗法可作为蕈样肉芽肿和Sézary综合征(CTCL的亚型)的治疗选择方案,尤其是当病变主要累及皮肤时。已有三种光疗法广泛用于治疗CTCL,并取得成功:①传统的广谱UVB照射;②系统口服光敏药物结合UVA照射,如8-甲氧补骨脂素;③局部给予光敏药物结合UVA照射。这些治疗方法通常结合其他全身治疗,如维A酸类药物和干扰素。已有研究结果表明,CTCL患者的成功光治疗,可达到病情长期的缓解,甚至可能治愈。

皮肤T细胞淋巴瘤(CTCL)指一组原发于皮肤的非霍奇金淋巴瘤[1,2]。通常,由于MF是该组疾病最常见的,因此术语CTCL被用来专指蕈样肉芽肿(MF)及MF罕见的白血病的变异型,Sézary综合征(SS)。两者都是低度恶性的T辅助细胞淋巴瘤。光疗及光化学疗法已成为CTCL中MF和SS型的治疗选择。因此,本章将重点研讨这两种疾病。

蕈样肉芽肿通常是一个长期演变的过程,皮肤最初表现为红斑或湿疹样斑片和斑块。最终,这些皮损会进展成肿块,然后形成溃疡,肿瘤细胞会扩散到淋巴结和内脏,预后较差。Sézary综合征是MF的白血病变异型,它表现为红皮病伴全身淋巴结肿大,循环系统出现非典型T淋巴细胞,这种非典型T淋巴细胞有大的扭曲的细胞核(Sézary细胞)。在最严重的病例,Sézary综合征表现为狮面,掌跖角化过度和裂纹,以及严重的瘙痒。

组织病理学检查,蕈样肉芽肿和Sézary综合征的特征是具有脑回状核的小T淋巴细胞在皮肤浸润,并显示辅助T细胞的表型(CD4+)。一旦诊断明确,患者要根据TNM系统进行分级,TNM系统是基于肿瘤细胞类型、皮损浸润程度以及淋巴结,血及内脏器官是否受累的情况来评价[3,4]。根据国家卫生研究院(NIH)的划分,MF的自然病程分为疾病早期(ⅠA,ⅠB,ⅡA期)和晚期(ⅡB,Ⅲ,Ⅳ期)[3,4]。这种划分与疾病对光疗及光化学疗法的反应很大程度上具有相关性。尽管早期阶段的反应良好并表现出长期的缓解,但普遍认为,一旦肿瘤恶化,那么预后显示完全缓解是罕见的,且只有的短暂的生存期。因此,CTCL分期不仅具有预后意义,还对于制定个体患者的治疗策略至关重要。

由于大多数早期MF患者的疾病局限于皮肤,单独局部治疗,包括紫外线(UVB和补骨脂素联合UVA)治疗,局部化疗(氮芥和卡莫司汀)和电子束治疗就足够了。

多年来一直有争论,是否应在疾病的进程中尽早积极治疗以诱导永久治愈,还是应该仅在 CTCL 晚期进行积极治疗。最终, Kaye 等[5], 在一个随机试验中, 对电子束疗法和化学疗法与保守局部治疗进行了比较。虽然早期积极治疗组的完全反应率显著高于局部治疗组, 但缓解期和总生存期在两组之间没有显著差异。因此, 根据疾病分期调整, 治疗积极性逐步递增的保守治疗方案, 已被广泛接受[6]。在过去的 31 年中, 除了局部化疗和使用全身皮肤电子束疗法, 光化疗和 UVB 光疗法已成为治疗早期 CTCL 患者有效且耐受性良好的治疗方式。

UVB 光疗

众所周知, MF 病变常发生在身体隐蔽处, 早期 MF 患者受益于阳光照射。正因如此, 早在现代高强度灯出现前, 传统 UV 灯已被长期用于治疗 MF。

口服光化学疗法于 1974 年推出, 它不仅开始了一个皮肤科治疗的新时代, 而且也引发了对光生物学研究的兴趣[7]。这接着又引发了高强度紫外线灯的研发, 从而极大地改善了 UVB 光治疗, 使得在相当短的照射时间内进行全身治疗变得可行。第一份家庭用 UVB 光疗法治疗早期 MF 的报道出现在 1982 年[8]: 31 例 I 期 MF 患者均采用荧光灯(WestinghouseFS40)治疗, 其发射的宽谱紫外线辐射介于 280~350nm 之间。每隔一天, 患者接受产生红斑的阈值剂量, 直至病灶清除。此后, 隔天一次的维持治疗持续数月。其中, 61% 的患者在 4 个月的中位治疗期后病灶完全清除, 23% 的患者反应率超过 50%。与明显的完全临床反应相比, 所有 18 例患者的皮肤活检, 均显示在真皮乳头有轻度的残余淋巴细胞浸润。4 例维持治疗相对较短(3~7 个月)的患者, 在停止治疗后数月内复发; 而超过 1 年以上的维持治疗则得到较长时间的缓解。

在长期随访中, 同一患者群的 74% 在中值 5 个月治疗后保持完全缓解[9]。湿疹样(斑片)期患者比斑块期患者对光治疗反应更好, 且皮肤受累范围不影响结果。停止维持治疗后, 23% 的患者在超过 90 个月没有出现病变。

Ramsay 等发现, 以相似的治疗方案治疗 CTCL 早期患者, 在中值 5 个月后, 83% 的患者病灶完全清除[10]。随着维持治疗时间的延长, 在观察期内中位缓解期是 22 个月。20% 有完全反应的患者出现疾病复发。4 例斑块期患者对 UVB 治疗没有反应。

一项初步研究中表明, 窄谱 UVB 疗法是有效的短期治疗方式, 但所有患者在平均 6 个月都出现复发[11]。在对 8 例斑期 MF 患者进行的小型研究中, 窄谱 UVB 光疗法, 诱导了 6 例患者病灶的完全清除, 在 4 例中延长了缓解期(平均 20 个月)[12]。相比之下, 伊朗对 16 例早期 MF 患者的研究中观察到的缓解期则更短[13]。75% 的患者在平均 28 次治疗后病灶清除; 然而, 一半患者在平均 4.5 个月后出现复发。在最近的一项窄谱 UVB 研究中, 长时间的维持治疗(最多达 30

个月)获得了 26±10 个月的无复发期[14]。

UVB 光疗法治疗 CTCL 的机制包括:表皮朗格汉斯细胞功能受损,角质形成细胞的细胞因子产生和黏附分子的表达发生改变[15]。近期,有观点指出窄谱 UVB 诱导的 T 淋巴细胞凋亡,可能是这种光源治疗特别有效的原因[16]。

综上所述,UVB 光疗法对早期湿疹样(斑片)期 CTCL 患者治疗有效,可在医生的指导下在家进行治疗。必须持续维持治疗,以防止早期复发。一般情况下,UVB 光疗法是 I 期 MF 的一种安全治疗选择。治疗结果取决于恶性浸润的深度,而不是体表受累的范围。UVB 治疗不适用于斑块期或更晚期的 CTCL 患者。

UVB 光疗法的实践操作

UVB 光疗法很容易进行,除了用紫外吸收护目镜保护眼睛外,不需要其他特殊的预防措施。治疗应给予产生红斑的阈值剂量,至少每周三次。建议使用所述最小红斑的 70% 剂量作为起始剂量;此后,逐渐递增剂量以诱导并保持微弱红斑反应。一旦病灶清除,应持续数月的隔日治疗。

UVB 治疗的急性副作用很少,主要表现为轻度过量反应或皮肤干燥。长期副作用,比如皮肤癌的风险,要比光化学疗法(PUVA)(见下文)低得多。另一方面,UVB 光疗法与 PUVA 相比,疗效明显较低,且清除和维持治疗持续时间较长,因此它需要较高的患者依从性。

有时建议增加 UVA 治疗,但患者是否会受益,则一直存在争议。尚未有使用窄谱 UVB(311~313nm 的辐射,飞利浦 TL-01 灯)疗法和宽谱 UVB 疗法治疗 MF 的比较。初步试验研究中已经证实了中高剂量 UVA-1 治疗 I A 期和 I B 期患者的有效性[17,18]。

光化学疗法(PUVA)

Gilchrest 等人在 1976 年,首次报道了成功应用补骨脂素加 UVA(PUVA)治疗 CTCL 的光化学疗法[19]。基于已知阳光照射在 MF 中的益处,这些研究者推测 PUVA 治疗将是有效的。9 例对其他治疗方法反应不佳,且组织学证实为斑块期,肿瘤期,或红皮期的 CTCL 患者接受了光化学疗法。这九例患者中,四例获得完全缓解,五例有显著改善。在治疗的整个初始阶段,屏蔽一前臂使其免受 UVA 曝光处理,当在所有其他部位病灶完全清除时,此对照臂疾病甚至出现恶化,从而清楚地显示了治疗的疗效,而排除了发生自发缓解的可能性。在对照臂没有出现任何治疗反应,也明确表明了 PUVA 对 CTCL 的治疗效果是局部而非全身的。

在这首次试验后有大量的临床、病理组织学和实验性的研究(为参考,见[20,21])致力于解决以下问题:初始反应率和平均缓解期持续时间与CTCL分期的关系,PUVA与其他已建立治疗方案的功效比较,联合治疗的疗效,疗效的机制,以及短期和长期危害的风险。

反应率和缓解期与CTCL分期的关系

数个大的队列研究已经提供了PUVA治疗的初始反应率与CTCL分期的关系的信息[22-27]。这些研究中,治疗方案,补骨脂的制剂,以及使用的光源的不同,可能造成了结果的不一致。据报道,在PUVA治疗的第一疗程中患者获得完全缓解的比例为,ⅠA期75%~100%,ⅠB期47%~100%,ⅡA期67%~83%,ⅡB期40%~100%为和Ⅲ期33%~100%。极少数Ⅳ期患者使用PUVA单一疗法,因为在这个阶段,PUVA仅具有姑息或辅助治疗价值。Herrmann等总结了共244例患者的五项研究的结果[21]。他们计算出下列平均的完全初步反应率:ⅠA期(90%),ⅠB期(76%),ⅡA期(78%),ⅡB期(59%)和Ⅲ期(61%)。

与预测长期预后主要相关的是复发率和平均缓解期的数据。在对44例接受PUVA治疗患者的平均44个月的随访研究中,56%(5/9)ⅠA期患者与和39%(10/26)ⅠB期患者仍处于缓解期[24]。经历复发的患者的缓解时间,在ⅠA期患者中是平均20个月,ⅠB期17个月。所有的ⅡB期患者(7/7)疾病有多次复发,2例Ⅲ期患者最初进入缓解期,1例在维持治疗期间复发,1例随访期失去联系。

最近对66例临床分期为ⅠA期至ⅡA期的患者的研究表明,在1979年至1995年间接受PUVA单独治疗达到完全缓解后,30%~50%的患者缓解期长达10年,但随后疾病确实复发。长期生存率并不受复发影响[23]。

对于不能全身施用补骨脂制剂的患者,PUVA水浴疗法可能是极有价值的替代选择。在对16例早期MF患者的回顾性分析中,8-MOP(1mg/L)水浴治疗,在平均29次治疗和平均累积的UVA曝光剂量33J/cm^{2}后,所有患者病灶全部清除[28]。然而,如果涉及头部,则PUVA疗法可能不可行。

总之,迄今发表的数据表明,由于PUVA具有高完全清除率,可使相当比例的患者保持疾病多年不复发,因此它是早期(ⅠA~ⅡA)CTCL患者极好的治疗选择。在晚期(ⅡB~ⅣB)患者中,PUVA不足以作为单一疗法,但可作为辅助治疗,它可以减少皮肤上的肿瘤负荷,提高患者的生活质量。PUVA是治疗MF有效的方法,可诱导长期缓解,也许在某些情况下可使疾病"痊愈"。

与其他既定的治疗方法比较

其他广泛使用的CTCL治疗方法包括外用氮芥(HN2),其他广泛使用的CTCL治疗方法包括外用氮芥(HN2),外用卡氮芥(BCNU),以及全身皮肤电子束放射治疗(EBRT)[29-32]。不幸的是,没有随机试验比较这些疗法在短期疗效,无复发期,和存活率上的不同。早期对42名患者的非随机研究发现,EBRT比HN2更有效,但其复发率显著更高[33]。近来,对ⅠA期患者的回顾性分析显示,在完全清除率和无复发期长短上,EBRT要优于HN2。但是,观察表明在10年的生存率上则没有显著差异[34]。在ⅠA期和ⅠB期患者中,使用PUVA疗法的结果与以往研究中使用HN2和BCNU疗法的相比,在完全缓解率和长期生存率上没有统计学的显著差异[21]。由于缺乏可比较的数据,不能比较HN2的缓解持续时间,但对ⅠA期和ⅠB期患者,PUVA的缓解持续时间在2年和5年,比BCNU更好。

联合治疗

联合维A酸(RePUVA)

维A酸治疗CTCL的有效性可能与其免疫调节能力,抗肿瘤,抗增殖和抗炎的性质有关。此外,经过维A酸治疗的皮肤表皮厚度减小,可增强UVA的皮肤渗透。

大量的临床研究已证实维A酸药物对MF和Sézary综合征的治疗有效[35-39]。当异维A酸和阿维A酯作为单药治疗时,两者都很少引起持久的缓解,迄今为止其主要用途是作为CTCL更成熟的方案,如全身化疗,干扰素或光化学疗法的辅助治疗。斯堪的纳维亚MF组对69例斑块期MF患者进行一个至关重要的问题的研究,即维A酸加PUVA联合治疗是否会比PUVA单独疗法效果更好。尽管到达缓解期时接受维A酸的患者,PUVA的累积剂量显著较低,但联合使用维A酸和PUVA与单独使用PUVA相比,并不能产生更高的反应率。然而,使用了维A酸的维持治疗似乎延长了缓解期[40]。阿维A酯以1.0~1.5mg/kg的剂量与PUVA联合治疗,在MF(ⅠB期至ⅣA期)患者中产生了80%(32/40)的完全清除率,在sézary综合征患者中为75%(6/8)[41]。然而,即使患者临床上病灶完全清除,活检组织病理学检查仍显示在真皮深层有异常淋巴细胞持续存在。

最近,贝沙罗汀已被批准在美国和欧洲作为单一口服的维A酸,用于治疗曾经接受过至少一种全身治疗而效果不佳的皮肤T细胞淋巴瘤患者。因此,人们尝试研究贝沙罗汀与PUVA联合治疗的疗效。singh和Lebwohl报道在所有八个患者中均出现最初的反应,其中五例完全缓解[42]。鉴于其良好的安全性,这种联合治疗可用于治疗其他难治的CTCL。还需要进一步研究以确定,以贝沙罗汀为基础的联合治疗的有效率是否比其他联合治疗更高[43,44]。

联合使用干扰素α

使用大剂量干扰素(IFN)-α成功治疗晚期难治性皮肤T细胞淋巴瘤的第一

次报告出现在 1984 年[45]。至今,数个临床试验,大多采用 IFN-α2a,证实了这种治疗方法在 CTCL 所有分期中的有效性。这些试验为疗效、剂量方案、反应的预测及其副作用提供了数据[46,47]。基于干扰素单一治疗取得了可喜的成效,结合 PUVA 和干扰素治疗,以增强两者疗效,这似乎顺理成章。在 Kuzel 等的 15 例 CTCL(分期ⅠB 至ⅣB)Ⅰ期临床试验中,联合使用 PUVA 和 IFN-α-2a 干扰素($6\times10^6 \sim 30\times10^6$ IU),每周三次,80% 获得完全缓解(12/15),总(完全或部分)有效率为 93%(14/15)。此外,联合治疗比单一使用 PUVA 或干扰素治疗,反应更快,更持久[48]。最近对这些患者及其随后加入的 24 例患者重新评估,IFN-α2a 最大剂量达 12×10^6 IU/m^2,完全反应率为 62%(24/39),总有效率为 90%(35/39)[49]。患者的完全反应率比初始试验较低,原因在于部分新加入患者的疾病更晚期。完全反应的中位缓解期为 60 个月,部分反应的中位缓解期为 13 个月。

对 11 例患者(1 例ⅠB 期,2 例ⅡA 期,5 例ⅡB 期,2 例Ⅲ期,1 例ⅣA 期),进行每周 4 次 PUVA,及 IFN-α-2a 初始剂量 9×10^6 IU,每周 3 次的治疗,疗效欠佳[50]。其中,45%(5/11)的患者肿瘤完全清除,55% 的患者(6/11)部分清除(改善 50%)。3 例患者在平均随访 7.5 个月内复发。在另一项研究中,PUVA 联合低剂量的 IFN-α($3\times10^6 \sim 6\times10^6$ IU/d)治疗,使 5 例以前对 PUVA 单一疗法无效的患者完全缓解,也减少了清除肿瘤所需的累积 UVA 剂量[51]。

最近一项随机多中心临床试验,调查了 IFN-α(9×10^6 IU,每周三次)联合 PUVA(每周 2～5 次)的疗效,与 IFN-α(9×10^6 IU,每周三次)联合阿维 A(0.5mg/kg 体重/d)的疗效对比[52]。对 40 例接受 IFN-α 和 PUVA 联合治疗的患者(30 例Ⅰ期,10 例Ⅱ期),和 38 例接受 IFN-α 和阿维 A 联合治疗的患者(30 例Ⅰ期,8 例Ⅱ期)进行了评估。在 IFN-α 和 PUVA 联合治疗的患者中,83% 的Ⅰ期患者(25/30)和 20% 的Ⅱ期患者(2/10)完全有效;在 IFN-α 和阿维 A 联合治疗的患者中,53%(16/30)的Ⅰ期患者和 0% 的Ⅱ期患者(0/8)完全有效。完全缓解的中位时间,在接受 IFN-α 加 PUVA 联合治疗的患者中是 21 周,在接受 IFN-α 加阿维 A 联合治疗的患者中是 62 周。在接受 IFN-α 加 PUVA 联合治疗的患者中,因为严重的副作用而终止治疗的 2 例,而在接受 IFN-α 加阿维 A 联合治疗的患者中有 8 例[52]。

最近的一项多中心研究(14 个月,低剂量 IFN-α 加 PUVA 联合治疗,与 IFN-α 单一疗法相比),显示出总有效率(98%:80%～92%)和完全反应率(84%:68%～75%),比所有其他 PUVA 和 IFN-α 联合治疗的疗效更高,且使用较低的 IFN-α2b 剂量,每周(6～18MU:18～90MU)[53]。

一个重要的方面是,患者可以在 IFN-α 治疗中产生抗干扰素抗体,这会降低疗效。已经有报道,PUVA 治疗抑制 MF 患者抗 IFN-α 抗体的生成[54]。一项最近的研究显示,中和 IFN-α 的干扰素抗体在接受 PUVA 的患者中显著降低;然而,检测发现与临床相关的结合 IFN-α 的干扰素抗体则高于预期[55]。因此,对进行 IFN-α 和 PUVA 联合治疗的患者,应定期监测 IFN-α 抗体。

光化学疗法的实践操作

在开始治疗前,需要进行完全的临床和病理组织学检查,包括免疫分型和分子生物学技术的应用,另外患者必须根据 TNM 分类法分期。对 ⅠA～ⅡA 期患者,我们通常开始 PUVA 单独治疗,其常常在可接受的时间内诱导完全和持久的缓解。与联合方案相比,PUVA 单独治疗具有低毒性特征的优势。下面所述治疗方案,需要平均 20～30 次照射和累积剂量 UVA 50～150J/cm²。联合治疗适用于,对 PUVA 单一疗法反应缓慢或不完全的患者,以及在维持治疗中或维持治疗停止后复发的患者。治疗晚期(ⅡB 至 Ⅳ)患者,我们建议 PUVA 作为一种辅助治疗,与电离辐射,全身化疗联合治疗,或在 Sézary 综合征患者进行体外光化学免疫疗法时作为辅助治疗。

CTCL 的光化学疗法指南通常与银屑病的相同(见第 3 章)。大多数研究使用 8-甲氧基补骨脂,因为 5-甲氧基补骨脂不易获取,尤其在美国。在斯堪的纳维亚,有用三甲沙林和 8-甲氧基补骨脂进行洗浴-PUVA 治疗 CTCL。洗浴 PUVA 可能不理想,因为面部和头皮几乎不能得到充分治疗,新病变可在治疗过程中出现在这些区域。8-甲氧基补骨脂和 5-甲氧基补骨脂都是合适的光敏剂,若提供有足够剂量的 UVA 辐射,它们的治疗效果相似。5-甲氧基补骨脂不良反应少,光毒性比 8-甲氧基补骨脂低,但需要更高的 UVA 剂量[56]。对于不耐受 8-甲氧基补骨脂的患者,建议使用 5-甲氧补骨脂素;而对光敏性显著的患者使用剂量测定。

因为没有可比数据,无法判断治疗 CTCL 患者是美国 PUVA 方案还是欧洲 PUVA 方案更好。在治疗银屑病方面,欧洲更积极的方法已被证明清除疾病更快,且 UVA 累积剂量较低[57]。两种治疗方案之间的主要区别在于,对患者 PUVA 敏感性的关注,初始 UVA 照射剂量的选择,随后剂量的递增,清除治疗和维持治疗阶段的治疗频率,和维持治疗阶段的长短(详见第 3 章)。

美国的治疗方案,采用的起始剂量基于患者治疗前的皮肤类型和色素沉着的程度,通常位于 1.5 和 3J/cm² 的范围[58]。每周治疗 2～3 次,UVA 剂量递增取决于红斑出现与否,为 0.5J/cm² 或更高。当在临床上获得完全缓解并由组织学确认后,则开始维持治疗,频率下降至每月一次,持续数月或一直持续下去。

在欧洲方案中,治疗前,给予每个病人光敏剂后,测试 MPD(最小的光毒性剂量)以确定其对光化学疗法的敏感性[59]。然后以 MPD,或仅低于 MPD 的剂量,作为起始剂量。每周治疗 4 次,并定期调整剂量以保持每个病人有微弱红斑的皮肤反应。与美国方案一样,在皮损完全清除后,从以前的皮损部位进行活检,以排除真皮深部的恶性浸润[60]。如何处理临床上没有皮损表现,但组织学存在皮肤浸润,则没有明确的答案。我们建议在这种情况下开始维持治疗。即每周两次持续一个月,然后每周一次再一个月。在这一治疗阶段中,UVA剂量通常保持恒定。如果病人2个月的维持治疗后保持不复发,则停止治疗。如果出现复发,则恢复初始的每周4次治疗,如果红斑不再明显,则增加UVA的剂量。到目前为止,还不能确定维持治疗期的长短,以及维持治疗能否延长生存期。

对CTCL患者治疗剂量必须谨慎,因为他们的红斑阈值往往非常低[60,61]。当MPD测试出现明显的光敏时,短疗程系统使用皮质类固醇激素(泼尼松龙或强的松)治疗,可让患者耐受PUVA治疗而不发生严重的光毒性反应[62]。光敏性增加也是公认的使用IFN-α的副作用[48,50]。

另一个特别的发现是在PUVA治疗的初始阶段,部分患者中以前看不到的亚临床病灶会出现。正是由于这个原因,患者即使只有少量皮损的也应接受全身治疗,并且洗浴-PUVA是不够的。需要特别重视和小心地暴露身体所有部位,包括间擦区域,进行UVA辐射。否则,遮光区域,如腹股沟和腋窝,病灶的清除将会延迟或不彻底[63]。UVA辐射无法到达的部位,如多毛的头皮或指间区,需要额外的处理,比如局部施用氮芥或电离辐射。当总UVA剂量超过1200J/cm^{2}或200次治疗时,保留病人的累积辐射剂量的记录,并考虑联合或间替疗法[64]。然而,这些是相当随意的数字,并且累积UVA剂量的长期副作用在恶性疾病的治疗中不那么重要,特别是,当其他治疗方法,如氮芥或电离辐射也是已知的致癌物。

对所有患者进行定期随访检查是必须的,随访应该包括仔细的临床评价有无皮肤恶性肿瘤的发展。可疑病变必须立即切除,并进行组织学检查。

PUVA治疗蕈样肉芽肿的作用机制

PUVA诱导的对恶性T细胞皮肤浸润的清除机制仍在研究中。PUVA影响皮肤各种不同标靶,治疗效果可能是由PUVA诱导数种细胞变化的相互作用产生。PUVA对浸润表皮和真皮浅层的T细胞施加细胞毒性作用。近期观察表明,PUVA通过诱导凋亡来选择性消除T淋巴细胞群,可能起主要作用[65]。PUVA也可能通过干扰表皮细胞因子的产生,直接下调亲表皮恶性T细胞的归巢受体而产生疗效。最后,CD1a+朗格汉斯细胞保持浸润T细胞对表皮的亲和力,参与了CTCL的发病机制,而PUVA治疗会导致CD1a+朗格汉斯细胞的功能障碍[15]。

光化学治疗的短期和长期危害

PUVA治疗CTCL患者的急性副作用,原则上与治疗其他对PUVA有效的疾病(如银屑病)患者相同。最常见的急性不良反应是光毒性,表现为疼痛性红斑、水肿、和偶尔水疱形成。银屑病因角化过度和表皮增厚可能降低UVA辐射的渗透，与银屑病皮损对比，其光侵蚀及浅表溃疡的发生率增加。在第一次治疗时出现以前看不见红斑和MF的湿疹样病变，并不罕见，且不归因于UVA的过量[66]。其他副作用包括皮肤瘙痒，对8-甲氧基补骨脂不耐受反应，如恶心或头晕，及罕见的播散性单纯疱疹。

最严重的问题，长期PUVA治疗的风险与罹患皮肤恶性肿瘤有关。现在根据众多对银屑病患者随访的研究认为，PUVA可作为完全的致癌物，与罹患鳞状细胞癌和角化棘皮瘤的风险增加呈剂量依赖性相关[67-69]。在PUVA治疗的CTCL患者中，也有报道比预期发生率更高的非黑素瘤皮肤癌和转移性鳞状细胞癌；然而，所有这些患者也接受了其他致癌性治疗，包括电离辐射，局部氮芥和全身化疗[70,72]。在赫尔曼等进行的长期随访研究中[72]，10%的患者出现慢性光化性损害，表现为PUVA诱导的色素斑和光化性角化病，82例患者中的3例（3.7%）发展为鳞状细胞癌。大多数这些慢性变化发生在已接受PUVA超过10年的患者中，且累积的UVA剂量超过2000J/cm^2[72]。

综合起来，有明确的证据表明，使用不同联合或序贯疗法治疗CTCL可以协同增加鳞状细胞癌的风险，而目前无法准确估算CTCL患者单独使用PUVA治疗的风险。有关长期使用PUVA的风险的更多信息可见第3章。当然，这种风险的影响，必须与治疗效果相比较，但如上所述，与银屑病相比，这对于潜在威胁生命的CTCL可能毫无意义。

展望

几个问题仍有待未来的对照研究来解答。目前，没有任何治疗方案可以防止晚期CTCL最终进展形成肿瘤，扩散和导致死亡。最重要的问题是，光化学疗法，单独给予或与其他治疗联合，能否诱导早期患者的永久缓解甚至治愈。20世纪70年代末，自推出PUVA治疗后，瑞典的MF死亡率显著下降。根据斯德哥尔摩的瑞典国家中央统计局的皮肤疾病死亡统计来看，很可能PUVA是使死亡率降低的原因[73]。还需要有更多的数据来改善最佳治疗CTCL的PUVA方案，它应是使用最低的UVA剂量并能提供最大功效。在这方面，联合治疗的优化必将使疗效大幅提高。最后，随着对CTCL免疫发病机制的认识进展，治疗的靶目标将被最终确定，以助实现治疗策略的个性化。

临床总结

光疗法和光化学疗法，对于治疗T淋巴细胞变异的蕈样肉芽肿和Sézary综

第6章 皮肤T细胞淋巴瘤的光(化学)疗法

合征患者是高度有效的,尤其当疾病局限于皮肤时。与其他全身疗法相结合,这些疾病的患者有望获得长期缓解。

(罗育武 译,李润祥 孟珍 校,朱慧兰 审)

参考文献

1. Willemze R, Jaffe ES, Burg G, Cerroni L, Berti E, Swerdlow SH, Ralfkiaer E, Chimenti S, Diaz-Perez JL, Duncan LM, Grange F, Harris NL, Kempf W, Kerl H, Kurrer M, Knobler R, Pimpinelli N, Sander C, Santucci M, Sterry W, Vermeer MH, Wechsler J, Whittaker S, Meijer CJ (2005) WHO-EORTC classification for cutaneous lymphomas. Blood 105:3768–3785
2. Querfeld C, Rosen ST, Guitart J, Kuzel TM (2005) The spectrum of cutaneous T-cell lymphomas: new insights into biology and therapy. Curr Opin Hematol 12:273–278
3. Foss F (2004) Mycosis fungoides and the Sézary syndrome. Curr Opin Oncol 16:421–428
4. Lamberg SI, Green SB, Byar DP et al (1984) Clinical staging for cutaneous T-cell lymphoma. Ann Intern Med 100:187–192
5. Kaye FJ, Bunn PA Jr, Steinberg S et al (1989) A randomized trial comparing combination electron-beam radiation and chemotherapy with topical therapy in the initial treatment of mycosis fungoides. N Engl J Med 321:1784–1790
6. Jörg B, Kerl H, Thiers BH, Bröcker EB, Burg G (1994) Therapeutic approaches in cutaneous lymphoma. Dermatol Clin 12:433–441
7. Parrish JA, Fitzpatrick TB, Tanenbaum L, Pathak MA (1974) Photochemotherapy of psoriasis with oral methoxsalen and longwave ultraviolet light. N Engl J Med 291:1207–1211
8. Milstein HI, Vonderheid EC, Van Scott EJ, Johnson WC (1982) Home ultraviolet phototherapy of early mycosis fungoides: preliminary observations. J Am Acad Dermatol 6:355–362
9. Resnik KS, Vonderheid EC (1993) Home UV phototherapy of early mycosis fungoides: long-term follow-up observations in thirty-one patients. J Am Acad Dermatol 29:73–77
10. Ramsay DL, Lish KM, Yalowitz CB, Soter NA (1992) Ultraviolet-B phototherapy for early-stage cutaneous T-cell lymphoma. Arch Dermatol 128:931–933
11. Hofer A, Cerroni L, Kerl H, Wolf P (1999) Narrowband (311-nm) UV-B therapy for small plaque parapsoriasis and early-stage mycosis fungoides. Arch Dermatol 135:1377–1380
12. Clark C, Dawe RS, Evans AT, Lowe G, Ferguson J (2000) Narrowband TL-01 phototherapy for patch-stage mycosis fungoides. Arch Dermatol 136:748–752
13. Ghodsi SZ, Hallaji Z, Balighi K, Safar F, Chams-Davatchi C (2005) Narrow-band UVB in the treatment of early stage mycosis fungoides: report of 16 patients. Clin Exp Dermatol 30:376–788
14. Boztepe G, Sahin S, Ayhan M et al (2005) Narrowband ultraviolet B phototherapy to clear and maintain clearance in patients with mycosis fungoides. J Am Acad Dermatol 53:242–246
15. Volc-Platzer B, Hönigsmann H (1995) Photoimmunology of PUVA and UVB therapy. In: Krutmann J, Elmets CA (eds) Photoimmunology. Blackwell Science, Oxford, pp 265–273
16. Ozawa M, Ferenczi K, Kikuchi T, et al (1999) 312-nanometer ultraviolet B light (narrow-band UVB) induces apoptosis of T cells within psoriatic lesions. J Exp Med 189:711–718
17. Plettenberg H, Stege H, Megahed M, Ruzicka T, Hosokawa Y, Tsuji T, Morita A, Krutmann J (1999) Ultraviolet A1 (340–400 nm) phototherapy for cutaneous T-cell lymphoma. J Am Acad Dermatol 41:47–50
18. Zane C, Leali C, Airo P, De Panfilis G, Pinton PC (2001) "High-dose" UVA1 therapy of widespread plaque-type, nodular, and erythrodermic mycosis fungoides. J Am Acad Dermatol 44:629–633
19. Gilchrest BA, Parrish JA, Tanenbaum L, Haynes HA, Fitzpatrick TB (1976) Oral methoxsalen photochemotherapy of mycosis fungoides. Cancer 38:683–689
20. Tanew A, Hönigsmann H (1997) Ultraviolet B and psoralen plus UVA phototherapy for cuta-

neous T-cell lymphoma. Dermatol Ther 4:38–46
21. Herrmann Jr, Roenigk HH Jr, Hönigsmann H (1995) Ultraviolet radiation for treatment of cutaneous T-cell lymphoma. Hematol Oncol Clin North Am 9:1077–1088
22. Abel EA, Sendagorta E, Hoppe RT, Hu CH (1987) PUVA treatment of erythrodermic and plaque-type mycosis fungoides. Arch Dermatol 123:897–901
23. Querfeld C, Rosen ST, Kuzel TM, Kirby KA, Roenigk HH Jr, Prinz BM, Guitart J (2005) Long-term follow-up of patients with early-stage cutaneous T-cell lymphoma who achieved complete remission with psoralen plus UV-A monotherapy. Arch Dermatol 141:305–311
24. Hönigsmann H, Brenner W, Rauschmeier W, Konrad K, Wolff K (1984) Photochemotherapy for cutaneous T cell lymphoma. J Am Acad Dermatol 10:238–245
25. Powell FC, Spiegel GT, Muller SA (1984) Treatment of parapsoriasis and mycosis fungoides: the role of psoralen and long-wave ultraviolet light A (PUVA). Mayo Clin Proc 59:538–546
26. Rosenbaum MM, Roenigk HH Jr, Caro WA, Esker A (1985) Photochemotherapy in cutaneous T cell lymphoma and parapsoriasis en plaques. J Am Acad Dermatol 13:613–622
27. Vella Briffa D, Warin AP, Harrington CI, Bleehen SS (1980) Photochemotherapy in mycosis fungoides. Lancet 2:49–53
28. Weber F, Schmuth M, Sepp N, Fritsch P (2005) Bath-water PUVA therapy with 8-methoxypsoralen in mycosis fungoides. Acta Derm Venereol 85:329–332
29. Holloway KB, Flowers FP, Ramos-Caro FA (1992) Therapeutic alternatives in cutaneous T-cell lymphoma. J Am Acad Dermatol 27:367–378
30. Hoppe R (1991) The management of mycosis fungoides at Stanford—standard and innovative treatment programs. Leukemia 5[Suppl 1]:46–48
31. Vonderheid EC, Tan ET, Kantor AF, Shrager L, Micaily B, van Scott EJ (1989) Long-term efficacy, curative potential, and carcinogenicity of topical mechlorethamine chemotherapy in cutaneous T cell lymphoma. J Am Acad Dermatol 20:416–428
32. Zackheim HS, Epstein EH Jr, Crain WR (1990) Topical carmustine (BCNU) for cutaneous T cell lymphoma: a 15-year experience in 143 patients. J Am Acad Dermatol 22:802–810
33. Hamminga B, Noordijk EM, van Vloten WA (1982) Treatment of mycosis fungoides. Total-skin electron-beam irradiation vs topical mechlorethamine therapy. Arch Dermatol 118:150–153
34. Kim YH, Jensen RA, Watanabe GL, Varghese A, Hoppe RT (1996) Clinical stage la (limited patch and plaque) mycosis fungoides. A long-term outcome analysis. Arch Dermatol 132:1309–1313
35. Claudy AL, Rouchouse B (1985) Treatment of cutaneous T cell lymphoma with retinoids. In: Saurat JH (ed) Retinoids: new trends in research and therapy. Retinoid symposium, Geneva, 1984. Karger, Basel, pp 335–340
36. Kessler JF, Jones SE, Levine N, Lynch PJ, Rohman Both A, Meyskens L Jr (1987) Isotretinoin and cutaneous helper T cell lymphoma (mycosis fungoides). Arch Dermatol 123:201–204
37. Mahrle G, Thiele B (1987) Retinoids in cutaneous T cell lymphomas. Dermatologica 175[Suppl 1]:145–150
38. Molin L, Thomsen K, Volden G et al (1987) Oral retinoids in mycosis fungoides and Sézary syndrome: a comparison of isotretinoin and etretinate. Acta Derm Venereol (Stockh) 67:232–236
39. Thomsen K, Molin L, Volden G, Lange Wantzin G, Hellbe L (1984) 13-cis-retinoic acid effective in mycosis fungoides. Acta Derm Venereol (Stockh) 64:563–566
40. Thomsen K, Hammar H, Molin L, Volden G (1989) Retinoids plus PUVA (RePUVA) and PUVA in mycosis fungoides, plaque stage. Acta Derm Venereol (Stockh) 69:536–538
41. Serri F, De Simone C, Venier A, Rusciani L, Marchetti E (1990) Combination of retinoids and PUVA (Re-PUVA) in the treatment of cutaneous T-cell lymphomas. Curr Probl Dermatol 19:252–257
42. Singh F, Lebwohl MG (2004) Cutaneous T-cell lymphoma treatment using bexarotene and PUVA: a case series. J Am Acad Dermatol 51:570–573

43. Coors EA, Von den Driesch P (2005) Treatment of mycosis fungoides with bexarotene and psoralen plus ultraviolet A. Br J Dermatol 152:1379–1381
44. Zhang C, Duvic M (2003) Retinoids: therapeutic applications and mechanisms of action in cutaneous T-cell lymphoma. Dermatol Ther 16:322–330
45. Bunn PA Jr, Foon KA, Ihde DC et al (1984) Recombinant leukocyte A interferon: an active agent in advanced cutaneous T-cell lymphomas. Ann Intern Med 101:484–487
46. Olsen EA, Bunn PA (1995) Interferon in the treatment of cutaneous T-cell lymphoma. Hematol Oncol Clin North Am 9:1089–1107
47. Thestrup-Pedersen K (1990) Interferon therapy in cutaneous T-cell lymphoma. Curr Probl Dermatol 19:258–263
48. Kuzel TM, Gilyon K, Springer E et al (1990) Interferon alfa-2a combined with phototherapy in the treatment of cutaneous T-cell lymphoma. J Natl Cancer Inst 82:203–207
49. Kuzel TM, Roenigk HH Jr, Samuelson E et al (1995) Effectiveness of interferon alfa-2a combined with phototherapy for mycosis fungoides and the Seizure syndrome. J Clin Oncol 13:257–263
50. Otte HG, Herges A, Stadler R (1992) Kombinationstherapie mit Interferon α2a und PUVA bei kutanen T-Zell-Lymphomen. Hautarzt 43:695–699
51. Mostow EN, Neckel SL, Oberhelman L, Anderson TF, Cooper KD (1993) Complete remissions in psoralen and UVA (PUVA)-refractory mycosis fungoides-type cutaneous T-lymphoma with combined interferon alfa and PUVA. Arch Dermatol 129:747–752
52. Stadler R, Otte HG, Luger T, Henz BM, Kuhl P, Zwingers T, Sterry W (1998) Prospective randomized multicenter clinical trial on the use of interferon-2α plus acitretin versus interferon-2α plus PUVA in patients with cutaneous T-cell lymphoma stages I and II. Blood 92:3578–3581
53. Rupoli S, Goteri G, Pulini S, Filosa A, Tassetti A, Offidani M, Filosa G, Mozzicafreddo G, Giacchetti A, Brandozzi G, Cataldi I, Barulli S, Ranaldi R, Scortechini AR, Capretti R, Fabris G, Leoni P (2005) Marche Regional Multicentric Study Group of Cutaneous Lymphomas. Long-term experience with low-dose interferon-alpha and PUVA in the management of early mycosis fungoides. Eur J Haematol 75:136–145
54. Kuzel TM, Roenigk HH Jr, Samuelson E, Rosen ST (1992) Suppression of anti-interferon α-2a antibody formation in patients with mycosis fungoides by exposure to longwave UV radiation in the A range and methoxsalen ingestion. J Natl Cancer Inst 84:119–121
55. Rajan GP, Seifert B, Prümmer O, Joller-Jemelka HI, Burg G, Dummer R (1996) Incidence and in-vivo relevance of antiinterferon antibodies during treatment of low-grade cutaneous T-cell lymphomas with interferon alpha-2a combined with acitretin or PUVA. Arch Dermatol Res 288:543–548
56. Tanew A, Ortel B, Rappersberger K, Hönigsmann H (1988) 5-Methoxypsoralen (Bergapten) for photochemotherapy. J Am Acad Dermatol 18:333–339
57. Henseler T, Wolff K, Hönigsmann H, Christophers E (1981) Oral 8-methoxypsoralen photochemotherapy of psoriasis. Lancet i:853–857
58. Roenigk HH Jr (1977) Photochemotherapy for mycosis fungoides. Arch Dermatol 113:1047–1051
59. Wolff K, Gschnait F, Hönigsmann H, Konrad K, Parrish JA, Fitzpatrick TB (1977) Phototesting and dosimetry for photochemotherapy. Br J Dermatol 96:1–10
60. Lowe NJ, Cripps DJ, Dufton PA, Vickers CFH (1979) Photochemotherapy for mycosis fungoides. A clinical and histological study. Arch Dermatol 115:50–53
61. Volden G, Thune PO (1977) Light sensitivity in mycosis fungoides. Br J Dermatol 97:279–284
62. Molin L, Volden G (1987) Treatment of light-sensitive mycosis fungoides with PUVA and prednisolone. Photodermatol Photoimmunol Photomed 4:106–107
63. Du Vivier A, Vollum DI (1980) Photochemotherapy and topical nitrogen mustard in the treatment of mycosis fungoides. Br J Dermatol 102:319–322

64. Whittaker SJ, Marsden JR, Spittle M, Russell Jones R (2003) British Association of Dermatologists; U.K. Cutaneous Lymphoma Group Joint British Association of Dermatologists and U.K. Cutaneous Lymphoma Group guidelines for the management of primary cutaneous T-cell lymphomas. Br J Dermatol 149:1095–1107
65. Johnson R, Staiano-Coico L, Austin L, Cardinale I, Nabeya-Tsukifuji R, Krueger JG (1996) PUVA treatment selectively induces a cell cycle block and subsequent apoptosis in human T-lymphocytes. Photochem Photobiol 63:566–571
66. Hönigsmann H, Tanew A, Wolff K (1987) Treatment of mycosis fungoides with PUVA. Photodermatol Photoimmunol Photomed 4:55–58
67. Maier H, Schemper M, Ortel B, Binder M, Tanew A, Hönigsmann H (1996) Skin tumors in photochemotherapy for psoriasis. A single center follow-up of 496 patients. Dermatology 193:185–191
68. Stern RS, Lunder EJ (1998) Risk of squamous cell carcinoma and methoxsalen (psoralen) and UV-A radiation (PUVA). A meta-analysis. Arch Dermatol 134:1582–1585
69. Studniberg HM, Weller P (1993) PUVA, UVB, psoriasis, and nonmelanoma skin cancer. J Am Acad Dermatol 29:1013–102
70. Abel EA, Sendagorta E, Hoppe RT (1986) Cutaneous malignancies and metastatic squamous cell carcinoma following topical therapies for mycosis fungoides. J Am Acad Dermatol 14:1029–1038
71. Smoller BR, Marcus R (1994) Risk of secondary cutaneous malignancies in patients with long-standing mycosis fungoides. J Am Acad Dermatol 30:201–204
72. Herrmann JJ, Roenigk HH Jr, Hurria A et al (1995) Treatment of mycosis fungoides with photochemotherapy (PUVA): long-term follow-up. J Am Acad Dermatol 33:234–242
73. Swanbeck G, Roupe G, Sandström MH (1994) Indications of a considerable decrease in the death rate in mycosis fungoides by PUVA treatment. Acta Derm Venereol (Stockh) 74:465–466

第7章　白癜风的光(化学)疗法

B. Ortel, V. Petronic-Rosic, P. Calzavara-Pinton

内容

引言	129
诊断	130
白癜风的社会心理影响	133
白癜风的治疗	134
白癜风复色的光疗选择	137
总结	150

要点

> 白癜风是一个以黑色素细胞为靶点的自身免疫性疾病,治疗难度较大。
> 目前,最好的单一疗法是窄谱 UVB(NB-UVB)光疗。
> 绝大部分治疗方案,包括光疗和联合治疗对于治疗白癜风均有一定疗效。

引言

　　以紫外线照射为基础的治疗白癜风方法是最有效的治疗选择。本章提供详细的光疗作用和应用方案。首先,明确疾病和鉴别于其他疾病。本章的主要部分将集中于紫外线光疗和光化学疗法,还会讨论辅助和联合治疗模式作为可选择的治疗方案。

诊断

白癜风是一种获得性色素障碍性疾病，临床特征为进展性白色斑点和斑片，是由于受影响的皮肤处黑色素细胞受到破坏引起[76,82,109]。据估计此病的发病率在美国和欧洲约为1%。女性患者占多数已经被提出，但这观察更可能反映出的是不同文化的女性对皮肤美容相关问题表示出的担忧。至少一半的患者在20岁之前出现这种疾病[89]。高龄发病并不常见，此时应该提高对潜在疾病或相关疾病的关注。泛发白癜风是最常见的临床表现，常累及面和肢端部分。这些外露部位的脱色导致美容上的毁容可能造成病人严重的心理压力。

临床特征

主要皮损是一种白色界限清楚的斑片，边缘色素加深。在白皙皮肤的个人，白癜风很难与色素减退及完全的黑色素缺乏（白斑病）区分。伍德灯的使用（见"鉴别诊断"）有助于区分色素减少和脱色的斑疹。伍德灯还有助于观察通常不被晒黑的深肤色人的太阳保护区的皮肤。偶尔，白癜风皮损出现红色隆起的边缘，可能会自觉瘙痒。这些变化是炎性细胞浸润的特征[12]。另一种罕见的白癜风为三色白癜风，以出现色素沉着、正常肤色、部分色素脱失、完全脱色渐变的三种色调来命名[58]。白癜风皮损区的头发可能保持色素，但在长期存在皮损区，通常为无黑色素（白发）。

分布

脱色发生有三个不同的模式。①泛发性白癜风是最常见的类型，脱色广泛且非常对称分布。斑疹发生于关节伸侧和骨突处及面部（特别是腔口周围区域，如口和眼周围）和颈部、肛门-生殖器区域，以及四肢肢端。②节段性白癜风特点是皮肤白斑沿单侧肢体皮节分布。③局限性白癜风表现为非皮节分布的局限性皮损。

病程和预后

白癜风是一种慢性疾病，它的病程是不可预测的。大多数时候，脱色是一个逐渐进展的过程，但在泛发性白癜风，患者可能几个月内会突然出现皮损迅速进展。随后，该病可能多年保持静止。多达30%的患者在夏季期间在毛囊周围和阳光暴露区皮损的边缘出现色素"自然"恢复。完全阳光诱导的色素恢复是极其罕见的。不同于疾病初期，白癜风可能停止发展，并保持稳定几十年。局限性和节段性白癜风通常不会超出他们最初的区域分布,一旦停止扩展,则相当稳定。节段型白癜风也可作为泛发性白癜风一个独特的部分,并可能先于其发病。

鉴别诊断

一些皮肤病可导致表皮黑色素沉着的减少或丧失(表7.1)[109,157]。因此,白癜风治疗之前首先也是最重要的一步是明确诊断。用紫外线(UVA)照射(320~400nm,如伍德灯或黑光)检查有利于鉴别色素减退和色素脱失[41]。UVA照射下,生物蝶呤代谢产物病理上的增加,使得正常和白斑区皮肤的荧光区别看起来更显著[132]。仔细检查肛门-生殖器区域有助于明确泛发性白癜风的诊断。这个区域色素沉着过度,泛发性白癜风常累及此区域。皮损边缘的多巴染色显示受损皮肤缺乏酪氨酸酶阳性的黑色素细胞。白癜风的黑色素细胞是缺失还是休眠仍有争议[84]。专门检测正常的黑色素细胞、痣、黑色素瘤细胞常表达的75kDa糖蛋白的Mel-5鼠单克隆抗体是一个量化研究表皮黑色素细胞的宝贵手段[19]。

表7.1提供了一个鉴别诊断的列表。泛发性白癜风的最重要临床诊断标准是对称的、肢端的、腔口周围分布的进展性皮损。先天性形式的白斑病和黑色素过少症往往呈一个典型的分布形态(如斑驳病)并且病变是稳定的。然而,他们不一定出生时就出现。炎症后色素脱失常出现在患特应性皮炎、红斑狼疮、或银屑病的皮肤黝黑的患者,常呈不规则色素沉着和色素减退区。

表7.1 白癜风的鉴别诊断

化学品诱发的白斑病	红斑狼疮
苯酚及其衍生物	特应性皮炎
感染	钱币状湿疹
花斑癣	脂溢性皮炎
密螺旋体病(品他病、梅毒)	白色糠疹
利什曼病	肿瘤
麻风	蕈样肉芽肿病
遗传综合征	特发性
斑驳病	特发性点滴状色素减少症
瓦尔敦堡综合征	进行性斑状色素减少症
伏格特-小柳-原田综合征	畸形
结节性硬化症	无色素/低色素痣
炎症后色素减退	贫血痣
银屑病	

因为麻木性斑疹可以模仿白癜风,排除由于麻风病引起的色素减退非常重要。麻风主要在美国德克萨斯、南部路易斯安那、夏威夷和加利福尼亚炎热潮湿的气候条件下流行。在大量来自麻风流行区的移民涌入的地区,也可能会发现麻风患者。后期梅毒性白斑已罕见,但诊断时必须要想到。色素减退的最常见的感染原因是引起花斑癣的糠秕马拉色菌。同样重要的是要排除化学品诱发的白斑病,其可帮助避免进一步接触致病物(如苯酚及其衍生物)。由于白癜风和化学性白斑病巨大的相似性,可能很难或不可能区分这两种病。

相关疾病

白癜风可以与一些现象相关联。有些对诊断很重要,而其他则提供发病机制的重要线索。有家族聚集性的报告,7%～20%白癜风患者至少有一个一级亲属也患有白癜风[92,6]。白斑病变可以在受到外伤的皮肤处出现,称为 Köbner 现象[100]。一个典型的特征是严重晒伤后白癜风会发生或加重。白癜风可能与患者或其亲属自身免疫性疾病相关,并且已经提出儿童期发病有强关联[52]。然而,自身抗体(如针对甲状腺抗原,线粒体,或胃黏膜壁细胞的)可以无临床相关性。因此,自身抗体的诊断意义就非常有限[131]。

表 7.2 显示了通常与白癜风有关的疾病。尽管大多数患者将会是健康的,最初的检查应包括个人史和潜在相关的自身免疫性疾病的临床症状的仔细评估。在缺乏临床证据时,广泛的血清学筛查是没有必要的。最近的一项来自英国和北美 2078 名白人白癜风患者的评估证明只有艾迪生病、炎症性肠病、恶性贫血、甲状腺疾病和系统性红斑狼疮与白癜风有关联[6]。

越来越多的证据表明,白癜风是一种影响整个色素系统的系统性疾病。多达 40% 的病人的视网膜和脉络膜的上皮出现色素脱失[111]。此外,白癜风患者的葡萄膜炎的发病率升高;因此,进行眼科检查是十分必要的[103]。已发现 14% 的患者有听力异常,但程度上很少达到影响日常生活[11]。

表 7.2 与白癜风相关的疾病

艾迪生病[a]	黑素瘤[a]
斑秃	局限性硬皮病
1 型糖尿病[a]	重症肌无力
晕痣	恶性贫血[a]
甲状旁腺功能减退[a]	系统性红斑狼疮
炎性肠病	甲状腺疾病[a]
慢性单纯苔癣	

[a] 可以检测到特异性自身抗体

黑素细胞痣周围同心环样脱色,称为晕痣(sutton),可能预示着白癜风的发病,但也可以是一个孤立的迹象。同时发生白癜风和黑色素瘤意味着一种自身免疫机制,被认为是转移性黑素瘤的一种变好的迹象[121]。同时,建议白癜风患者应仔细检查有无黑色素瘤,特别是老年发病患者。

发病机制

传统上,有三个学说来解释白癜风发病:免疫,神经,自体细胞毒素。科学证据有利于自身免疫学说[32,85,104]。血清学、自身免疫现象的临床表现,以及免疫调节治疗的有效性,均支持这一学说。节段型白癜风似乎是主要基于神经障碍[5,72]。支持这一学说的是节段型白癜风患者的临床过程不同于泛发性白癜风患者[57]。化学诱导的白斑病和泛发性白癜风相似的临床表现支持自体细胞毒素学说,其提出黑色素细胞会被正常的黑素生物合成时形成的有毒中间产物破坏。在这样的背景下,它会被认定是四氢生物喋呤的一个特定的代谢物抑制苯丙氨酸羟化酶反应并最终引发白癜风色素脱失[132]。此外,角化细胞的钙失衡也被提出[130]。考虑到多种机制在白癜风的发病中起作用是非常重要的[83]。

白癜风的社会心理影响

白癜风不仅是一个美容问题。尽管缺乏自然发病率和死亡率的显著相关性,但白癜风会导致严重的心理和社会障碍[123,124,10]。虽然没有种族倾向性,白癜风往往在肤色较深人群或种族更易造成毁容。大多数的患者在青春期发病,在这样一个重视美容的年龄,会严重的抑制个性的发展。肉眼可见的病灶,经常出现在影响社交互动的部位,如面部和手指,使患者感到他们是经常被注视的对象。他们的痛苦可能造成他们与别人不合群,患者通常被认为缺乏理解和同情心。有些病例报告严重的心理创伤,比如家庭成员的去世,会导致疾病的发作和恶化。

医生尊重白癜风患者的感受是非常重要的,否则她或他可能会增加痛苦。同等重要的是告诉病人疾病是良性的和不危及生命的。然而,咨询不应该止于这一点,应考虑到我们今天提供的许多有用的治疗方案[48,49]。患者可能会发现与其他白癜风患者相聚并交流经验会助于恢复。全球支持组织为患者提供信息。

白癜风的治疗

尽管脱色区易受光损伤,但白癜风对患者的生命没有威胁。为了预防晒伤的极端不良后果,如皮肤癌,必须进行严密的防晒。治疗的主要目标是改善美容外观,可利用三种方法:遮盖皮损、诱导皮损色素恢复或使非皮损区脱色。虽然光疗方法是最有效的,但治疗白癜风经常联合或连续使用几种方法[42,8,35],如下面的总结。

防晒

避免阳光照射皮肤,持续使用 SPF 为 25 或更高的防晒霜对每个白癜风患者来说非常重要。由于缺乏黑色素保护,白斑区皮肤更容易受到紫外线辐射损伤,即使短暂的太阳暴露也可能会引起很痛的日晒伤。易出现 Koebner 反应的患者,这种晒伤可能导致疾病的恶化。太阳光引起的正常皮肤变黑也增强了与受影响的皮肤的对比度。因此,不透明的或同时对 UVA 和 UVB 有保护作用的防晒霜更为可取。全面防晒的信息包括建议选择适当的服装和避免日晒的策略。白肤色的个体做好认真的防晒就足够了。

化妆遮瑕

本身皮肤低黑色素的患者,使用普通化妆品就足以掩饰白癜风。如未受影响的皮肤和白癜风区肤色对比很明显,则需要特别准备。专业化妆产品有效的掩饰可适用于大多数皮肤色调,即使有季节性的颜色变化。这些医疗化妆品的另一个良好的特性是防水。这可减少化妆频率,这一过程非常耗时。有些病人偏爱使用电影或舞台上使用的那些专业化妆品。"无光性"晒黑剂含有二羟基丙酮(dihydroxyacetone,DHA),可诱导与角层蛋白发生化学反应,从而生成一种洗不掉的橙棕色。由于在表皮更新过程中角质层不断脱落,维持效果需要重复使用。化学美黑并不能提供足够的光保护能力,因此应结合常规的防晒措施。

某种橙色或褐色皮肤的颜色也可以通过服用 β-胡萝卜素和(或)角黄素获得。虽然这个特定的颜色可能不被认为是最优的,如果加上防晒,口服胡萝卜素可能是 I 和 II 型皮肤人群的一种替代治疗。

恢复色素的治疗

表 7.3 列出了恢复白癜风正常色素的治疗策略。

表7.3 恢复白癜风正常色素的治疗方法

方法	系统性	局部性
光疗		+
光化学疗法		
-补骨脂素	+	+
-凯林	+	+
-苯丙氨酸	+	
免疫抑制剂和免疫调节剂		
-皮质激素	+	+
-环磷酰胺	+	
-环孢霉素	+	
-他克莫司、吡美莫司		+
-异丙肌苷	+	
-左旋咪唑	+	
抗氧化剂		
-水龙骨提取物	+	
-假过氧化氢酶		+
-银杏	+	
维生素 D 类似物		
-5-氟尿嘧啶		+
-Melagenin*		+
-黑素细胞移植		+

*在美国、加拿大和意大利禁止使用

免疫调节和免疫抑制

使用免疫抑制剂治疗是基于白癜风是一种自身免疫性疾病的假设,其有效率也支持了这一观点。可以局部[80]和系统[70,114,125]使用皮质类固醇。所有形式的类固醇使用有一定的副作用。局部外用3类或4类糖皮质激素往往是从未治疗患者的一线治疗选择。当系统使用时,糖皮质激素通常用冲击疗法或结合细胞毒性药物使用,以减少副作用[125]。环磷酰胺[45],5-氟尿嘧啶[146,152],左旋咪唑[115],和异丙肌苷等免疫调节剂都被用于治疗白癜风,疗效相差较大。系统性免疫抑制治疗方案可能发生严重的副作用,需要仔细分析获益与风险。因为白癜风是只是一种色素障碍,长期使用系统性类固醇和免疫抑制引起的潜在的严重副作用可能无法支持他们在这种情况下使用。

非甾体类钙调磷酸酶抑制剂局部免疫抑制治疗开创了新时代,如他克莫司和吡美莫司等,对白癜风的治疗影响深大[30,75,87,139]。预期风险-效益比要比类固醇和其他免疫调制剂好[64]。直到最近动物实验发现大剂量使用这些药物可能引起某些淋巴瘤,才告诫人们长期使用的风险。这些药物没有小于 2 岁儿童的使用说明。

卡泊三醇一直作为单一疗法治疗[73],疗效不大,但很适合用于联合方案,特别是结合光疗[151]。

黑素细胞移植

该疗法的原理是将病人正常皮肤的自体黑色素细胞移植到白斑区[40]。这种方式可能被用于稳定、非进展性节段或局限性白癜风。肢端或口周皮肤经过非手术治疗未能恢复色素的是黑素细胞移植的最好适应证。治疗原则是去除皮损区的表皮,用正常的自体表皮替代。已经开发了多种技术用于除去白癜风的皮肤和采集、移植正常表皮,或者在体外培养的黑素细胞[38,39,88]。在头皮上、眉毛和眼睑,单株毛发移植已经可以成功地用于复色[98]。相反,自体移植逆转了白发[4]。

替代治疗方式

在开始或通过现代医学治疗失败后,许多患者可能寻求替代疗法。互联网是一个永无止境"治愈"白癜风的来源,相当多的网站还引用大量满意的顾客。复色方法包括维生素和矿物质的置换,中医和其他草药,印度传统医学派生的药物,顺势疗法,和胎盘制剂。这些补救措施可以外用,口服,肌注,或联合。很多情况下,太阳的或人工紫外线照射都增加了一个很好的措施。整体疗法尝试个体化治疗,经常将白癜风患者的心理需求与他们的药物治疗结合起来。这些治疗效果异常好的报告通常推荐给个人或没有同行审核的出版物。缺乏对照研究使得绝大多数替代方法难以或不可能公正或定量评价。

脱色

通常,化学诱导白斑病通常是不可逆的,因此我们应该仔细考虑挑选患者。此选择只适用于面积达 50% 以上的泛发性型的白癜风患者,且是复色治疗失败、拒绝或不能使用者[97]。除了使用化学脱色,冷冻疗法可用于小面积残留的色素[126]。Q-开关红宝石激光可以使局部区域未受到影响的皮肤永久脱色[102,71]。

白癜风复色的光疗选择

历史

光疗用于白癜风是基于观察到许多患者在夏季的几个月里阳光暴露部位出现复色的毛囊。最早关于白癜风光化学疗法的描述可以追溯到大约4000年前,这最古老的治疗原则,仍在21世纪使用[120]。在世界的一些地区可观察到局部外用植物提取物随后配合太阳照射后良好效果。其中一些光疗的治疗方案仍在印度次大陆和北非的流行/民族医学沿用。可以推断这些口服和局部制剂含有补骨脂素或相关光敏剂,因为UVA照射后可见光毒性反应(图7.3e)。大半世纪前,当El Mofty发表他成功的治疗试验和随后确定了补骨脂素是活性化合物,白癜风光化学疗法因现代医学而复兴[37]。用补骨脂素光化学疗法仍是治疗白癜风最有效的方法之一。仅仅数年前PUVA仍是白癜风治疗的黄金标准。最近资料显示,窄谱UVB的高效性及优越的安全性已经取代PUVA作为光疗的首选方案。

开始治疗前

一旦明确了白癜风的诊断,病人决定尝试复色治疗,可以考虑光疗。光疗或光化学疗法启动之前,病人需要广泛咨询有关的具体治疗方法。医生应该为病人提供有关疾病的书面信息、光疗和治疗选择。需要仔细评估双方的期望。患者也需要了解对治疗反应的部位差异,这是所有光疗是常见的问题。尤其口周和肢端的病变是最难好的。

除非患者强烈要求,否则依从性差,就不应该开始治疗。患者需要知道有关治疗的不便,以应付这些不便。白癜风的光疗和光化学疗法需要高达300次照射,需花费大量的时间以及相当大的成本。长期缺失治疗不利,因为可能引起复色进展过程停止。另一个问题是涉及较深肤色个体:正常表皮光疗引起的晒黑会加剧皮损与周围未受影响皮肤之间的反差,以至于直到复色之前都会使皮损看起来更明显。在此期间,额外的措施,例如化妆品掩盖暴露的部位是有用的。但是,在每次治疗前,需要除去任何阻挡物质或吸收紫外线的物质。讨论光线疗法相关问题后,病人被要求签署一份同意书来总结这些信息,包括具体的方案和可能的不利影响。

光疗

太阳光光疗

在夏季期间许多患者在阳光暴露区毛囊出现色素恢复。这种太阳光紫外线的效应通常是短暂的,但可重复。一项局部凯林和阳光的研究显示,只有阳光照射区域取得满意的治疗效果[105]。阳光强度在温和的气候中依赖季节性和天气的变化,太阳作为唯一的光源可能不足以诱导完全复色。另外,白癜风对晒伤和自然光无法预知的剂量测定的敏感性增加,单独太阳能光疗还没有成为一个真正的治疗选择。一个例外是在死海可以照射太阳光。那里,负海拔增加了大气短波紫外线辐射的吸收并创造一个更利于光疗的光谱。然而,没有多少人能够花足够多的时间在这个地方获得最佳效益。

人工紫外线光疗

在2000年前,只有少数关于UVB治疗白癜风的报告发表。一项由Koster和Wiskemann[74]的研究显示全身宽谱UVB光疗取得良好效果。一项对照研究显示局部UVB光疗在节段性白癜风取得非常好的结果[90]。在一项比较全身窄谱(311nm)UVB(NB-UVB)射线和使用局部未被取代的补骨脂素的PUVA的研究中发现311nm UVB和PUVA一样有效,但副作用较少[156]。这个开创性的报告之后,许多研究证实了其在几个不同的人群(包括儿童)的有效性和安全性[20,67,99,67,99,150]。UVB也被用作联合疗法的一部分将在本章的结束处讨论。UVA本身疗效有限,主要与光敏剂联用或用于联合疗法。

光试验和开始治疗

为以最佳剂量进行白癜风光疗,有必要暴露在狭窄的剂量范围以获取引起最小可察觉的红斑。更强烈的红斑不仅会引起不适或疼痛,还可能导致疾病恶化。为了避免不必要的UVB引起受损皮肤的光毒性,光疗开始时必须小心。红斑阈值在阳光保护地区可能会大幅减少。因此,通过确定最小红斑量(minimal erythema dose,MED)来评估个体最初UVB敏感性非常重要。用来做MED的地方是白斑区域应该选择在正常情况下不是太阳暴露的部位(通常臀部、下背部或腹部-反之如前臂)。重复日晒导致甚至脱色区在内的皮肤适应性变化,导致UVB灵敏度降低(高MED)[93,148]。为了避免早期治疗阶段的光毒性反应,初始剂量不应在这些可变性区域测量。MED试验剂量的测定选择通常用于Ⅰ型皮肤的较低范围内。有明显的光敏历史的白癜风患者,仍然会选择低剂量。当使用固定剂量方案时,应该选择剂量为或低于Ⅰ型皮肤类型的范围。

治疗方案和剂量

首次以50%~70% MED量照射皮损的皮肤。随后根据白癜风区域的临床反应选择剂量。目的是诱导刚可察觉到的红斑。红斑是用于确定个体增加剂量的唯一参数。增量为10%~30%。应该避免更强烈或持续不退的红斑。根据过度红斑的程度,随后的剂量不增加或减少 10% ~ 20%。不应该连续照光以避免累积光毒性。通常,每周三次治疗,但已有每周两次 NB-UVB 治疗有效的报道[99,101,156]。用固定剂量的 NB-UVB 光疗方案也获得了成功。起始剂量为100 ~ 280mJ/cm^2,以后每次剂量增加 50mJ/cm$^{2[20]}$。这两种方法,累积 NB-UVB 的剂量可达 30 ~ 100J/cm^2。

准分子 308nm 激光的治疗方案非常相似。起始剂量低至 50mJ/cm^2 剂量的增量同荧光管发射的 NB-UVB 一样。激光发射的 NB-UVB 的一个优点是能单独根据解剖位置予不同的能量。例如,肢端的病变有较厚的角质层,可以比面部或躯干皮肤耐受更高的剂量[63]。大多数研究者使用每周治疗两次取得良好的效果,每周治疗三次效果也很好。已有累积剂量达 100J/cm^2 的报告,与传统 NB-UVB 累积照射剂量类似。最近的一项每周一次、两次和三次照射 308nm 激光的评估表明,每周三次起效更快。然而,似乎在这项研究中,照射的总数比每周的频率对于复色更加相关[62]。

如果选择宽谱 UVB 治疗白癜风,强烈建议光试验。固定剂量方案的起始剂量应该是 NB-UVB 值的十分之一,因为宽谱 UVB 更易引起红斑反应。宽谱 UVB 一年光疗累积剂量为 30J/cm$^{2[74]}$。

光源

一般情况下,任何适合光线疗法的光源(如治疗银屑病)都可以用于治疗白癜风。荧光灯应用最频繁,但金属卤化物灯和选择性紫外线光疗灯(SUP)也可以使用。最近的一系列研究证明 NB-UVB 辐射有极好的有效性和安全性。大量的出版物已记录了飞利浦 TL-01 荧光灯已经成功地用于全身照射[99,101,135,156](图 7.1)。

对临床上有用的准分子激光(308nm)装置的发展及其在治疗局限性银屑病的疗效[9]促使一系列这样的单色紫外线照射治疗白癜风的应用研究[13,141,147]。整体效果非常好,往往少量治疗就出现复色。一项直接比较发射 NB-UVB 的荧光灯和准分子激光治疗韩国患者的研究发现激光治疗要优于传统 NB-UVB[63]。准分子激光设备发出每个脉冲几毫焦到直径 1 ~ 2cm 的圆形区域。照射区域看起来小,但高达 200Hz 的重复频率,每点的照射治疗可以在几秒钟内完成。一种可能替代昂贵的激光系统的是使用一种发光峰值在 308±1nm 的单色准分子灯(MEL)[86]。这盏灯的另一个优点是照射面积可宽达 500cm^2 的皮肤区域。

对于红斑和抗银屑病活性紫外线作用光谱的不同已经在理论上和实践上证明 NB-UVB 在银屑病中的作用。白癜风光疗的作用光谱仍未知道,但最近关于 NB-UVB 的一系列报道提出这一波长范围的卓越功效。在一个小型研究 NB-UVB 与宽谱 UVB 的直接比较中发现前者有优势[60]。

白癜风对 UVB 剂量要求更高,因为其白斑区皮肤比其他病的光敏性增加。初始治疗阶段是最关键的,因为 UVB 诱导白癜风部位光耐受从而降低其敏感度。重要的是控制基础单位辐射的输出剂量和保持仔细记录,不仅仅是曝光时间。许多商业照射机器内置测试仪,但并不能替代手持剂量计定期检查校准[65]。特别要注意治疗程序的任何更改。灯泡更换、单位内更换机器,或者到不同的治疗中心均会带来过量照射与光毒副作用的风险。

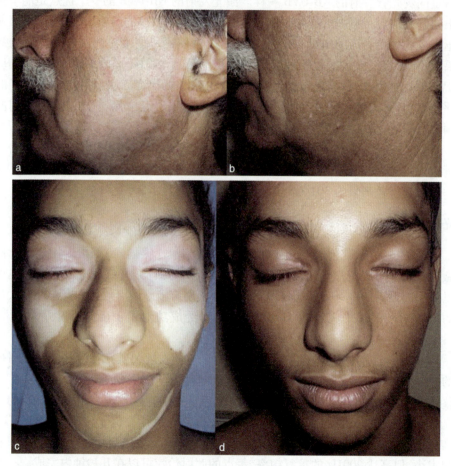

图 7.1 使用 TL-01 荧光管进行 NB-UVB 光疗取得极好的效果的患者的面部皮损。**a.** 治疗前。**b.** 36 次照光之后,累积剂量为 26.2J/cm²。**c.** 治疗前。**d.** 54 次照光之后,累积剂量为 48.3J/cm²

副作用

最常见的副作用是 UVB 诱导的红斑。自然环境中 UVB 照射可以是巨大的,因此建议在治疗期间防晒。由于 Köbner 反应,强烈的光毒反应可能会导致疾病的恶化。定期监测临床反应、光毒性的早期症状,如瘙痒和烧灼的感觉,有助于避免严重急性副作用。UVB 诱导的烧伤的治疗包括对症处理和局部外用类固醇。对可能发生严重的光毒性的意外照光过度,可能需要用系统性非甾体类和糖皮质激素。一些患者的白癜风复色区周围可能有几个月的皮肤变黑,这一现象更常见于 PUVA 治疗。长期 UVB 治疗诱导光老化加速[23],皮肤及全身免疫抑制[16,17],及皮肤癌风险的增加[154]。因为无法详细调查大范围的白癜风患者,因此我们无法得到这些影响的确切数据,只能推测。少数报告表明在长期接受 UVB 治疗患者中,这些风险没有很大的临床意义[143,145,155]。

光化学疗法

光敏剂配合 UVA 辐射提供了比 UVB 光疗更多的治疗方案,提供了额外的多样性。可根据局部或全身性选择不同光敏剂和不同光源。如上所述,病人和医生形成一个明确的共识和评估关于预期的疗效是否值得投入时间和费用非常重要。只有患者目的强烈,且病变是在已知会对光化学疗法起反应的位置,治疗才能开始。肢端型白癜风和所谓的唇尖型对光化学疗法反应最小[81]。

开始治疗

详细解释治疗是必需的。理想情况下,患者应该获得一些了解光化学疗法的原则,使他们体会到治疗相关的风险。除了医生的解释,病人应获得详细的关于治疗、色素恢复的几率及短期和长期的副作用的文字信息。这些信息可以"知情同意"的形式签署。病人必须按指示佩戴可吸收 UVA 的太阳镜,治疗后 24 小时避免照射直接和过滤的阳光。同其他疾病的光化学疗法一样,相同的预防措施也适用于白癜风。禁忌证也相同,包括低于 12 岁,怀孕和哺乳。

表7.4 光敏剂的选择

	普通人群		儿童		配合日光	
光敏剂	外用的	口服的	局部的	口服的	局部的	口服的
8-MOP	+	+	+			
5-MOP	+	+				+
TMP	+	+		+		+
凯林	+	+	+		+	+
苯丙氨酸		+		+		+

至关重要的是,患者应明白像其他白癜风疗法一样 PUVA 疗法可能会需要几个月,甚至几年才达到令人满意的效果。应避免有关时限和疗效太乐观的预后。患者必须意识到,最初的治疗刺激正常的皮肤色素沉着,这将提高正常和白斑皮肤之间的反差。随着白癜风区毛囊周围点状的色素增多,治疗效果渐明显。同时可以看到边缘带状色素恢复。通常,这些色素恢复区域的颜色比周围的正常皮肤黑。最佳的反应是 20~50 次照光后开始出现毛囊点状色素恢复,并且逐渐扩大,甚至全部恢复色素。然而,治疗反应可能会停止,即使继续治疗也无法达到完全色素恢复。

系统性光化学疗法

在系统性光化学疗法,光敏剂一般靠口服摄入,尽管也寻找过其他给药途径。呋喃香豆素补骨脂素,8-甲氧补骨酯素(8-MOP,图 7.2),5-甲氧补骨酯素(5-MOP)和三甲补骨脂内酯(TMP)已经被成功使用[55,118-118]。以及其他几个光敏剂可用于白癜风治疗。凯林是一种色酮(1,4-苯并吡喃酮)和呋喃衍生物,具有补骨脂素相似结构,可被 UVA 激活[96]。氨基酸中的 L-苯丙氨酸结合 UVA 照射在治疗白癜风也取得了一些成功[7]。近似"PUVA"为补骨脂素加 UVA,首字母缩写为的"KUVA"和"PAUVA"的规则已经被建议采用。

PUVA

治疗白癜风口服剂量通常小于银屑病(8-MOP 0.3~0.6mg/kg)。5-MOP 和 TMP 的剂量为 0.6~0.8mg/kg。摄入光敏剂和照射之间的时间取决于所使用的药物,也取决于剂型。例如,8-MOP 有结晶形式、微晶化及液体胶囊。所有这些制剂会对绝对值、延迟时间、血浆峰值水平的重现性产生不同的影响。

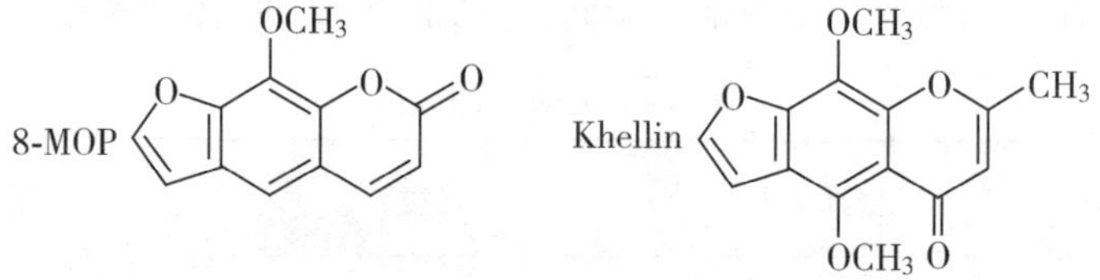

图 7.2 光敏剂的化学结构,8-甲氧补骨脂素(甲氧沙林,8-MOP)和凯林

使用 8-MOP 和 5-MOP,强烈建议测定 MPD 以避免光毒性的副作用。与 UVB MED 的测定一样,这种测试应优先在最敏感的皮损处进行。

以 50% MPD 的低 UVA 剂量开始治疗。增量应该非常谨慎(之前剂量的 10%~20%)及使用比其他曝光低的频率。每周治疗 2~3 次,每周 1 次的 PUVA 治疗白癜风的相对疗效尚未确定。使用 5-MOP 和 8-MOP 时,UVA 的剂量应增加直至白斑区出现浅粉色红斑,并且进一步的剂量增加仅为维持这个最小红斑反应。尽管目前尚不清楚的最小红斑是否为最佳剂量的良好指标,但它似乎是适合个体的 UVA 剂量的唯一临床参数。进一步增加没有用。此剂量依赖于皮肤光类型,范围在 $5\sim15J/cm^2$。

应该避免产生症状性红斑,因为过多的光毒性可能产生的 Koebner 反应。如果 PUVA 诱发过度红斑反应,治疗应该中断,直到这些过大剂量的迹象消退。恢复治疗时应该用较低剂量 UVA。反复发作的光毒性是一个补骨脂素剂量需要降低的指征。

口服 TMP 不会引起临床光毒性反应,因为相比其他补骨脂素其血液水平非常低,没有达到急性的光毒性水平[144]。因此,MPD 测试没必要像 TMP 那样遵循一个固定剂量的方案。照射从 $1\sim2J/cm^2$ 开始,每周增加 $1J/cm^2$,直到 $10\sim15J/cm^2$ 的维持剂量。

KUVA

凯林(Khellin)(图 7.2)是在埃及发明的现代光化学疗法,最初与太阳光照射结合用于治疗白癜风[1]。用人造光源每周三次频率的这种改进的光化学疗法已被确认有效[107]。KUVA 最近已被证明在体外可以刺激黑素细胞增殖和黑素合成[26]。

口服 100mg 凯林标准剂量 2½ 小时后达到可靠的血浆水平。口服凯林最大的优点之一是从未引起临床光毒性反应[107]。因此,可以比 PUVA 的 UVA 更高剂量开始和可以更快速的增加能量。另一个优势是,太阳可以作为光源。在夏季,治疗可以在户外完成。以太阳为光源,UVB 诱导的红斑独立于凯林成为一个受曝光时间影响有限的因素。UVB 防晒霜可能有利于延长太阳光 UVA 照射。目前,没有可用的纯凯林的药物制剂。凯林是不可能被批准用于治疗白癜风的。此外,约 30% 的白癜风患者发生可逆性肝脏转氨酶增加仍有待解释[107]。在特殊情况下,监测肝功能参数,如果有系统性的凯林,也可被当作为一种传统光敏剂的替代品[61],可以理解,这是一个没有得到学会批准的治疗方式。

PAUVA

PAUVA 是氨基酸中的 L-苯丙氨酸结合 UVA 照射。使用生理而不是异物性光敏剂使这种形式的光化学疗法在概念上富有吸引力[29]。照射前 $0.5\sim1$ 小时摄入 $50\sim200mg/kg$ 固定剂量的 L-苯丙氨酸是有效的。每周进行三次治疗[29,138]。没有 L-苯丙氨酸严重的副作用研究报告,但如此高剂量的潜在副作用已被提出[22]。

类似于凯林,L-苯丙氨酸没有产生任何临床光毒性的副作用。因此,UVA 剂量和太阳光照射是不成问题的。UVA剂量可增加到最大水平12J/cm^2。一些报道描述了良好的治疗效果,但总体疗效仍存在争议[129,149]。

外用光化学疗法

外用8-甲氧补骨脂素的光化学疗法可用于病变局限的患者(少于15%体表总面积)或禁忌用系统性PUVA的12岁以下的儿童。该疗法只能在诊所进行,因为家里治疗具有很高的光毒性的严重副作用的风险。已有用浓度高达1%的8-MOP外用制剂。如此高的浓度导致光毒性的副作用的发生率较高,但治疗效果却不见得比低浓度范围(0.1%)好[47]。因此,推荐用0.1% 8-MOP或更低的醇溶液或软膏。已有外用含有0.006% 8-MOP成功治疗白癜风的报道[77]。

治疗的频率为每周1~3次。为了避免皮肤中的8-MOP浓度差异,必须小心将光敏剂制剂均匀涂于治疗区域。外用20到30分钟后,UVA照射暴露的皮肤,最初剂量为0.25~0.5J/cm^2。照光时间每周小剂量增加(0.12~0.25J/cm^2)。一旦达到5J/cm^{2}的最大剂量,稍微增加外用补骨脂素的浓度,照射仍用同一剂量方案。重复这个过程,直到获得一个产生红斑但无烧灼感的剂量和照射时间。照射后病人需要立即用肥皂和水洗掉剩余的8-MOP和应用UVA防晒物以避免自然环境中阳光照射引起的光毒性副作用。未被取代的补骨脂素也被制成0.005%凝胶外用配合人工UVA照射[156]。TMP和5-MOP也可以用于局部PUVA[106]。然而,相比之下使用口服的光毒性较低,TMP和5-MOP外用时比8-MOP光毒性大。

另一方面,局部凯林的光化学疗法不会导致临床光毒性。这使得外用KUVA与太阳照射形成低风险的组合。口服凯林,必须考虑阳光中的UVB部分。5%和10%浓度外用制剂的被证明是有效的[107,153]。有证据表明,这种药物的利用率和临床反应并不仅取决于凯林的浓度,还可能与载体有非常重要的关系[26,105]。已有一个研究证明,凯林被并入用苯丙氨酸作为稳定剂的卵磷脂脂质体制剂中。在一个对照的单中心研究中,这个外用喷雾型凯林的浓度为0.005%,以UVA和UVB为照射源,效果非常显著[34]。因为外用KUVA的病人没有光毒性的风险,可以试着在夏天用太阳紫外线照射。与其他方案相比,长期外用KUVA疗效仍未确定。

局部PAUVA本身尚未成为治疗的选择。一项研究发现,口服PAUVA和外用10%苯丙氨酸霜均增加皮损的光活性[7]。另一组报告配合外用丙酸氯倍他索,口服和外用10%苯丙氨酸合并UVA均取得良好疗效[25]。

照射源和剂量测定法

用于PUVA疗法的常规UVA灯,也可作为白癜风光化学疗法的光源。这些是荧光灯或金属卤化物灯。如果使用金属卤化物灯,需要用 UVB 过滤器消除部分较短波长的发射光谱。正如已经讨论过的光疗,白癜风的光化学疗法的剂量需要特别小心,因为过度照光可能导致严重不良反应。已有少数研究评估了使用 NB-UVB 激活补骨脂素。这样的方案已成功地治疗了局部和系统补骨脂素光敏化后的银屑病[108]。一份报告为口服 0.7mg/kg 的 8-MOP 致敏化后,半侧比较使用 UVA 和宽谱 UVB 照射白癜风的治疗。作者发现两种光源照射 30 次后,疗效和光毒性的副作用发生率均类似。UVA 累积剂量大约比 UVB 高 10 倍[94]。

用太阳光线进行光化学疗法(PUVASol)

PUVASol 是以太阳光为 UVA 照射光源并结合补骨脂素[118]的疗法。对于这种治疗方式,至关重要的一点是病人必须彻底的遵从指示。治疗通常没有医生在一旁监督,所以患者需要了解治疗的原理和可能来自补骨脂素的非治疗性光毒性就很重要。治疗开始前,处理同常规 PUVA 的推荐。

TMP 和低剂量 5-MOP(0.6mg/kg)是口服药物的选择。因为系统性 8-MOP 摄入后的光毒性太高,如没有密切观察,就不能推荐使用。然而,谨慎的方法,定期随访,可获得良好的治疗效果[118]。由于其光毒性的可能性高,不应使用外用补骨脂素结合自然的阳光。然而,凯林可以配合阳光外用或口服[1,34]。系统用 *L*-苯丙氨酸和系统加局部 *L*-苯丙氨酸也被用来与阳光照射配合[78]。

太阳光谱中的 UVB 部分可导致独立于治疗作用的晒伤。这可以应用 UVB 防晒霜来避免,而 UVA 辐射仍可穿透。大多数病人都知道他们可以在阳光下待多久而没有被灼伤。特别是在头几个周,当建立治疗诱导日光耐受后,照光时间应缓慢增加,两侧身体开始 5 分钟的照光(在温和气候上午 11 点和下午 3 点之间),接着的每周增加 2~5 分钟,直到任意一侧最大值 45 分钟为止。

日晒较强烈的地区必须调整照光时间。用补骨脂素治疗时应该采用一周两到三次而不是连续数天。应该定期检查患者,记录患者确切给药方法、照光时间和副作用。

家庭治疗

仅动机适当和充分理解治疗的患者可以在家中利用人工辐射源进行治疗。类似于 PUVASol,低剂量 8-MOP、TMP、5-MOP、凯林和 *L*-苯丙氨酸可以作为光敏剂。因为光毒性的危险,我们强烈反对应用任何外用补骨脂素。在一些国家(如意大利),补骨脂素被认为是化疗药物只能在医院使用。家庭晒黑用的 UVA 荧光管可以用作 UVA 辐射源。剂量和剂量的增量必须仔细地讨论和执行。不应该依赖设备生产商提供的能量输出信息。输出水平低或设备较小,需要长时间有效的照光治疗。金属卤化物灯的 UVA 设备,通常输出能量高,但是它们价格昂贵,并且需要过滤 UVB。这些灯照射面积小和欠均匀,但这些可以满足面积小的,如节段或局限性白癜风。在最初的治疗阶段,定期复诊能帮助患者避免光毒性的副作用而且仍能在合理的时间达到治疗相关剂量。

不良反应

光疗或光化学疗法最重要的急性副作用是过度的光毒性。症状为瘙痒、红斑、水肿、水疱,PUVA 大量过量时出现皮肤坏死。治疗包括局部类固醇、非甾体类抗炎药物,严重光毒性时系统性用类固醇。出现不良反应时光化学疗法必须中断,并待过量的迹象已解决后才以较低剂量继续治疗。

如其他光疗方式长期使用一样,PUVA 的长期副作用包括皮肤过早老化。这可能与凯林、L-苯丙氨酸和系统性 TMP 相关性更大,因为这些方案中使用了高剂量 UVA。长期用 PUVA 治疗白癜风可能诱发干燥症、角化病以及黑子("PUVA 黑子")[59]。已有少量 PUVA 诱导多毛症的报道[31]。

美国和欧洲的研究证明用 8-MOP 的长期 PUVA 治疗银屑病后,鳞状细胞癌的发生率增加。在银屑病治疗中,鳞状细胞癌的发病率与 UVA 累积剂量相关,但在白癜风治疗中,累积剂量通常低得多。因此,进行光化学疗法的白癜风患者发生皮肤癌的风险较低。已有白癜风 PUVA 治疗患者患角化病和皮肤癌的报告[21,110,159],这可能提示部分白癜风患者可能更容易受到 PUVA 诱导的致癌作用。一些回顾性研究无法证明光化学疗法对白癜风患者有增加皮肤癌的风险[51,158]。

已经在银屑病患者处证明了足够防护措施可避免严重的眼部副作用[128]。如果病人要照射眼周的皮肤,眼部损害可能会成为一个问题。在这种情况下,照射过程中眼睛需要一直闭着,治疗后需要佩戴 UVA 防护眼镜。标准光化学疗法病人的治疗后建议包括治疗初始进行眼科检查,之后至少每年复查一次。

除了那些与光化学有关的副作用,个体治疗模式可能导致治疗方案特定的不良反应。由于接触周围的正常皮肤,局部 PUVA 会引起周边地区色素过度沉着。口服的光敏剂可能导致胃肠道和中枢神经症状,相比 5-MOP 或 TMP,8-MOP 和凯林在这方面更常见。对于 L-苯丙氨酸,目前为止尚未见其具体的副作用的报道。多达 30% 口服凯林疗法的患者产生可逆的肝功能指标增高(见 KUVA)。

光化学疗法的治疗效果

没有任何参数可以预测单独一个病人可能的预后。皮肤光类型与治疗的反应在一定程度上关联,深肤色患者更容易获得可以接受程度的色素恢复。面部、颈部和躯干的皮损比肢端的起效快。即使经过长时间的治疗获得良好的总体效应,但甲周、瘢痕、生殖器、乳头、手掌和脚底仍倾向于保持脱色(图 7.3c 和 d)。存在已久的白癜风对治疗的反应比近期发生的差。复色的初始速率与整体治疗成功无关联,因此不能被用作预后因素。

第7章 白癜风的光(化学)疗法

光疗和光化学疗法复色的过程中非常相似。开始时,只有不受影响的皮肤显示对治疗起反应,导致与白斑区皮肤对比提高,使疾病更明显。使用补骨脂素时这种效应最为明显,因为其可提高晒黑反应。KUVA 和 PAUVA 不导致临床光毒性,所以这种效果不显著。同时,白斑区的皮肤形成一种与色素沉着无关的辐射保护。这种保护作用常见于光疗和光化学疗法,导致对太阳光灵敏度降低,深受患者喜爱。在德国被称为"Lichtschwiele"(译者注:光硬化),这种对紫外线的屏障作用来自表皮增生伴角化过度。

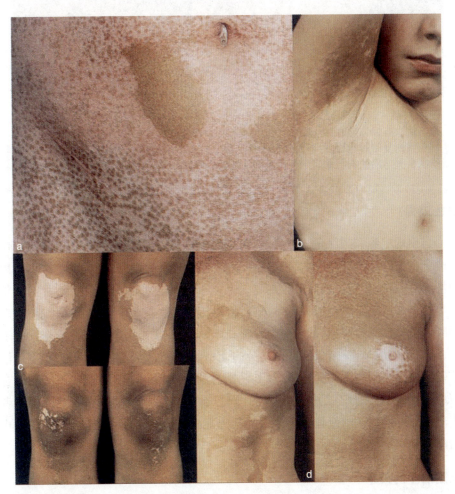

图7.3 光疗和光化学疗法的临床效果。(a)使用口服三甲补骨脂内酯(TMP)的 PUVA 致毛囊复色。(b)经过四个月的窄带紫外线光疗几乎完全复色。(c)使用 5-甲氧基补骨脂素的 PUVA 进行复色,治疗 12 个月后右膝盖的瘢痕无复色。(d)PUVA 诱发的白癜风大面积复色,引起少量空隙

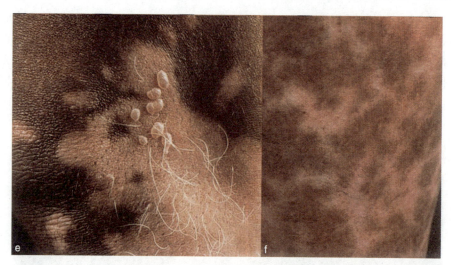

图7.3(续) （e）口服凯林联合UVA治疗的患者出现红斑、水肿和水疱的光毒性反应。他没有报告同时自行服用从利比亚来的含有补骨脂素的中药制剂。（f）小腿下部色素恢复的静止程度，即使延长光疗也不会改善。这些病人图片来自奥地利维也纳医科大学皮肤病与性病学科光疗部（CHAir，Herbert Hönigsmann，MD）

复色过程

当出现毛囊和边缘色素恢复时，可以在15～20照射后首次看到白癜风确切的改善（图7.3）。新形成的色素比不受影响的晒黑的皮肤暗（图7.3a,b）。理想情况下，紧接着首次治疗效果的是一个相对快速蔓延的复色，经过数月至数年会导致色素区完全融合（图7.3b,c）。然而初始复色起效后至完全复色前，更多的时候是复色逐渐减速，或者完全停滞（图7.3d,f）。如果遇到这种治疗反应下降，进一步增加UVA剂量通常是徒劳的，因为这将导致光毒性的反应，而不是治疗效果改善。调整不同的光敏剂（如从凯林、8-MOP到5-MOP）或使用药物组合（如8-MOP加上TMP）是值得考虑的[118]。通常，对治疗效果进展的看法，患者比治疗师更乐观。即使延续治疗实际上未能成功，这些病人可能也不希望终止治疗。

长期治疗的结果

记录到白癜风治疗的长期疗效，包括光疗方式的报道并不多。PUVA诱导的复色在大多数患者可以持续很多年[69]。直到复色发生停滞，对治疗的患者来说似乎是很真实的。其他研究报道40%的白癜风病人PUVA治疗后复发，考虑PUVA疗效有限[158,81]。没有足够的数据来严格评估UVB光疗和其他光化学疗法方案的长期疗效。

机制

白癜风的发病机制和光疗诱导复色的机制仍未完全理解。UVB 和 PUVA 可刺激正常皮肤的黑色素细胞的黑素生成,导致晒黑。然而,诱发的白斑区皮肤复色这种效果似乎是独立的机制。口服 KUVA 治疗的对照实验表明,单独 UVA 和 KUVA 均可刺激正常皮肤的色素沉着,但只有 KUVA 可诱导受影响的皮肤毛囊复色。这表明局部光毒性的机制对治疗效果来说可能是至关重要的,或假定的单独的系统性效应的光化学疗法并不足以诱导复色[107]。

免疫抑制治疗白癜风的疗效支持自身免疫的发病机制的概念。UVB 和 PUVA 的局部和系统性免疫抑制作用已经很确切,这本书包含了其对皮肤免疫的影响的广泛回顾。UVB 和 PUVA 会调节生长因子表达,这可能有助于治疗效应。NB-UVB 和 PUVA 都已经被证明能高效诱导淋巴细胞的凋亡及白癜风自身免疫反应介质。

儿童的光化学疗法

12 岁以下儿童不应该接受口服 PUVA 治疗,因为 UVA 可进入眼睛前部。由于高危的光毒副作用,使用 PUVA 时只能外用 8-MOP 来治疗白癜风,且由一位有经验的光治疗专家操作。使用 0.0002% 8-MOP 洗澡后光疗已被证明有效,但这一药物不易购得[91]。凯林可以用于外用治疗且没有光毒性作用,也可以较大范围使用且没有显著危害[107,105,26]。因为它可能导致肝毒性、口服凯林时应非常小心和常规监控肝功能指标。还没有遇到过系统性凯林光毒性。联合口服 L-苯丙氨酸和 UVA 治疗被推荐用于儿童,未见有严重的毒副作用的报道[136]。系统性 TMP 致敏已成功用于联合医院光疗设备治疗,也可联合阳光治疗[137]。近来,NB-UVB 已用于儿童取得满意效果,将有可能取代儿童白癜风的大部分光化学疗法[101,66,20]。

联合疗法

联合疗法旨在获得更高的功效,这可能会得到更快的治疗效果和/或减少副作用。在联合治疗白癜风时,光疗法通常被许多皮肤科医生考虑是联合方案的一个必要组成部分。光疗和光化学疗法有效且副作用相对较少。PUVA 对正常皮肤的色素沉着和白癜风复色有良好的刺激效应。在联合治疗中,光疗成分有对黑素细胞的刺激作用。目前为止,在大型随机研究结果中,还没有确立有显著优势的光疗联合疗法,但观测报告十分丰富。几种组合策略在日常实践中找到了一席之地。

在阳光足够充裕的地方，太阳能光疗可能与例如皮质类固醇等物质外用联合[53]。

局部钙调磷酸酶抑制剂已与传统和准分子激光发射的 NB-UVB 光疗联合使用[27,68,68]。

卡泊三醇可能是联合疗法中的一个较为重要的局部辅助性的药物。几项研究显示其活性与太阳辐射相关[113]。添加钙泊三醇到以医院为主的光疗方案是否受益是有争议的。在对照研究中，卡泊三醇联合 PUVA 或 NB-UVB 治疗优于单用光疗法[112,79,28]。然而，其他研究发现单用 PUVA 或 NB-UVB 治疗效果与联合疗法效果大致相当[15,2]。

小群体患者的研究也显示，PUVA 与米诺地尔的组合有效[142]。

一种外用制剂包含所谓假过氧化氢酶和钙是由于发现白斑皮肤过氧化氢水平增加和体内钙稳态改变，局部应用联合 UVB 或太阳照射。第一次报告的结果是可喜的[133]。但随后一个独立的小组的研究并没有成功[117]，但其他人未得到最初制备的抗氧化剂化合物，除了描述的原始结果的小组。除非有市售的活性制剂，否则不可能进行严格的评价和优化光疗组合。

Anapsos 是植物来源的一种药物。200 年前，南美医学流行从水龙骨属蕨类植物中提取治疗各种疾病的药物。最近一段时间以来，水龙骨（PLE）水性提取免疫调节作用已经被描述[18]。水龙骨属提取物 anapsos（7~10mg/kg）已经应用于白癜风的治疗具有相当长的一段时间，初步结果显示疗效较好[95,127]，但仍需大量的对照实验研究验证其确切的疗效性。这也表明，结合阳光，尤其是 PUVA 可提高 PLE 诱导的免疫调节和增加治疗效果。冈萨雷斯证明了局部以及全身 PLE 增加皮肤的 UVB 和 PUVA 反应阈值，从而建立了光保护作用[46]。这将使 PLE 加光疗成为极好的组合，但需更大规模的研究以证明他们的疗效，例如单独与 NB-UVB 比较疗效。

最后，光疗法治疗方案同样也是适用于配合外科治疗白癜风。白癜风在自体表皮移植时，移植黑色素细胞受 PUVA 刺激在加速离心扩散，引起复色加快[56,140,14]。同样的方法可以用于 NB-UVB 光疗法，而对照研究也正在进行中[122]。

总结

使用 NB-UVB 光疗和补骨脂素光化学疗法是治疗白癜风最有效的方法。光疗治疗方案的选择主要取决于患者的范围、年龄、光敏剂的有效性和辐射源的敏

第7章 白癜风的光(化学)疗法

感性等临床参数。目前,尽管 NB-UVB 光疗法的治疗效果的持久性和长期安全性尚未建立,但是仍为绝大多数病人的首选。光疗法治疗方案可以单独使用,亦可以联合使用。新的容易获得的药物如卡泊三醇和钙调磷酸酶抑制剂已经拓宽了白癜风患者的联合治疗方案。

(李润祥 译,唐亚平　陈荃 校,朱慧兰 审)

参考文献

1. Abdel-Fattah A, Aboul-Enein MN, Wassel GM, El-Menshawi BS (1982) An approach to the treatment of vitiligo by khellin. Dermatologica 165:136–140
2. Ada S, Sahin S, Boztepe G, Karaduman A, Kolemen F (2005) No additional effect of topical calcipotriol on narrow-band UVB phototherapy in patients with generalized vitiligo. Photodermatol Photoimmunol Photomed 21:79–83
3. Africk J, Fulton J (1971) Treatment of vitiligo with topical trimethylpsoralen and sunlight. Br J Dermatol 84:151–156
4. Agrawal K, Agrawal A (1995) Vitiligo: surgical repigmentation of leukotrichia. Dermatol Surg 21:711–715
5. Al'Abadie MS, Senior HJ, Bleehen SS, Gawkrodger DJ (1994) Neuropeptide and neuronal marker studies in vitiligo. Br J Dermatol 131:160–165
6. Alkhateeb A, Fain PR, Thody A, Bennett DC, Spritz RA (2003) Epidemiology of vitiligo and associated autoimmune diseases in Caucasian probands and their families. Pigment Cell Res 16:208–214
7. Antoniou C, Schulpis H, Michas T, Katsambas A, Frajis N, Tsagaraki S, Stratigos J (1989) Vitiligo therapy with oral and topical phenylalanine with UVA exposure. Int J Dermatol 28:545–547
8. Antoniou C, Katsambas A (1992) Guidelines for the treatment of vitiligo. Drugs 43:490–498
9. Asawanonda P, Anderson RR, Chang Y, Taylor CR (2000) 308-nm excimer laser for the treatment of psoriasis: a dose-response study. Arch Dermatol 136:619–624
10. Austin M (2004) Fighting and living with vitiligo. J Am Acad Dermatol 51:S7–8
11. Aydogan K, Turan OF, Onart S, Karadogan SK, Tunali S (2006) Audiological abnormalities in patients with vitiligo. Clin Exp Dermatol 31:110–113
12. Badri AM, Todd PM, Garioch JJ, Gudgeon JE, Stewart DG, Goudie RB (1993) An immunohistological study of cutaneous lymphocytes in vitiligo. J Pathol 170:149–155
13. Baltas E, Csoma Z, Ignacz F, Dobozy A, Kemeny L (2002) Treatment of vitiligo with the 308-nm xenon chloride excimer laser. Arch Dermatol 138:1619–1620
14. Barman KD, Khaitan BK, Verma KK (2004) A comparative study of punch grafting followed by topical corticosteroid versus punch grafting followed by PUVA therapy in stable vitiligo. Dermatol Surg 30:49–53
15. Baysal V, Yildirim M, Erel A, Kesici D (2003) Is the combination of calcipotriol and PUVA effective in vitiligo? J Eur Acad Dermatol Venereol 17:299–302
16. Beissert S, Schwarz T (1999) Mechanisms involved in ultraviolet light-induced immunosuppression. J Investig Dermatol Symp Proc 4:61–64
17. Beissert S, Schwarz T (2002) Role of immunomodulation in diseases responsive to phototherapy. Methods 28:138–144
18. Bernd A, Ramirez-Bosca A, Huber H, Diaz Alperi J, Thaci D, Sewell A, Quintanilla Almagro E, Holzmann H (1995) In vitro studies on the immunomodulating effects of polypodium leucotomos extract on human leukocyte fractions. Arzneimittelforschung 45:901–904
19. Bhawan J (1997) Mel-5: a novel antibody for differential diagnosis of epidermal pigmented

lesions of the skin in paraffin-embedded sections. Melanoma Res 7:43–48
20. Brazzelli V, Prestinari F, Castello M, Bellani E, Roveda E, Barbagallo T, Borroni G (2005) Useful treatment of vitiligo in 10 children with UV-B narrowband (311nm). Pediatr Dermatol 22:257–261
21. Buckley DA, Rogers S (1996) Multiple keratoses and squamous carcinoma after PUVA treatment of vitiligo. Clin Exp Dermatol 21:43–45
22. Burkhart CG, Burkhart CN (1999) Phenylalanine with UVA for the treatment of vitiligo needs more testing for possible side effects. J Am Acad Dermatol 40:1015
23. Calanchini-Postizzi E, Frenk E (1987) Long-term actinic damage in sun-exposed vitiligo and normally pigmented skin. Dermatologica 174:266–271
24. Calzavara-Pinton PG, Carlino A, Manfredi E, Semeraro F, Zane C, De Panfilis G (1994) Ocular side effects of PUVA-treated patients refusing eye sun protection. Acta Derm Venereol Suppl (Stockh) 186:164–165
25. Camacho F, Mazuecos J (1999) Treatment of vitiligo with oral and topical phenylalanine: 6 years of experience. Arch Dermatol 135:216–217
26. Carlie G, Ntusi NB, Hulley PA, Kidson SH (2003) KUVA (khellin plus ultraviolet A) stimulates proliferation and melanogenesis in normal human melanocytes and melanoma cells in vitro. Br J Dermatol 149:707–717
27. Castanedo-Cazares JP, Lepe V, Moncada B (2003) Repigmentation of chronic vitiligo lesions by following tacrolimus plus ultraviolet-B-narrow-band. Photodermatol Photoimmunol Photomed 19:35–36
28. Cherif F, Azaiz MI, Ben Hamida A, Ben O, Dhari A (2003) Calcipotriol and PUVA as treatment for vitiligo. Dermatol Online J 9:4
29. Cormane RH, Siddiqui AH, Westerhof W, Schutgens RB (1985) Phenylalanine and UVA light for the treatment of vitiligo. Arch Dermatol Res 277:126–130
30. Coskun B, Saral Y, Turgut D (2005) Topical 0.05% clobetasol propionate versus 1% pimecrolimus ointment in vitiligo. Eur J Dermatol 15:88–91
31. Cox NH, Jones SK, Downey DJ, Tuyp EJ, Jay JL, Moseley H, Mackie RM (1987) Cutaneous and ocular side-effects of oral photochemotherapy: results of an 8-year follow-up study. Br J Dermatol 116:145–152
32. Cui J, Bystryn JC (1995) Melanoma and vitiligo are associated with antibody responses to similar antigens on pigment cells. Arch Dermatol 131:314–318
33. de Gruijl FR (1999) Skin cancer and solar UV radiation. Eur J Cancer 35:2003–2009
34. de Leeuw J, van der Beek N, Maierhofer G, Neugebauer WD (2003) A case study to evaluate the treatment of vitiligo with khellin encapsulated in l-phenylalanin stabilized phosphatidylcholine liposomes in combination with ultraviolet light therapy. Eur J Dermatol 13:474–477
35. Drake LA, Dinehart SM, Farmer ER, Goltz RW, Graham GF, Hordinsky MK, Lewis CW, Pariser DM, Skouge JW, Turner ML, Webster SB, Whitaker DC, Lowery BJ, Nordlund JJ, Grimes PE, Halder RM, Minus HR (1996) Guidelines of care for vitiligo. American Academy of Dermatology. J Am Acad Dermatol 35:620–626
36. Duschet P, Schwarz T, Pusch M, Gschnait F (1989) Marked increase of liver transaminases after khellin and UVA therapy. J Am Acad Dermatol 21:592–594
37. El Mofty (1948) A preliminary clinical report on the treatment of leukoderma with *Ammi majus Linn*. J Royal Egypt Med Assoc 31:651–655
38. Falabella R (1988) Treatment of localized vitiligo by autologous minigrafting. Arch Dermatol 124:1649–1655
39. Falabella R (2003) Surgical treatment of vitiligo: why, when and how. J Eur Acad Dermatol Venereol 17:518–520
40. Falabella R (2005) Surgical approaches for stable vitiligo. Dermatol Surg 31:1277–1284
41. Fitzpatrick TB, Ortonne J-P (2003) Normal skin color and general considerations of pigmentary disorders. In: Freedberg IM, Eisen AZ, Wolff K et al (eds) Dermatology in general medicine. McGraw-Hill, New York

42. Frenk E (1986) Treatment of vitiligo. Hautarzt 37:1–5
43. Gargoom AM, Duweb GA, Elzorghany AH, Benghazil M, Bugrein OO (2004) Calcipotriol in the treatment of childhood vitiligo. Int J Clin Pharmacol Res 24:11–14
44. Gauthier Y, Andre MC, Taieb A (2003) A critical appraisal of vitiligo etiologic theories. Is melanocyte loss a melanocytorrhagy? Pigment Cell Res 16:322–332
45. Gokhale BB, Parakh AP (1983) Cyclophosphamide in vitiligo. Indian J Dermatol 28:7–10
46. Gonzalez S, Pathak MA, Cuevas J, Villarrubia VG, Fitzpatrick TB (1997) Topical or oral administration with an extract of Polypodium leucotomos prevents acute sunburn and psoralen-induced phototoxic reactions as well as depletion of Langerhans cells in human skin. Photodermatol Photoimmunol Photomed 13:50–60
47. Grimes PE, Minus HR, Chakrabarti SG, Enterline J, Halder R, Gough JE, Kenney JA Jr (1982) Determination of optimal topical photochemotherapy for vitiligo. J Am Acad Dermatol 7:771–778
48. Grimes PE (2004) White patches and bruised souls: advances in the pathogenesis and treatment of vitiligo. J Am Acad Dermatol 51:S5–7
49. Grimes PE (2005) New insights and new therapies in vitiligo. JAMA 293:730–735
50. Grundmann-Kollmann M, Ludwig R, Zollner TM, Ochsendorf F, Thaci D, Boehncke WH, Krutmann J, Kaufmann R, Podda M (2004) Narrowband UVB and cream psoralen-UVA combination therapy for plaque-type psoriasis. J Am Acad Dermatol 50:734–739
51. Halder RM, Battle EF, Smith EM (1995) Cutaneous malignancies in patients treated with psoralen photochemotherapy (PUVA) for vitiligo. Arch Dermatol 131:734–735
52. Halder RM (1997) Childhood vitiligo. Clin Dermatol 15:899–906
53. Handa S, Pandhi R, Kaur I (2001) Vitiligo: a retrospective comparative analysis of treatment modalities in 500 patients. J Dermatol 28:461–466
54. Handa S, Dogra S (2003) Epidemiology of childhood vitiligo: a study of 625 patients from north India. Pediatr Dermatol 20:207–210
55. Hann SK, Cho MY, Im S, Park YK (1991) Treatment of vitiligo with oral 5-methoxypsoralen. J Dermatol 18:324–329
56. Hann SK, Im S, Bong HW, Park YK (1995) Treatment of stable vitiligo with autologous epidermal grafting and PUVA. J Am Acad Dermatol 32:943–948
57. Hann SK, Lee HJ (1996) Segmental vitiligo: clinical findings in 208 patients. J Am Acad Dermatol 35:671–674
58. Hann SK, Kim YS, Yoo JH, Chun YS (2000) Clinical and histopathologic characteristics of trichrome vitiligo. J Am Acad Dermatol 42:589–596
59. Harrist TJ, Pathak MA, Mosher DB, Fitzpatrick TB (1984) Chronic cutaneous effects of long-term psoralen and ultraviolet radiation therapy in patients with vitiligo. Natl Cancer Inst Monogr 66:191–196
60. Hartmann A, Lurz C, Hamm H, Brocker EB, Hofmann UB (2005) Narrow-band UVB 311 nm vs. broad-band UVB therapy in combination with topical calcipotriol vs. placebo in vitiligo. Int J Dermatol 44:736–742
61. Hofer A, Kerl H, Wolf P (2001) Long-term results in the treatment of vitiligo with oral khellin plus UVA. Eur J Dermatol 11:225–229
62. Hofer A, Hassan AS, Legat FJ, Kerl H, Wolf P (2005) Optimal weekly frequency of 308-nm excimer laser treatment in vitiligo patients. Br J Dermatol 152:981–985
63. Hong SB, Park HH, Lee MH (2005) Short-term effects of 308-nm xenon-chloride excimer laser and narrow-band ultraviolet B in the treatment of vitiligo: a comparative study. J Korean Med Sci 20:273–278
64. Hultsch T, Kapp A, Spergel J (2005) Immunomodulation and safety of topical calcineurin inhibitors for the treatment of atopic dermatitis. Dermatology 211:174–187
65. Ibbotson SH, Bilsland D, Cox NH, Dawe RS, Diffey B, Edwards C, Farr PM, Ferguson J, Hart G, Hawk J, Lloyd J, Martin C, Moseley H, McKenna K, Rhodes LE, Taylor DK (2004) An update and guidance on narrowband ultraviolet B phototherapy: a British Photodermatol-

ogy Group Workshop report. Br J Dermatol 151:283–297
66. Kanwar AJ, Dogra S, Parsad D (2004) Topical tacrolimus for treatment of childhood vitiligo in Asians. Clin Exp Dermatol 29:589–592
67. Kanwar AJ, Dogra S (2005) Narrow-band UVB for the treatment of generalized vitiligo in children. Clin Exp Dermatol 30:332–336
68. Kawalek AZ, Spencer JM, Phelps RG (2004) Combined excimer laser and topical tacrolimus for the treatment of vitiligo: a pilot study. Dermatol Surg 30:130–135
69. Kenney JA Jr (1971) Vitiligo treated by psoralens. A long-term follow-up study of the permanency of repigmentation. Arch Dermatol 103:475–480
70. Kim SM, Lee HS, Hann SK (1999) The efficacy of low-dose oral corticosteroids in the treatment of vitiligo patients. Int J Dermatol 38:546–550
71. Kim YJ, Chung BS, Choi KC (2001) Depigmentation therapy with Q-switched ruby laser after tanning in vitiligo universalis. Dermatol Surg 27:969–970
72. Koga M, Tango T (1988) Clinical features and course of type A and type B vitiligo. Br J Dermatol 118:223–228
73. Kose O, Riza Gur A, Kurumlu Z, Erol E (2002) Calcipotriol ointment versus clobetasol ointment in localized vitiligo: an open, comparative clinical trial. Int J Dermatol 41:616–618
74. Koster W, Wiskemann A (1990) Phototherapy with UV-B in vitiligo. Z Hautkr 65:1022–1024, 1029
75. Kostovic K, Pasic A (2005) New treatment modalities for vitiligo: focus on topical immunomodulators. Drugs 65:447–459
76. Kovacs SO (1998) Vitiligo. J Am Acad Dermatol 38:647–666; quiz 667–668
77. Kreuter A, Gambichler T, Avermaete A, Jansen T, Altmeyer P, von Kobyletzki G (2001) Localized vitiligo successfully treated with cream-psoralen+ultraviolet A. J Eur Acad Dermatol Venereol 15:357–358
78. Kuiters GR, Hup JM, Siddiqui AH, Cormane RH (1986) Oral phenylalanine loading and sunlight as source of UVA irradiation in vitiligo on the Caribbean island of Curacao NA. J Trop Med Hyg 89:149–155
79. Kullavanijaya P, Lim HW (2004) Topical calcipotriene and narrowband ultraviolet B in the treatment of vitiligo. Photodermatol Photoimmunol Photomed 20:248–251
80. Kumari J (1984) Vitiligo treated with topical clobetasol propionate. Arch Dermatol 120:631–635
81. Kwok YK, Anstey AV, Hawk JL (2002) Psoralen photochemotherapy (PUVA) is only moderately effective in widespread vitiligo: a 10-year retrospective study. Clin Exp Dermatol 27:104–110
82. Le Poole C, Boissy RE (1997) Vitiligo. Semin Cutan Med Surg 16:3–14
83. Le Poole IC, Das PK, van den Wijngaard RM, Bos JD, Westerhof W (1993) Review of the etiopathomechanism of vitiligo: a convergence theory. Exp Dermatol 2:145–153
84. Le Poole IC, van den Wijngaard RM, Westerhof W, Dutrieux RP, Das PK (1993) Presence or absence of melanocytes in vitiligo lesions: an immunohistochemical investigation. J Invest Dermatol 100:816–822
85. Le Poole IC, Wankowicz-Kalinska A, van den Wijngaard RM, Nickoloff BJ, Das PK (2004) Autoimmune aspects of depigmentation in vitiligo. J Investig Dermatol Symp Proc 9:68–72
86. Leone G, Iacovelli P, Paro Vidolin A, Picardo M (2003) Monochromatic excimer light 308 nm in the treatment of vitiligo: a pilot study. J Eur Acad Dermatol Venereol 17:531–537
87. Lepe V, Moncada B, Castanedo-Cazares JP, Torres-Alvarez MB, Ortiz CA, Torres-Rubalcava AB (2003) A double-blind randomized trial of 0.1% tacrolimus vs 0.05% clobetasol for the treatment of childhood vitiligo. Arch Dermatol 139:581–585
88. Lerner AB, Halaban R, Klaus SN, Moellmann GE (1987) Transplantation of human melanocytes. J Invest Dermatol 89:219–224
89. Liu JB, Li M, Yang S, Gui JP, Wang HY, Du WH, Zhao XY, Ren YQ, Zhu YG, Zhang XJ (2005) Clinical profiles of vitiligo in China: an analysis of 3742 patients. Clin Exp Dermatol

30:327–331
90. Lotti TM, Menchini G, Andreassi L (1999) UV-B radiation microphototherapy. An elective treatment for segmental vitiligo. J Eur Acad Dermatol Venereol 13:102–108
91. Mai DW, Omohundro C, Dijkstra JW, Bailin PL (1998) Childhood vitiligo successfully treated with bath PUVA. Pediatr Dermatol 15:53–55
92. Majumder PP, Nordlund JJ, Nath SK (1993) Pattern of familial aggregation of vitiligo. Arch Dermatol 129:994–998
93. Miescher G (1930) Das Problem des Lichtschutzes und der Lichtgewöhnung. Strahlentherapie 35:403
94. Mofty ME, Zaher H, Esmat S, Youssef R, Shahin Z, Bassioni D, Enani GE (2001) PUVA and PUVB in vitiligo—are they equally effective? Photodermatol Photoimmunol Photomed 17:159–163
95. Mohammad A (1989) Vitiligo repigmentation with anapsos (Polypodium leucotomos). Int J Dermatol 28:479
96. Morliere P, Honigsmann H, Averbeck D, Dardalhon M, Huppe G, Ortel B, Santus R, Dubertret L (1988) Phototherapeutic, photobiologic, and photosensitizing properties of khellin. J Invest Dermatol 90:720–724
97. Mosher DB, Parrish JA, Fitzpatrick TB (1977) Monobenzylether of hydroquinone. A retrospective study of treatment of 18 vitiligo patients and a review of the literature. Br J Dermatol 97:669–679
98. Na GY, Seo SK, Choi SK (1998) Single hair grafting for the treatment of vitiligo. J Am Acad Dermatol 38:580–584
99. Natta R, Somsak T, Wisuttida T, Laor L (2003) Narrowband ultraviolet B radiation therapy for recalcitrant vitiligo in Asians. J Am Acad Dermatol 49:473–476
100. Njoo MD, Das PK, Bos JD, Westerhof W (1999) Association of the Kobner phenomenon with disease activity and therapeutic responsiveness in vitiligo vulgaris. Arch Dermatol 135:407–413
101. Njoo MD, Bos JD, Westerhof W (2000) Treatment of generalized vitiligo in children with narrow-band (TL-01) UVB radiation therapy. J Am Acad Dermatol 42:245–253
102. Njoo MD, Vodegel RM, Westerhof W (2000) Depigmentation therapy in vitiligo universalis with topical 4-methoxyphenol and the Q-switched ruby laser. J Am Acad Dermatol 42:760–769
103. Nordlund JJ, Taylor NT, Albert DM, Wagoner MD, Lerner AB (1981) The prevalence of vitiligo and poliosis in patients with uveitis. J Am Acad Dermatol 4:528–536
104. Norris DA, Kissinger RM, Naughton GM, Bystryn JC (1988) Evidence for immunologic mechanisms in human vitiligo: patients' sera induce damage to human melanocytes in vitro by complement-mediated damage and antibody-dependent cellular cytotoxicity. J Invest Dermatol 90:783–789
105. Orecchia G, Perfetti L (1992) Photochemotherapy with topical khellin and sunlight in vitiligo. Dermatology 184:120–123
106. Orecchia G, Malagoli P (1995) Topical photochemotherapy with 5-methoxypsoralen in vitiligo. J Invest Dermatol 104:694
107. Ortel B, Tanew A, Honigsmann H (1988) Treatment of vitiligo with khellin and ultraviolet A. J Am Acad Dermatol 18:693–701
108. Ortel B, Perl S, Kinaciyan T, Calzavara-Pinton PG, Honigsmann H (1993) Comparison of narrow-band (311nm) UVB and broad-band UVA after oral or bath-water 8-methoxypsoralen in the treatment of psoriasis. J Am Acad Dermatol 29:736–740
109. Ortonne J-P, Bahadoran P, Fitzpatrick TB, Mosher DB, Hori Y (2003) Hypomelanoses and hypermelanoses. In: Freedberg IM, Eisen AZ, Wolff K et al (eds) Dermatology in general medicine. McGraw-Hill, New York
110. Park HS, Lee YS, Chun DK (2003) Squamous cell carcinoma in vitiligo lesion after long-term PUVA therapy. J Eur Acad Dermatol Venereol 17:578–580

111. Park S, Albert DM, Bolognia JL (1992) Ocular manifestations of pigmentary disorders. Dermatol Clin 10:609–622
112. Parsad D, Saini R, Verma N (1998) Combination of PUVAsol and topical calcipotriol in vitiligo. Dermatology 197:167–170
113. Parsad D, Saini R, Nagpal R (1999) Calcipotriol in vitiligo: a preliminary study. Pediatr Dermatol 16:317–320
114. Pasricha JS, Khaitan BK (1993) Oral mini-pulse therapy with betamethasone in vitiligo patients having extensive or fast-spreading disease. Int J Dermatol 32:753–757
115. Pasricha JS, Khera V (1994) Effect of prolonged treatment with levamisole on vitiligo with limited and slow-spreading disease. Int J Dermatol 33:584–587
116. Passeron T, Ostovari N, Zakaria W, Fontas E, Larrouy JC, Lacour JP, Ortonne JP (2004) Topical tacrolimus and the 308-nm excimer laser: a synergistic combination for the treatment of vitiligo. Arch Dermatol 140:1065–1069
117. Patel DC, Evans AV, Hawk JL (2002) Topical pseudocatalase mousse and narrowband UVB phototherapy is not effective for vitiligo: an open, single-centre study. Clin Exp Dermatol 27:641–644
118. Pathak MA, Mosher DB, Fitzpatrick TB, Parrish JA (1980) Relative effectiveness of three psoralens and sunlight in repigmentation of 365 vitiligo patients. J Invest Dermatol 74:252
119. Pathak MA, Mosher DB, Fitzpatrick TB (1984) Safety and therapeutic effectiveness of 8-methoxypsoralen, 4,5′,8-trimethylpsoralen, and psoralen in vitiligo. Natl Cancer Inst Monogr 66:165–173
120. Pathak MA, Fitzpatrick TB (1992) The evolution of photochemotherapy with psoralens and UVA (PUVA): 2000 BC to 1992 AD. J Photochem Photobiol B 14:3–22
121. Phan GQ, Attia P, Steinberg SM, White DE, Rosenberg SA (2001) Factors associated with response to high-dose interleukin-2 in patients with metastatic melanoma. J Clin Oncol 19:3477–3482
122. Pianigiani E, Risulo M, Andreassi A, Taddeucci P, Ierardi F, Andreassi L (2005) Autologous epidermal cultures and narrow-band ultraviolet B in the surgical treatment of vitiligo. Dermatol Surg 31:155–159
123. Porter J, Beuf AH, Lerner A, Nordlund J (1987) Response to cosmetic disfigurement: patients with vitiligo. Cutis 39:493–494
124. Porter JR, Beuf AH, Lerner AB, Nordlund JJ (1990) The effect of vitiligo on sexual relationships. J Am Acad Dermatol 22:221–222
125. Radakovic-Fijan S, Furnsinn-Friedl AM, Honigsmann H, Tanew A (2001) Oral dexamethasone pulse treatment for vitiligo. J Am Acad Dermatol 44:814–817
126. Radmanesh M (2000) Depigmentation of the normally pigmented patches in universal vitiligo patients by cryotherapy. J Eur Acad Dermatol Venereol 14:149–152
127. Reyes E, Jaen P, Heras Ede L, Eusebio E, Carrion F, Cuevas J, Gonzalez S, Villarrubia VG, Alvarez-Mon M (2006) Systemic immunomodulatory effects of Polypodium leucotomos as an adjuvant to PUVA therapy in generalized vitiligo: a pilot study. J Dermatol Sci 41:213–216
128. Ronnerfalt L, Lydahl E, Wennersten G, Jahnberg P, Thyresson-Hok M (1982) Ophthalmological study of patients undergoing long-term PUVA therapy. Acta Derm Venereol 62:501–505
129. Rosenbach T, Wellenreuther U, Nurnberger F, Czarnetzki BM (1993) [Treatment of vitiligo with phenylalanine and UV-A]. Hautarzt 44:208–209
130. Schallreuter KU, Pittelkow MP (1988) Defective calcium uptake in keratinocyte cell cultures from vitiliginous skin. Arch Dermatol Res 280:137–139
131. Schallreuter KU, Lemke R, Brandt O, Schwartz R, Westhofen M, Montz R, Berger J (1994) Vitiligo and other diseases: coexistence or true association? Hamburg study on 321 patients. Dermatology 188:269–275
132. Schallreuter KU, Wood JM, Pittelkow MR, Gutlich M, Lemke KR, Rodl W, Swanson NN, Hitzemann K, Ziegler I (1994) Regulation of melanin biosynthesis in the human epidermis

by tetrahydrobiopterin. Science 263:1444–1446
133. Schallreuter KU, Wood JM, Lemke KR, Levenig C (1995) Treatment of vitiligo with a topical application of pseudocatalase and calcium in combination with short-term UVB exposure: a case study on 33 patients. Dermatology 190:223–229
134. Schallreuter KU, Moore J, Behrens-Williams S, Panske A, Harari M (2002) Rapid initiation of repigmentation in vitiligo with Dead Sea climatotherapy in combination with pseudocatalase (PC-KUS). Int J Dermatol 41:482–487
135. Scherschun L, Kim JJ, Lim HW (2001) Narrow-band ultraviolet B is a useful and well-tolerated treatment for vitiligo. J Am Acad Dermatol 44:999–1003
136. Schulpis CH, Antoniou C, Michas T, Strarigos J (1989) Phenylalanine plus ultraviolet light: preliminary report of a promising treatment for childhood vitiligo. Pediatr Dermatol 6:332–335
137. Sehgal VN (1971) Oral trimethylpsoralen in vitiligo in children: a preliminary report. Br J Dermatol 85:454–456
138. Siddiqui AH, Stolk LM, Bhaggoe R, Hu R, Schutgens RB, Westerhof W (1994) L-phenylalanine and UVA irradiation in the treatment of vitiligo. Dermatology 188:215–218
139. Silverberg NB, Lin P, Travis L, Farley-Li J, Mancini AJ, Wagner AM, Chamlin SL, Paller AS (2004) Tacrolimus ointment promotes repigmentation of vitiligo in children: a review of 57 cases. J Am Acad Dermatol 51:760–766
140. Skouge J, Morison WL (1995) Vitiligo treatment with a combination of PUVA therapy and epidermal autografts. Arch Dermatol 131:1257–1258
141. Spencer JM, Nossa R, Ajmeri J (2002) Treatment of vitiligo with the 308-nm excimer laser: a pilot study. J Am Acad Dermatol 46:727–731
142. Srinivas CR, Shenoi SD, Balachandran C (1990) Acceleration of repigmentation in vitiligo by topical minoxidil in patients on photochemotherapy. Int J Dermatol 29:154–155
143. Stern RS, Laird N (1994) The carcinogenic risk of treatments for severe psoriasis. Photochemotherapy Follow-up Study. Cancer 73:2759–2764
144. Stolk L, Siddiqui AH, Cormane RH (1981) Serum levels of trimethylpsoralen after oral administration. Br J Dermatol 104:443–445
145. Studniberg HM, Weller P (1993) PUVA, UVB, psoriasis, and nonmelanoma skin cancer. J Am Acad Dermatol 29:1013–1022
146. Szekeres E, Morvay M (1985) Repigmentation of vitiligo macules treated topically with Efudix cream. Dermatologica 171:55–59
147. Taneja A, Trehan M, Taylor CR (2003) 308-nm excimer laser for the treatment of localized vitiligo. Int J Dermatol 42:658–662
148. Tham SN, Gange RW, Parrish JA (1987) Ultraviolet-B treatment of psoriasis in patients with concomitant vitiligo. Arch Dermatol 123:26–27
149. Thiele B, Steigleder GK (1987) Repigmentation treatment of vitiligo with L-phenylalanine and UVA irradiation. Z Hautkr 62:519–523
150. Tjioe M, Otero ME, van de Kerkhof PC, Gerritsen MJ (2005) Quality of life in vitiligo patients after treatment with long-term narrowband ultraviolet B phototherapy. J Eur Acad Dermatol Venereol 19:56–60
151. Travis LB, Silverberg NB (2004) Calcipotriene and corticosteroid combination therapy for vitiligo. Pediatr Dermatol 21:495–498
152. Tsuji T, Hamada T (1983) Topically administered fluorouracil in vitiligo. Arch Dermatol 119:722–727
153. Valkova S, Trashlieva M, Christova P (2004) Treatment of vitiligo with local khellin and UVA: comparison with systemic PUVA. Clin Exp Dermatol 29:180–184
154. van der Leun JC (1984) UV-carcinogenesis. Photochem Photobiol 39:861–868
155. Weischer M, Blum A, Eberhard F, Rocken M, Berneburg M (2004) No evidence for increased skin cancer risk in psoriasis patients treated with broadband or narrowband UVB phototherapy: a first retrospective study. Acta Derm Venereol 84:370–374

156. Westerhof W, Nieuweboer-Krobotova L (1997) Treatment of vitiligo with UV-B radiation vs topical psoralen plus UV-A. Arch Dermatol 133:1525–1528
157. Westerhof W, Njoo MD, Schallreuter KU (1997) Vitiligo. Hautarzt 48:677–693; quiz 693
158. Wildfang IL, Jacobsen FK, Thestrup-Pedersen K (1992) PUVA treatment of vitiligo: a retrospective study of 59 patients. Acta Derm Venereol 72:305–306
159. Yagi S, Hanawa S, Morishima T (1983) Bowen disease and bowenoid lesion arising on vitiliginous skin during longterm phototherapy. Nippon Hifuka Gakkai Zasshi 93:741–745

第8章　移植物抗宿主病（GvHD）的光（化学）疗法

B. Volc-Platzer

内容

引言 ·· 159
移植物抗宿主病 ·································· 160
UVA 光疗（光化学疗法）·························· 164
UVA1 光疗 ······································· 168
UVB 光疗 ·· 168
总结和展望 ······································ 169

要点

> 光疗对扁平苔藓样慢性 GvHD 和迟发性急性 GvHD 的疗效最好。
> 标准的 PUVA 疗法与体外光化学免疫疗法疗效基本相当。
> 基于未直接暴露于光化学疗法的黏膜皮损仍有效缓解的发现,认为光化学疗法具有系统性效应。
> PUVA 浴疗或许可以作为治疗局限初发的 GvHD 的播散性硬斑样皮损的选择。
> PUVA 浴疗和 UVA1 对泛发硬皮病样 GvHD 是最合适的光疗方案。
> 对于急性 GvHD,PUVA 和体外光疗的疗效仍需进行大样本的对照实验。

引言

　　异源干细胞移植（stem cell transplantation,SCT）,即骨髓或外周血干细胞移植,已经越来越多地用于治疗致命性血液恶性肿瘤、血液病、自身免疫性疾病以及某些代谢性疾病[1,2]。这些异源干细胞可以由亲属或非亲属提供,与宿主的人类白细胞抗原(human leukocyte antigen,HLA)相配或者不相配。随着支持性护理技术、组织相容性的分子匹配、预防以及标准治疗模式的不断提高和进展,异源干细胞移植在过去数十年间已经取得了明显的进步。但移植物抗宿主反应仍是异源干细胞移植后影响整个过程的主要并发症,约有50%的患者可出现[3,4]。非亲属供者的干细胞和与宿主HLA不匹配的干细胞的应用增加了严重移植物抗宿主病(GvHD)的发生概率[5,6]。还有几种危险因素可诱发GvHD,即供者和宿主年龄不符、移植物聚集的T淋巴细胞数量、供者和宿主性别匹配不当(其中,女性供者与男性宿主的配对模式具有较高的风险)等,均可使GvHD更易发生。

急性GvHD患者若存在中毒性表皮坏死、肝衰竭、严重的内脏受累以及使用高剂量免疫抑制剂,均使得出现机会性感染的可能显著增加[7],或提高了潜在疾病复发的风险,严重威胁患者生命。免疫抑制本质上与慢性GvHD相关。环孢素A和激素是分别用于预防和治疗GvHD的标准免疫抑制疗法,但它不但增加了感染的风险,同时也会诱发继发性恶性肿瘤[9]。

基于紫外线照射的免疫调节效应,随着辅助和替代治疗手段的应用及发展,使得紫外线照射可以减少甚至替代标准免疫抑制疗法如激素的使用,在急慢性GvHD的治疗上有着迫切的需求。此外,紫外线照射移植物进行免疫调节的方案也可考虑用于预防GvHD的发生。

移植物抗宿主病

定义和免疫病理学概念

1966年,Billingham提出了三个发生GvHD的先决条件:
1. 移植物中存在具有免疫活性的T淋巴细胞;
2. 与宿主HLA不相配的供者;
3. 宿主无力对移植物发动有效的免疫攻势[10]。

免疫抑制严重的宿主,体内具有不同的主要与次要组织相容性抗原(minor histocompatibility antigens,miHA),它可以导致一系列免疫反应,对靶器官(如皮肤、胃肠道和肝脏)造成损伤,这其中包括了效应T细胞的活化和克隆扩增。目前有研究证实,急慢性GvHD的特征至少有一部分是由于单核细胞和T淋巴细胞相继激活时产生的失调细胞因子所致。预处理方案对宿主组织的损伤导致IL-1、IL-6以及TNF-α等炎症因子释放,促进Ⅱ类异抗原和黏附分子的构建和异常表达,从而增加了供者的活化T淋巴细胞[11]。T淋巴细胞主要分泌IL-2和IFN-α,诱导细胞毒性T细胞和NK细胞反应,使单核细胞产生TNF-α和IL-1[12]。皮肤和肠道GvHD的特征改变,如表皮细胞分化不良和凋亡等[13],可能是由细胞因子通过TNF-α所介导,亦可能是由Fas/Fasl系统激活所产生[15],或者由CTL和NK细胞效应分子所介导[16]。

临床症状、组织学表现和免疫病理

急性GvHD通常发生在移植后的第14天到21天之间,即外周血中第一次出现反应性白细胞的时间前后。当宿主与供者HLA不匹配或患者没有行任何预防措施时,急性GvHD也可以发生在SCT后的数天内。50%的患者可发生急性GvHD,受累器官包括皮肤、肝脏和其他内脏。皮疹特征主要为密集分布的斑疹、丘疹,有时需与药物疹及病毒疹相鉴别。皮损可能逐渐加重,累及全身(红斑水肿),伴水疱形成和表皮剥脱(中毒性表皮坏死样)。Glucksherg等提出根据受累脏器的症状,可以对皮肤、肝脏、肠道急性GvHD进行分期以及分级[17],而最终由组织病理来确诊[18]。尽管近年来尝试对这个分级和分期系统进行修改,以便更适用于生物统计评估和分析,但所有的移植中心仍将使用Glucksherg分级和分期来评估患者预后和紫外线疗法等新治疗手段的效果。急性GvHD可以在移植后第2~3个月出现症状,这与在移植后100天左右环孢素A(CSA)的减量或停药有关。这种迟发的急性皮肤型GvHD,在临床以及组织学上多为扁平苔藓样改变,并且有着更高的发生率。

慢性皮肤型GvHD可表现为扁平苔藓样皮疹,约55%左右的移植宿主可出现,最早于移植后的第60天左右出现[19],该病也可以表现为湿疹样皮疹[20]。此外,皮肤和口腔、生殖器黏膜可出现苔藓硬化样或硬皮病样皮损(如局限性硬化病),同时也是慢性GvHD其他器官受累的主要表现[21]。其中,皮肤和黏膜受累占90%以上[21,22],但其他器官如眼、肠道、肝脏、肌肉-骨骼系统、中枢神经系统、脾、胰腺以及肺亦可受累,这在一定程度上类似于自身免疫性疾病(Sjögren综合征、自身免疫性肝炎、红斑狼疮、皮肌炎、硬皮病等)。

皮肤型轻型GvHD,若表现为斑丘疹,且受累少于体表面积的25%,且组织学上为基底层角质细胞空泡形成,此类型一般不增加患者预后的风险,目前认为,可以将它作为与移植物抗宿主反应密切相关的移植物抗白血病(GVL)效应的进展指标。GVL反应由供体的T淋巴细胞所介导(最低量为1×10^7 $CD3^+T$细胞),尽管研究数据显示体外激活的NK细胞起重要作用,但目前尚无明确的表型标志物可以识别以及分离GVL的效应细胞[23-25]。即便是自体骨髓移植,在使用大剂量化疗药物、CSA或撤药时,仍会经常诱发轻度GvHD,

这可能与 GVL 或移植物抗肿瘤效应相关[25]，然而，其发展为扁平苔藓样 GvHD 的风险也增高。

目前仅有少量评估 GvHD 疗效的研究报道。免疫抑制剂 CSA、FK506、吗替麦考酚酯以及大剂量糖皮质激素[26]或在激素抵抗时使用的抗人胸腺细胞球蛋白[27]，这些基础治疗原本用于治疗慢性 GvHD，现在认为同样适用于急性皮肤 GvHD Ⅱ 期或以上。此外，沙利度胺可以选择性用于慢性 GvHD[28]。近 15 年来，紫外线疗法，如 UVB、口服补骨脂素后 UVA 照射（PUVA）[29-37]、PUVA 浴疗[38]、体外光化学免疫疗法（extracorporeal photochemotherapy，ECP）[41]以及长波紫外线 A（UVA1）[39,40]已经成为治疗激素抵抗、慢性以及较小范围的急性 GvHD 的方法。近期数据显示（表 8.1），ECP 似乎可以作为激素抵抗的急性以及慢性 GvHD 的一种有效辅助治疗手段[42,43,89-94]，而 PUVA（表 8.2）、PUVA 浴疗以及 UVA1，对慢性 GvHD 更具疗效[44]。口腔 PUVA 治疗也已成功用于治疗疼痛性口腔皮损[30,37]。窄波 UVB（UVB-311）则是针对轻型慢性 GvHD 的一种相对保守以及技术上相对简单的治疗方案[86]。

表 8.1 ECP 治疗激素抵抗的急性和慢性 GvHD

参考文献	病例数	GvHD 类型	预后
sniecinski I et al.,1994[68]	20	5 例急性 GvHD（无分型）	未缓解
		15 例慢性 GvHD	其中 6 例改善
Besnier DP et al.,1997[65]	7	2 例急性 GvHD（Glucksberg Ⅳ级）	死亡
		5 例慢性泛发性 GvHD	其中 4 例改善
Richter HI et al.,1997[67]	1	急性 GvHD（Glucksberg Ⅲ级）	完全缓解
Greinix HT et al.,1998[42]	21	6 例急性 GvHD（Glucksberg Ⅱ-Ⅲ级）	其中 5 例完全缓解
		15 例慢性泛发性 GvHD	其中 12 例皮肤完全缓解，挛缩部分缓解
			口腔均完全缓解；10 例肝脏受累患者中 7 例完全缓解
Owsianowski M et al.,1994[69]	1	慢性泛发性 GvHD	皮肤完全缓解，干燥症部分缓解
Rossetti F et al.,1995[70]	1	慢性泛发性 GvHD	改善
Balda BR et al.,1996[71]	1	慢性泛发性 GvHD	部分缓解
Gerber M et al.,1997[66]	1	慢性泛发性皮肤型 GvHD	完全缓解

续表

参考文献	病例数	GvHD 类型	预后
Dall'Amico R et al. ,1997[72]	4	慢性泛发性 GvHD	其中 3 例改善
Abhyankars et al. ,1998[73]	53	慢性泛发性 GvHD	81% 皮肤改善;77% 口腔改善
sniecinski I et al. ,1998[68]	48	11 例急性 GvHD 37 例慢性泛发性 GvHD	其中 1 例部分缓解 80% 皮肤完全或部分缓解
Bishop MR et al. ,1998[74]	14	慢性 GvHD	其中 4 例完全缓解;2 例部分缓解
GreinixHAT et al. , 2000[43]	21	严重激素抵抗的急性 GvHD	60% 完全缓解(皮肤);67%(肝脏)
Apisarnthanarax N et al. ,2003[89]	32	激素抵抗和激素依赖性慢性 GvHD	其中 7 例完全缓解;其中 11 例部分缓解
Bisaccia E et al. ,2003[90]	6	激素抵抗性慢性 GvHD	均改善;其中 4 例皮肤软化
Messina C et al. ,2003[91]	44	GvHD 患儿	55% 改善;29% 稳定(肺部受累的病例中 30% 完全缓解,14% 部分缓解;肝脏受累的病例中 40% 完全缓解,20% 部分缓解)
Seaton ED et al. ,2003[92]	28	慢性 GvHD	53% 的病例硬化和苔藓样变有所改善
Foss FM et al. ,2005[93]	25	激素抵抗的慢性泛发性 GvHD	其中 20 例改善;其中 6 例口腔溃疡治愈
Couriel DR et al. ,2006[94]	71	激素抵抗的慢性 GvHD	其中 14 例完全缓解;皮肤、肝脏、口腔黏膜、眼睛改善明显

表 8.2　PUVA 治疗激素抵抗的急性和慢性 GvHD

参考文献	病例数	GvHD 类型	预后
Hymes R et al. ,1985[29]	1	进展期苔藓样慢性皮肤型 GvHD	完全缓解
Atkinson K et al. ,1986[31]	4	3 例顽固性慢性皮肤型 GvHD;1 例急性皮肤型 GvHD	其中 4 例在进行全身以及口腔 PUVA 治疗后完全缓解
Volc-Platzer B et al. ,1990[30]	4	泛发性慢性 GvHD(皮肤、口腔黏膜、肝脏受累)	其中 2 例完全缓解;1 例未缓解;1 例未评估
Eppinger T et al. ,1990[32]	11	7 例泛发性慢性 GvHD;4 例急性 GvHD(Glucksberg Ⅲ-Ⅳ级)	慢性 7 例中有 3 例完全缓解;急性 4 例中有 2 例完全缓解;剩余 6 例部分缓解

续表

参考文献	病例数	GvHD 类型	预后
Jampel RM et al. ,1991[33]	6	慢性局限性 GvHD	其中 3 例完全缓解;1 例部分缓解;1 例改善;1 例未缓解
Kapoor N et al. ,1992[34]	15	泛发性慢性 GvHD	其中 12 例得以评估:4 例完全缓解;4 例部分缓解;2 例改善;2 例稳定
Reinauer S et al. ,1993[35]	6	急性皮肤型 GvHD(Glucksberg Ⅱ-Ⅲ级)	其中 4 例完全缓解;2 例转为慢性 GvHD
Aubin F et al. ,1995[36]	11	7 例泛发性慢性 GvHD;4 例急性 GvHD(GlucksbergⅢ-Ⅳ级)	其中 6 例完全缓解(3 例为急性,3 例为慢性);2 例部分缓解(慢性);3 例未评估
Vogelsang GB et al. ,1996[37]	40	35 例难治性慢性 GvHD;5 例高风险慢性 GvHD	31 例有所改善(其中 16 例完全缓解;15 例部分缓解)
Jubran RF, Dinndorf PA, 1998[87]	1	难治性 GvHD,他克莫司和 PUVB 联合治疗	完全缓解
Wiesmann A et al. ,1999[88]	20	急性 GvHD(其中 7 例累及其他脏器),强的松和 PUVB 联合治疗	其中 15 例有效果

UVA 光疗(光化学疗法)

PUVA(8-甲氧补骨脂素+UVA)

慢性 GvHD 的治疗

PUVA 在银屑病治疗中的广泛应用激发了人们对非电离辐射在其他皮肤病的疗效评估研究,如特应性皮炎、蕈样肉芽肿、白癜风、斑秃以及扁平苔藓[45]。基于特发性扁平苔藓与苔藓样 GvHD 的临床与组织学相似性,我们以及其他学者尝试运用 PUVA 治疗苔藓样 GvHD[29,30]。在 1985 年至 2007 年间,除基本免疫抑制治疗外,PUVA 成功治疗苔藓样 GvHD 的案例报道逐年递增[20,29-37]。

关于 PUVA 治疗硬皮病样亚型的皮肤 GvHD 的结果报道存在争议。根据治疗经验,我们发现局限性的皮损似乎对 PUVA 治疗更为敏感,治疗过程中纤维化、硬化的结缔组织随之出现软化。然而,泛发性的皮损对 PUVA 则反应欠佳[44]。近年来,部分研究显示 PUVA 浴疗可以更快使皮肤厚度更快地变薄[38],而 UVA1 则可以改善关节活动性以及硬化程度[40,44,45]。

有报道指出 PUVA 可能不止发挥出局部效应，还可以发挥出系统性效应。我们观察到一例用 PUVA 治疗慢性苔藓样 GvHD 时黏膜糜烂改善并逐渐愈合的案例 GvHD 患者在治疗过程中，其他脏器如肝脏并无任何改善。尽管如此，在使用了经肝脏代谢的补骨脂素进行治疗后，并无肝脏型 GvHD 加重的案例报道。

慢性 GvHD 的治疗原则与银屑病或蕈样肉芽肿基本一致。患者在摄取 5 甲氧补骨脂素或 8 甲氧补骨脂素（5-MOP，8-MOP）后 1~2 小时，进行 UVA 照射。治疗前、治疗中及治疗后，患者需使用遮光镜对眼睛进行遮挡。

UVA 的初始剂量可以根据 Fitzpatrick 分型进行经验制定，或者根据最小光毒量（MPD）制定。初始剂量为 MPD 的 50%~70%。因此，UVA 剂量一般为 0.5~2.0J/cm^2[29-37]。UVA 辐射剂量不应增加过快，以避免红斑和 GvHD 加重的可能。UVA 剂量在每 2~4 次治疗后一个月增加 0.5J/cm^2，每周治疗 3~4 次。皮损缓解后，可减量至每周 2 次，维持一个月，最后减至每周一次（维持治疗）。

其中一个关注点是，皮肤型 GvHD 进行紫外线治疗存在导致皮肤肿瘤的风险。Kelley 等通过动物模型对紫外线介导的免疫抑制药物的致癌性进行了研究[46]。Altwan 和 Adler[47] 报道了 PUVA 治疗慢性皮肤型 GvHD 过程中多发皮肤鳞状细胞癌的案例及其发生发展，但紫外线诱发皮肤癌仍缺乏决定性证据。个别患者尽管遵循 PUVA 治疗原则，却患上了鳞状细胞癌。尽管 PUVA 仍不能明确是否为诱发肿瘤的原因之一，也应考虑到其他危险因素的影响，如移植前的日常生活中患者长期暴露于 UVB 下的；身体电离辐射总量与大剂量静脉使用环磷酰胺的相互作用的、在慢性骨髓白血病（CML）严重危险期进行移植的、捐赠者为非亲属的、皮肤和内脏的急性皮肤型 GvHD、用激素和 ATG 治疗的急性 GvHD；起病急的、慢性硬皮病样 GvHD 使用激素治疗的；CSA、咪唑硫嘌呤和沙利度胺等。然而，PUVA 治疗时使用推荐剂量，治疗时间不超过 3 个月，UVA 的光化学疗法引起继发性恶性肿瘤的可能性极小。但是，所有骨髓/外周血干细胞受者，不管他们是否出现皮肤型 GvHD 或是否接受过 UVA 的光化学疗法，都应由有经验的皮肤科医生进行定期检查，因为他们继发性恶性肿瘤的风险可能增加，尤其是在皮肤和黏膜处[9]。

急性 GvHD 的治疗

近几年内，PUVA 已经逐渐成为对激素抵抗的急性 GvHD 患者的辅助治疗手段。然而，不管是单一疗法或是联合治疗，包括与激素联用，与激素和 CSA 联用，或与 MTX 联用，均不能证明 PUVA 的任何优势[48]。Reinauer 等[35]对 6 例 II 期-III 期急性皮肤型 GvHD 患者给予 CSA 的基础免疫抑制疗，并同时进行 PUVA 治疗，所有患者均在第 5~12 次光疗后症状有所改善。第 8~12 次光疗后基本痊愈。然而，6 例患者中有 2 例发展为慢性皮肤型 GvHD，表现为扁平苔藓样皮损,皮肤异色症以及干燥综合征。Eppinger 等[32]报道了 4 例急性皮肤型 GvHD,只有 2 例为 70 天左右出现的迟发急性皮肤型 GvHD,并在使用 PUVA 治疗的第 28~40 天后皮损得到改善。这些患者在 4~20 个月间,无急性复发,也没有慢性皮肤型 GvHD 症状。最大样本量研究来自 Fred Hvtchinson 癌症研究中心的西雅图组(Seattle Group)[49],他收集了 103 例对激素抵抗的急性 GvHD 患者(其中 29 例来自亲属供者,74 例非亲属供者)进行 PUVA 治疗,治疗后第 6 周激素用量按体重给药从平均 1.6mg/kg 减量至 0.7mg/kg,其中 59 个患者在进行 PUVA 治疗后不需要进一步治疗。然而,92% 的患者发展为慢性 GvHD,在第 129~1883 天有 51% 患者仍存活。因此,PUVA 对急性 GvHD 的治疗效果是有限的,使得其他治疗如 ECP 的应用增加。

慢性 GvHD 的治疗原则基本相同。尽管 Reinauer 等报道在使用初始剂量为 2.5J/cm^2 的情况下并无任何不良反应[35],无皮肤恶化或 PUVA 促发皮肤外病变等,但仍要注意初始 UV 辐射的初始剂量不能太高。

PUVA 浴疗

PUVA 浴疗在局限性硬皮病[50]和扁平苔藓[51]等疾病的治疗上均有成功案例的报道,引起学者们开始对其在选择性扁平苔藓样和硬皮病样 GvHD 上的疗效进行研究。该疗法的优势是可以避免系统应用补骨脂素所引起的不良反应,需要的 UVA 剂量也相对较低。早期,我们使用 0.001% 的 8-MOP 的水溶液对 2 例儿童慢性 GvHD 和 1 例成人慢性 GvHD 进行治疗[未发表],患者需在水溶液中保持 20min,初始的 UV 剂量为 0.5J/cm^2。Leiter 等[38]在近期的研究中提出,UVA 剂量由个体的 Fizpatrick 皮肤分型决定,治疗次数为每周 3-4 次,皮损改善后可减至每周 2 次,最后 4 次的治疗可每周进行 1 次。对强的松或吗替麦考酚酯等免疫抑制疗法耐药的,或系统性激素减量后复发的 6 例严重慢性皮肤型 GvHD 患者,按照标准方案每周治疗 3 次,平均 14.5 次治疗后,皮损均得到改善。其中 3 名患者完全缓解。所有患者的免疫抑制治疗均可减药[38]。Luftl 等[44]观察到苔藓样和硬皮病样 GvHD 患者通过该治疗可得到明显改善。

事实上,目前只有小样本的病例报道,缺乏标准患者评估、录入标准评估以及标准治疗方案评估,使得无法对该疗法进行全面评估。然而,该治疗可以对症状有一定缓解,且根据 Leiter 等[38]的报道,使用 PUVA 浴疗可以减少免疫抑制治疗。

体外光化学免疫疗法

体外光化学免疫疗法(extracorporeal photopheresis,ECP)是一种针对细胞的免疫调节疗法。先将白细胞分离出来,并体外暴露于光敏剂,随后进行 UVA 照射,再将其输注回体内。已有成功运用 ECP 治疗皮肤 T 细胞淋巴瘤(CTCL)[53]以及选择性自身免疫性疾病如天疱疮[54]和系统性硬皮病[55]的相关报道。目前,食品药品监督管理局仅批准将该疗法用于治疗 CTCL。

通过临床和实验室观察,ECP 的作用机制可能是其免疫调节效应。但仍有很多方面需被证实。下面简要讨论其可能机制。

1. 经过体外光活化后,补骨脂素与白细胞 DNA 连接,从而抑制了 DNA 复制[56]。然而,1 次 ECP 治疗期间只有约 2%~5% 的患者单核细胞数量受影响[57],该直接作用不能完全解释 ECP 的免疫调节效应。

2. 经过光分离置换法后的淋巴细胞分泌 IL-1、IL-6 以及 TNF-α 等细胞因子,影响整个免疫系统,出现一系列分子和生物学效应。

3. ECP 治疗过程中,会出现淋巴细胞凋亡,这可能会导致移植反应 T 细胞的清除。

4. 另一种可能性是光活化 8-MOP 可能改变了个体基因(如 T 细胞受体 HLA、Ⅰ类相关肽),这些基因型是由Ⅰ类表达上调而引起的已知或未知的特异性自体反应 T 细胞克隆所表达[52]。Ⅰ类分子数量的增多可能诱发特异性自体调节 T 细胞的减少,其中最常见的是具有抑制功能和细胞毒性的 $CD8^+$ T 细胞[60]。一种可能存在的抗个体基因型 T 细胞因此增多,引起非辐射自体反应细胞溶解,因而其表达的反应性抗原减少。相关动物模型的研究支持上述观点。

近来,Gatza 等[64]利用一个运用广泛的小鼠模型,对已经建立的 GvHD 模型逆转的可能性进行研究,其方法为:在移植了经过 ECP 治疗的细胞后,供体的调节性 T 淋巴细胞增多,从而间接地减少了供体未暴露于补骨脂素和 UVA 的效应淋巴细胞数量。然而,ECP 对免疫系统的影响仍有很多未知之处需要进一步阐明。

关于此技术的详细内容会在本书其他章节有所介绍。ECP 治疗是在 UVAR 光分离置换系统上进行的(Therakos,West Chester,PA),每次光分离置换的平均时间为 3.5 小时,治疗通常连续两天,进行两次。最初,用维也纳大学医院皮肤科的光分离置换装置进行 ECP 治疗,间隔时间为 1~4 周。使用甲氧补骨脂素(甲氧沙林®)进行白细胞光激活治疗,比使用 8-MOP 系统毒性更低。

最初,我们以及其他研究者曾报道 ECP 是治疗激素抵抗的急性和慢性 GvHD 患者的辅助治疗[65-75]。然而,仍需完善双盲对照研究,使用标准参数来评估 ECP 对各器官系统的效应,从而清楚证明此辅助治疗的优势。在我们的经验看来,早期发病的苔藓样皮肤型 GvHD 患者,一般可观察到较好的反应[66],而硬皮病样 GvHD 患者则反应较差[42]。对耐激素的急性皮肤型 GvHD 反应也较好[75]。

Searisbrick 等针对近年来的文献进行了回顾,阐述了 ECP 对 CTCL 和慢性

GvHD 的应用指南以及其安全性资料,使得人们对此类疾病达成了一定的共识。

然而,尽管几个大型的回顾性研究显示了初步结果,但仍需要收集大样本的患者资料,进行相关研究,以建立该病的治疗原则,明确 ECP 治疗的间隔时间以及时间范围。此外,通过随机对照研究,正确评估 GvHD 治疗效果和对潜在疾病复发的影响之间的利弊尤为重要。

最近,运用 ECP 治疗 CTCL 和慢性 GvHD 的共识已经达成[41]。作者对最重要的已发表的研究进行了回顾总结,对患者的选择也给出了一些建议:只有那些难治的、对糖皮质激素依赖的或不能耐受糖皮质激素的慢性 GvHD 患者,可以考虑使用 ECP 治疗。该建议看起来有些严格,然而,需要开展 ECP 治疗对急性 GvHD 的对照研究,从而探讨 ECP 对该病激素抵抗类型的作用。

UVA1 光疗

从 1995 年起,长波紫外线 A(UVA1)已经作为一种对治疗硬化性皮肤病有效的手段[44]。尽管尚无标准的 UVA1 治疗方案,临床上通常每周行 3~5 次 UVA1 治疗,并依次提高剂量,直到接近最大反应。各类 UVA1 的每日剂量有着不同的范围,如低剂量 UVA1($10\text{-}20J/cm^2$),中等剂量 UVA1($30\sim50J/cm^2$),以及大剂量 UVA1(最大 $130J/cm^2$)。对硬皮病样结缔组织疾病的治疗,一般使用传统的宽谱 UVA 灯进行治疗,因为 UVA1 相对比较贵。

与 PUVA 浴疗一样,硬皮病样 GvHD 患者的相关研究仅有小样本研究和病例报道。其中一例患者使用 UVA_1 和 PUVA 浴疗联合治疗[38]。目前尚无治疗急性 GvHD 的相关报道。UVA1 每日剂量为 $20\sim50J/cm^2$ 不等,治疗次数为 15~30 次[44]。尽管资料有限,UVA1 在治疗硬皮病样 GvHD 患者时,其关节灵活性和硬化改善还是显示出一定疗效,而 PUVA 治疗则更容易使皮损变薄。因此,UVA1 光疗被认为是硬皮病样 GvHD 的一个有效的治疗选择,也可与系统性免疫抑制剂联用。

UVB 光疗

关于 UVB 在延长移植物生存率方面的作用的相关研究已在进行[76-78],还有研究显示 UVB 对预防移植物排斥和 GvHD 有着重要作用[79]。UVB 的作用机制,似乎是基于 UVB 诱导了外周血淋巴细胞的凋亡[80],而正常骨髓干细胞可在类似的剂量中得以保存[81]。使用 280~320nm(窄谱 UVB)的光疗是治疗炎症性皮肤病的一种重要手段[82]。

目前,UVB 光疗对皮肤型 GvHD 的治疗只局限于部分患者[83,84]。即使 UVB

成功治疗了一例湿疹样 GvHD 患者[85]，但使用标准窄谱 UVB 治疗皮肤 GvHD 的经验仍较欠缺。310~315nm 单色 UV 的窄谱 UVB，目前可用于治疗银屑病、特应性皮炎、白癜风和其他疾病[82]，并取得良好的效果。Grundmann-Kollmann 在一小样本系列中对 10 例激素抵抗 GvHD 患者使用窄谱 UVB 治疗[86]，其中有 7 例(7/10)反应完全。若要对 UVB 治疗皮肤型 GvHD 进行循证医学评估，需要进行对照研究。

总结和展望

目前研究表明：

1. 进展的扁平苔藓样皮肤改变、静止的局限性慢性皮肤型 GvHD 以及在 CSA 减量或撤药后引发的迟发急性 GvHD，对光化学疗法反应良好。

2. 标准 PUVA 和 ECP 同样有效。

3. 基于黏膜皮损(无直接暴露于光化学疗法)的疗效，提出了系统性效应的作用。

4. PUVA 浴疗似乎可以作为初发的慢性 GvHD 播散性硬斑样皮损光疗的选择。

5. PUVA 浴疗和 UVA1 是治疗对泛发硬皮病样 GvHD 的最好的选择。

6. 目前已有大型的临床试验针对 PUVA 和 ECP 治疗对急性 GvHD 的效果进行评估。我们通过初步的实验，发现使用 ECP 治疗的患者比未使用 ECP 治疗的患者更早地出现了免疫抑制反应的减弱或消除，证实了 ECP 治疗在急性皮肤型 GvHD 上的作用。但其防止疾病向慢性 GvHD 转变以及防止疾病的复发的长期效应作用机制目前尚不完全明确。

目前关于光化学疗法治疗该病的相关临床经验仅出自于少量的临床病例，且这些患者同时使用了其他的系统治疗。尽管近 8 年期间，相关的数据逐渐完善，我们仍需尽快地对各种不同的光化学疗法对该病的治疗进行大量的实验评估。近日，来自英国以及斯堪的纳维亚的光分离置换法专家学组对 ECP 在治疗皮肤型 GvHD 上达成了一致的观念，从而在对英国的该病患者的诊断、评估以及治疗的选择等方面制定了标准化方案。我们希望更多的光化学疗法在该病上的运用的相关研究可以紧随而上，可以向评估生物疗法一样对光化学疗法进行评估。换而言之，我们希望可以对某个患者适合进行哪一种光化学疗法进行评估。

但是，我们仍需要对短波长 UVP 照射(311nm 或 312nm)的疗效进行评估。目前，研究较为广泛地仍为基于 UVA 照射的光疗功效的相关研究。

尽管越来越多的皮肤病学家对 GvHD 的治疗研究逐渐深入，我们仍需要记住，UV 光疗对预防实质脏器、造血干细胞移植的排斥反应具有一定效果。接下来我们需要研究的方面主要针对防止接受了骨髓移植或外周血干细胞移植的患者发生 GvHD 的可能性。这可能需要通过阻止细胞群体介导的 GvHD 的发生，或者抑制外周血细胞介导的 GvL 效应才能完成。

(梁碧华 译,叶倩雯　陈荃 校,朱慧兰 审)

参考文献

1. Thomas ED, Storb R, Clift RA, Fefer A, Buckner CD, Neimann PE, Lerner KC. Bone marrow transplantation. N Engl J Med (1975) 292: 832–843, 895–902
2. Armitage JO. Bone marrow transplantation. N Engl J Med (1994) 330: 827–838
3. Clift RA, Buckner CD, Thomas ED, Bensinger WI, Bowden R, Bryant E, Deeg HJ, Doney KC, Fisher LD, Hansen JA, Martin P, McDonald GB, Sanders JE, Schoch G, Singer J, Storb R, Sullivan KM, Witherspoon RP, Appelbaum FR. Marrow transplantation for chronic myeloid leukemia: a randomized study comparing cyclophosphamide and total body with busulfan and cyclophosphamide. Blood (1994) 84: 2036–2043
4. Greinix HAT, Reiter E, Keil F, Fischer G, Lechner K, Dieckmann K, Leitner G, Schulenburg A, Höcker P, Haas OA, Knöbl P, Mannhalter C, Fonatsch C, Hinterberger W, Kalhs P. Leukemia-free survival and mortality in patients with refractory or relapsed acute leukemia given marrow transplants from sibling and unrelated donors. Bone Marrow Transplantation (1998) 21: 673–678
5. Hansen JA, Gooley TA, Martin PJ, Appelbaum F, Chauncey TR, Clift RA, Petersdorf EW, Radich J, Sanders JE, Storb RF, Sullivan KM, Anasetti C. Bone marrow transplants from unrelated donors for patients with chronic myeloid leukemia. N Engl J Med (1998) 338: 962–968
6. Lee SJ, Kuntz KM, Horowitz MM, McGlave PB, Goldman JM, Sobocinski KA, Hegland J, Kollmann C, Parsons SK, Weinstein MC, Weeks JC, Antin JH. Unrelated donor bone marrow transplantation for chronic myeloid leukemia: a decision analysis. Ann Int Med (1997) 127: 1080–1088
7. Bowden RA. Infections in patients with graft-vs.-host disease. In: Graft-vs.-host disease. Eds: Burakoff SJ, Deeg HJ, Ferrara J, Atkinson K. Marcel Dekker, New York (1990), pp 525–538
8. Socie G, Stone JV, Wingard JR, Weisdorf D, Henslee-Downey PJ, Bredeson C, Cahn JY, Passweg JR, Rowlings PA, Schouten HC, Kolb HJ, Klein JP. Long-term survival and late deaths after allogeneic bone marrow transplantation. N Engl J Med (1999) 341: 14–21
9. Curtis RE, Rowlings PA, Deeg HJ, Shriner DA, Socie G, Travis LB, Horowitz MM, Witherspoon RP, Hoover RN, Sobocinski KA, Fraumeni JF Jr, Boice JD Jr. Solid cancer after bone marrow transplantation. N Engl J Med (1997) 336: 897–904
10. Billingham RE. The biology of graft-versus-host reactions. Harvey Lect (1966) 62: 21–72
11. Ferrara JLM, Deeg HJ. Graft-versus-host disease. N Engl J Med (1991) 324: 828–834
12. Ferrara JL. The cytokine modulation of acute graft-versus-host disease. Bone Marrow Transplant (1998) 21: S13–15
13. Gilliam AC, Whitaker-Menezes D, Korngold R, Murphy GF. Apoptosis is the predominant form of epithelial target cell injury in acute experimental graft-versus-host disease. J Invest Dermatol (1996) 107: 377–383
14. Piguet PF, Grau GE, Allet B, Vassalli P. Tumor necrosis factor/cachectin is an effector of skin and gut lesions of the acute phase of the graft-vs-host disease. J Exp Med (1987) 166: 1280–1289
15. Kagi D, Vignaux F, Ledermann B, Burki K, Depraetere V, Nagata S, Hengartner H, Golstein P. Fas and perforin pathways as major mechanisms of T cell-mediated cytotoxicity. Science

(1994) 265: 528–530
16. Braun MY, Lowin B, French L, Acha-Orbea H, Tschopp J. Cytotoxic T cells deficient in both functional Fas ligand and perforin show residual cytolytic activity yet lose their capacity to induce lethal acute graft-versus-host disease. J Exp Med (1996) 183: 657–661
17. Glucksberg H, Storb R, Fefer A, Buckner CD, Neiman PE, Clift RA, Lerner KG, Thomas ED. Clinical manifestations of graft-versus-host disease in human recipients of marrow from HLA-matched siblings. Transplantation (1974) 18: 295–304
18. Lerner KG, Kao GF, Storb R, Buckner CD, Clift RA, Thomas ED. Histopathology of graft-versus-host reaction (GVHR) in human recipients of marrow from HLA-matched siblings. Transplant Proc (1974) 367–371
19. Horn TD, Zahurak ML, Atkins D, Solomon AR, Vogelsang GB. Lichen planus-like histopathologic characteristics in the cutaneous graft-vs-host reaction. Arch Dermatol (1997) 133: 961–965
20. Tanasescu E, Boullie MC, Vannier JP, Tron P, Joly P, Lauret P. Eczema-like cutaneous graft versus host disease treated by UV-B therapy in a 2 year old child. Ann Dermatol Venereol (1999) 126: 51–53
21. Shulman HM, Sale GE, Lerner KG, Barker EA, Weiden PL, Sullivan K, Gallucci B, Thomas ED, Storb R. Chronic cutaneous graft-versus-host disease. Am J Pathol (1980) 91: 545–570
22. Sullivan KM, Shulman HM, Storb R, Weiden PL, Witherspoon RP, McDonald GB, Schubert MM, Atkinson K, Thomas ED. Chronic graft-versus-host disease in 52 patients: adverse natural course and successful treatment with combination immunosuppression. Blood (1981) 57: 267–276
23. Sullivan KM, Storb R, Buckner CD, Fefer A, Fisher L, Weiden PL, Witherspoon RP, Appelbaum FR, Banaji M, Hansen J et al. Graft-versus-host disease as adoptive immunotherapy in patients with advanced hematologic neoplasms. N Engl J Med (1989) 320: 828–834
24. Xun CQ, Thompson JS, Jennings CD, Brown SA. The effect of human IL-2-activated natural killer and T cells on graft-versus-host disease and graft-versus-leukemia in SCID mice bearing human leukemic cells. Transplantation (1995) 60: 821–827
25. Elmaagacli AH, Beelen DW, Trenn G, Schmidt O, Nahler M, Schaefer UW. Induction of graft-versus-leukemia reaction by cyclosporin A withdrawal as immunotherapy for leukemia relapsing after allogeneic bone marrow transplantation. Bone Marrow Transplant (1999) 23: 771–777
26. Martin PJ, Schoch G, Fisher L, Byers V, Anasetti C, Appelbaum FR, Beatty PG, Doney K, McDonald GB, Sanders JE, Sullivan KM, Storb R, Thomas ED, Witherspoon RP, Lomen P, Hannigan J, Hansen JA. A retrospective analysis of therapy for acute graft-versus-host disease: initial treatment. Blood (1990) 76: 1464–1472
27. Doney KC, Weiden PL, Storb R, Thomas ED. Treatment of graft-versus-host disease in human allogeneic marrow graft recipients: a randomized trial comparing antithymocyte globulin and corticosteroids. Am J Hematol (1981) 11: 1–8
28. Vogelsang GB, Farmer ER, Hess AD, Altamonte V, Beschorner WE, Jabs DA, Corio RL, Levin LS, Colvin OM, Wingard JR et al. Thalidomide for the treatment of chronic graft-versus-host disease. N Engl J Med (1992) 326: 1055–1058
29. Hymes SR, Morison WL, Farmer ER, Walters LL, Tutschka PJ, Santos GW. Methoxypsoralen and ultraviolet A radiation in treatment of chronic graft-versus-host reaction. J Am Acad Dermatol (1985) 12: 30–37
30. Volc-Platzer B, Hönigsmann H, Hinterberger W, Wolff K. Photochemotherapy improves chronic cutaneous graft-versus-host disease. J Am Acad Dermatol (1990) 23: 220–228
31. Atkinson K, Weller P, Ryman W, Biggs J. PUVA therapy for drug-resistant graft-versus-host disease. Bone Marrow Transplant (1986) 1: 227–236
32. Eppinger T, Ehninger G, Steinert M, Niethammer D, Dopfer R. 8-Methoxypsoralen and ultraviolet A therapy for cutaneous manifestations of graft-versus-host disease. Transplantation (1990) 50: 807–811

33. Jampel RM, Farmer ER, Vogelsang GB, Wingard J, Santos GW, Morison WL. PUVA therapy for chronic cutaneous graft-vs-host disease. Arch Dermatol (1991) 127: 1673–1678
34. Kapoor N, Pelligrini AE, Copelan EA, Cunningham I, Avalos BR, Klein JL, Tutschka PJ. Psoralen plus ultraviolet A (PUVA) in the treatment of chronic graft versus host disease: preliminary experience in standard treatment resistant patients. Sem Hematol (1992) 29: 108–112
35. Reinauer S, Lehmann P, Plewig G, Heyll A, Söhngen D, Hölzle E. Photochemotherapie (PUVA) der akuten Graft-versus-Host Erkrankung. Hautarzt (1993) 44: 708–712
36. Aubin F, Brion A, Deconinck E, Plouvier E, Herve P, Humbert P, Cahn JY. Phototherapy in the treatment of cutaneous graft-versus-host disease. Transplantation (1995) 59: 151–155
37. Vogelsang GB, Wolff D, Altomonte V, Farmer E, Morison WL, Corio R, Horn T. Treatment of chronic graft-versus-host disease with ultraviolet irradiation and psoralen (PUVA). Bone Marrow Transplant (1996) 17: 1061–1067
38. Leiter U, Kaskel P, Krähn G, Gottlöber P, Bunjes D, Peter R-U, Kerscher M. Psoralen plus ultraviolet-A-bath photochemotherapy as an adjunct treatment modality in cutaneous chronic graft versus host disease. Photodermatol Photoimmunol Photomed (2002) 18: 183–190
39. Grundmann-Kollmann M, Behrens S, Gruss C, Gottlöber P, Peter R-U, Kerscher M. Chronic sclerodermic graft-versus-host disease refractory to immunosuppressive treatment responds to UVA1 phototherapy. J Am Acad Dermatol (2000) 42: 134–136
40. Ständer H, Schiller M, Schwarz T. UVA1 therapy for sclerodermic graft-versus-host disease of the skin. J Am Acad Dermatol (2002) 46: 799–800
41. Scarisbrick JJ, Taylor P, Holtick U, Makar Y, Douglas K, Berlin G, Juvonen E, Marshall S on behalf of the Photopheresis Expert Group. U.K. consensus statement on the use of extracorporeal photopheresis for treatment of cutaneous T-cell lymphoma and chronic graft-versus-host disease. Br J Dermatol (2008) 158: 659–678
42. Greinix HT, Volc-Platzer B, Rabitsch W, Gmeinhart B, Guevara-Pineda C, Kalhs P, Krutmann J, Hönigsmann H, Ciovica M, Knobler RM. Successful use of extracorporeal photochemotherapy in the treatment of severe acute and chronic graft-versus-host disease. Blood (1998) 92: 3098–3104
43. Greinix HAT, Volc-Platzer B, Kalhs P et al. Extracorporeal photochemotherapy in the treatment of severe steroid-refractory acute graft-versus-host disease: a pilot study. Blood (2000) 96: 2426–2431
44. Brenner M, Herzinger T, Berking C, Plewig G, Degitz K. Phototherapy and photochemotherapy of sclerosing skin diseases. Photodermatol Photoimmunol Photomed (2005) 21: 157–165
45. Hönigsmann H, Fitzpatrick TB, Pathak MA, Wolff K. Oral photochemotherapy with psoralens and UVA (PUVA): principles and practice. In: Dermatology in general medicine. Eds: Fitzpatrick TB, Eisen K, Wolff K, Freedberg IM, Austen KF. McGraw-Hill, New York (1993), pp 1728–1775
46. Kelly GE, Meikle W, Sheil AG. Effects of immunosuppressive therapy on the induction of skin tumors by ultraviolet irradiation in hairless mice. Transplantation (1987) 44: 429–433
47. Altman JS, Adler SS. Development of multiple cutaneous squamous cell carcinomas during PUVA treatment for chronic graft-versus-host disease. J Am Acad Dermatol (1994) 31: 505–507
48. Aschan J. Treatment of moderate to severe acute graft-versus-host disease: a retrospective analysis. Bone Marrow Transplant (1994) 14: 601–607
49. Furlong T, Leisenring W, Storb R, Anasetti C, Appelbaum FR, Carpenter PA, Deeg HJ, Doney K, Kiem HP, Nash RA, Sanders JE, Witherspoon R, Thompson D, Martin PJ. Psoralen and ultraviolet A irradiation (PUVA) as therapy for steroid-resistant cutaneous acute graft-versus-host disease. Bone Marrow Transplant (2002) 8: 206–212
50. Kerscher M, Volkenandt M, Meurer M, Lehmann P, Plewig G, Röcken M. Treatment of localized scleroderma with PUVA bath photochemotherapy. Lancet (1994) i: 1233

51. Kerscher M, Volkenandt M, Meurer M, Lehmann P, Plewig G, Röcken M. PUVA-bath photochemotherapy of lichen planus. Arch Dermatol (1995) 131:1210–1211
52. Lüftl M, Degitz K, Plewig G, Röcken M. Psoralen bath plus UV-A therapy. Possibilities and limitations. Arch Dermatol (1997) 1597–1603
53. Edelson R, Berger C, Gasparro F, Jegasothy B, Heald P, Wintroub B, Vonderheid V, Knobler R, Wolff K, Plewig G, McKiernan G, Christiansen I, Oster M, Hönigsmann H, Wilfert H, Kokoschka E, Rehle T, Perez M, Stingl G, Laroche L. Treatment of leukemic cutaneous T cell lymphoma with extracorporeally-photoactivated 8-methoxypsoralen. N Engl J Med (1987) 316: 297–303
54. Rook AH, Heald PW, Nahass GT, Macey W, Witmer WK, Lazarus GS, Jegasothy BV. Treatment of autoimmune disease with extracorporeal photochemotherapy: pemphigus vulgaris—preliminary report. The Yale J Biol Med (1989) 62: 647–652
55. Rook AH, Freundlich B, Nahass GT, Washko R, Macelis B, Skolnicki M, Bromley P, Witmer WK, Jegasothy BV. Treatment of autoimmune disease with extracorporeal photochemotherapy: progressive systemic sclerosis. The Yale J Biol Med (1989) 62: 639–645
56. Lüftl M, Röcken M, Plewig G, Degitz K. PUVA inhibits DNA replication, but not gene transcription at nonlethal dosages. J Invest Dermatol (1998) 111: 399–405
57. Lee KH, Garro J Jr. Engineering aspects of extracorporeal photochemotherapy. The Yale J Biol Med (1989) 62: 621
58. Vowels BR, Cassin M, Boufal MH, Walsh L, Rook AH. Extracorporeal photochemotherapy induces the production of tumor necrosis factor-α by monocytes: implications for the treatment of cutaneous T-cell lymphoma and systemic sclerosis. J Invest Dermatol (1992) 98: 686–692
59. Yoo EK, Rook AH, Elenitsas R, Gasparro FP, Vowels BR. Apoptosis induction by ultraviolet light A and photochemotherapy in cutaneous T-cell lymphoma: relevance to mechanism of therapeutic action. J Invest Dermatol (1996) 107: 235–242
60. Lambert M, Ronai Z, Weinstein IB, et al. Enhancement of major histocompatibility class I protein synthesis by DNA damage in cultured human fibroblasts and keratinocytes. Mol Cell Biol (1989) 9: 847
61. Ware R, Jiang H, Braunstein N, Kent J, Wiener E, Pernis B, Chess L. Human CD8+ T lymphocyte clones specific for T cell receptor V beta families expressed on autologous CD4+ T cells. Immunity (1995) 2: 177–184
62. Berger CL, Perez M, Laroche L, Edelson R. Inhibition of autoimmune disease in a murine model of systemic lupus erythematosus induced by exposure to syngeneic photoinactivated lymphocytes. J Invest Dermatol (1990) 94: 52–97
63. Girardi M, Herreid P, Tigelaar RE. Specific suppression of lupus-like graft-versus-host disease using extracorporeal photochemical attenuation of effector lymphocytes. J Invest Dermatol (1995) 104: 177–182
64. Gatza E, Rogers CE, Clouthier SG, Lowler KP, Tawara I, Liu C, Reddy P, Ferrara JLM. Extracorporeal photopheresis reverses experimental graft-versus-host disease through regulatory T cells. Blood (2008) April 14.
65. Besnier DP, Chabannes D, Mahe B, Mussini JMG, Baranger TAR, Muller JY, Milpied N, Esnault VLM. Treatment of graft-versus-host disease by extracorporeal photochemotherapy. Transplantation (1997) 64: 49
66. Gerber M, Gmeinhart B, Volc-Platzer B, Kalhs P, Greinix H, Knobler R. Complete remission of lichen-planus-like graft-versus-host disease (GVHD) with extracorporeal photochemotherapy (ECP). Bone Marrow Transplant (1997) 19: 517–519
67. Richter HI, Stege H, Ruzicka T, Söhngen D, Heyll A, Krutmann J. Extracorporeal photopheresis in the treatment of acute graft-versus-host disease. J Am Acad Dermatol (1997) 36: 787
68. Sniecinski I, Parker P, Dagis A, Collier T, Wang S, Rickard K, Snyder D, Nademanee A, Spielberger R, Rodriguez R, Krishnan A, Fung H, Stein A, O'Donnell M, Rosenthal J, Sa-

hebi F, Kogut N, Falk P, Molina A, Loui W, Planas I, Niland J, Forman S. Extracorporeal photopheresis (ECP) is an effective treatment of chronic refractory graft-versus-host disease (GvHD). Blood (1998) 92S: 454a

69. Owsianowski M, Gollnick H, Siegert W, Schwerdtfeger R, Orfanos CE. Successful treatment of chronic graft-versus-host disease with extracorporeal photopheresis. Bone Marrow Transplant (1994) 14: 845–848

70. Rossetti F, Zulian F, Dall'Amico R, Messina C, Montini G, Zacchello F. Extracorporeal photochemotherapy as single therapy for extensive, cutaneous, chronic graft-versus-host disease. Transplantation (1995) 59: 149–151

71. Balda BR, Konstantinow A, Starz H, Gnekow A, Heidemann P. Extracorporeal photochemotherapy as an effective treatment modality in chronic graft-versus-host disease. J Eur Acad Dermatol Venereol (1996) 7: 155

72. Dall'Amico R, Rossetti R, Zulian F, Montini G, Murer L, Andreetta B, Messina C, Baraldi E, Montesco MC, Dini G, Locatelli F, Argiolu F, Zaccello G. Photopheresis in paediatric patients with drug-resistant chronic graft-versus-host disease. Br J Haematol (1997) 97: 848

73. Abhyankar S, Bishop M. Adjunctive treatment of resistant chronic graft versus host disease with extracorporeal photopheresis using UVADEX sterile solution. Blood (1998) 92S1: 454a

74. Bishop MR, Ketcham M, Lynch J, Tarantolo SR, Pavletic ZS, Oria N, Morris M, Reddy RL, Armitage JO, Kessinger A. Extracorporeal photopheresis permits steroid withdrawal in steroid-resistant chronic graft-versus-host disease. Blood (1998) 92S1: 455a

75. Greinix HAT, Volc-Platzer B, Kalhs P et al. Extracorporeal photochemotherapy in the treatment of severe steroid-refractory acute graft-verus-host disease: a pilot study. Blood (2000) 96: 2426–2431

76. Hill JC, Sarvan J, Maske R, Els WJ. Evidence that UV-B irradiation decreases corneal Langerhans cells and improves corneal graft survival in the rabbit. Transplantation (1994) 57:1281–1284

77. De Fazio SR, Gozzo J. Prolongation of skin allograft survival by co-transplantation of ultraviolet B-irradiated skin. Transplantation (1994) 58:1044–1057

78. Habibullah CM, Ayesha Q, Khan AA, Naithani R, Lahiri S. Xenotransplantation of UV-B-irradiated hepatocytes. Survival and immune response. Transplantation (1995) 59: 1495–1497

79. Ohajewke OA, Hardy MA, Oluwole SF. Prevention of graft-versus-host disease and the induction of transplant tolerance by low-dose UV-B irradiation of BM cells combined with cyclosporine immunosuppression. Transplantation (1995) 60: 1510–1516

80. Yaron I, Yaron R, Oluwole SF, Hardy MA. UVB irradiation of human-derived peripheral blood lymphocytes induces apoptosis but not T-cell anergy: additive effects with various immunosuppressive agents. Cell Immunol (1996) 168: 258–266

81. Gowing H, Lawler M, Hagenbeek A, McCann SR, Pamphilon DH, Hudson J, van Weelden H, Braakman E, Martens ACM. Effect of ultraviolet-B light on lymphocyte activity at doses at which normal bone marrow stem cells are preserved. Blood (1996) 87: 1635–1643

82. Berneburg M, Brod C, Benedix F, Röcken M. New and established indications for phototherapy with narrowband UVB. JDDG (2005) 3: 874–882

83. Van Dooren-Greebe RJ, Schattenberg A, Koopman RJJ. Chronic cutaneous graft-versus-host disease: successful treatment with UVB. Br J Dermatol (1991) 125: 498–499

84. Torinuki W, Mauduit G, Guyotat D, Archimbaud E, Fiere D, Thivolet J. Effect of UVB radiation on the skin after allogeneic bone-marrow transplantation in man. Arch Dermatol Res (1987) 279: 424–426

85. Creamer D, Martyn-Simmons CL, Osborne G, Kenyon M, Salisbury JR, Devereux S, Pagliuca A, Ho AY, Mufti GJ, du Vivier AWP. Eczematoid graft-vs-host disease: a novel form of chronic cutaneous graft-vs-host disease and its response to psoralen–UV-A therapy. Arch Dermatol (2007) 143: 1157–1162

86. Grundmann-Kollmann M, Martin H, Ludwig R, Klein S, Boehncke WH, Hoelzer D, Kaufmann R, Podda M. Narrowband UV-B phototherapy in the treatment of cutaneous graft ver-

sus host therapy. Transplant (2002) 74: 1631–1634
87. Jubran RF, Dinndorf PA. Successful therapy of refractory graft versus host disease with tacrolimus and psoralen plus ultraviolet light. Ther Drug Monit (1998) 20: 236–239
88. Wiesmann A, Weller A, Lischka G, Klingbiel T, Kanz L, Einsele H. Treatment of acute graft-versus-host disease with PUVA (psoralen and ultraviolet irradiation): results of a pilot study. Bone Marrow Transplant (1999) 23: 151–155
89. Apisarnthanarax N, Donato M, Korbling M et al. Extracorporeal photopheresis therapy in the management of steroid-refractory or steroid-dependent cutaneous chronic graft-versus-host disease after allogeneic stem cell transplantation: feasibility and results. Bone Marrow Transplant (2003) 31: 459–465
90. Bisaccia E, Palangio M, Gonzalez J et al. Treating refractory chronic graft-versus-host disease with extracorporeal photochemotherapy. Bone Marrow Transplant (2003) 31: 291–294
91. Messina C, Locatelli F, Lanino E et al. Extracorporeal photochemotherapy for pediatric patients with graft-versus-host disease after haematopoietic stem cell transplantation. Br J Haematol (2003) 122: 118–127
92. Seaton ED, Szydlo RM, Kanfer E et al. Influence of extracorporeal photopheresis on clinical and laboratory parameters in chronic graft-versus-host disease and analysis of predictors of response. Blood (2003) 102: 1217–1223
93. Foss FM, DiVenuti GM, Chin K et al. Prospective study of extracorporeal photopheresis in steroid-refractory or steroid-resistant extensive chronic graft-versus-host disease: analysis of response and survival incorporating prognostic factors. Bone Marrow Transplant (2005) 35: 1187–1193
94. Couriel DR, Hosing C, Saliba R et al. Extracorporeal photochemotherapy for the treatment of steroid-resistant chronic GVHD. Blood (2006) 107: 3074–3080

9 第9章 少见适应证的光(化学)疗法

T. schwarz, J. Hawk

内容

引言	177
扁平苔藓	177
苔藓样糠疹和淋巴瘤样丘疹病	178
玫瑰糠疹	179
脂溢性皮炎	179
掌跖皮肤病	180
慢性苔藓样角化病	181
色素性紫癜	181
硬皮病	181
环状肉芽肿	182
肥大细胞增多症	183
硬化性黏液性水肿	184
组织细胞增多症 X	184
嗜酸性粒细胞增多性皮肤病	185
瘙痒症	185
人类免疫缺陷病毒(HIV)相关性皮肤病	185
斑秃	186
寻常痤疮	187
红斑狼疮	188
其他皮肤病	188
总结	189

要点

- 因其抗炎和免疫抑制特性,光疗常用于治疗许多难治性炎症性皮肤病。
- 硬皮病、色素性荨麻疹以及特殊类型扁平苔藓已经成为光疗的明确适应证。
- 大部分其他罕见适应证是基于个案病例报道。
- 总之,光疗总体不良反应较少且短暂,对很多炎症性皮肤病尤其是难治性皮肤病仍然是有用的治疗选择。

引言

紫外线光疗,无论宽谱 UVB(broadband UVB,BB-UVB)、较新的窄谱 UVB(narrowband UVB,NB-UVB),还是补骨脂光化学疗法(psoralen photochemotherapy,PUVA),在近几十年已经成为治疗皮肤疾病的重要方法。除了经典适应证如寻常型银屑病、特应性皮炎、蕈样肉芽肿、多形性日光疹以及白癜风等有确切疗效,也显示出了对多种其他皮肤病的治疗前景[33]。然而,这些疾病经常是尝试性或试验性地进行治疗,成功率并无有效证实。无论如何,光疗毫无疑问可用于治疗的皮肤病数目稳步增加并被认为是一确切的治疗选择。包括某些类型硬皮病、色素性荨麻疹和扁平苔藓。此外,尽管部分报道大多是单个病例,大量的病例报道也显示光疗在各种其他皮肤病中的疗效。但也不能下绝对的结论,光疗对这些疾病的真正效果需要更多的报道或对照研究结果才能更加清楚。此外,新的紫外线设备也在逐渐发展,尤其是 UVA-1(340~380nm)灯和 308nm 氙激光。随着这些新设备使用经验的增长,它们可能取代目前可用于治疗这些少见适应证的技术。尽管大部分缺乏正确的方法学,该章节回顾了光疗对这些少见适应证疗效的证据。如需考虑使用该疗法时,建议读者咨询原文献作者。

扁平苔藓

PUVA 对扁平苔藓(lichen planus,LP)的明显疗效首次报道是在该疗法推出后不久。在该研究中[12],15 例泛发性 LP 在接受 6 次系统性 PUVA 治疗后缓解。Ortonne 等[109]发现 7 例泛发 LP 有 6 例达到同样缓解。然而,之后的研究报道的成功率较之前更不确定,约为 50%~90%,比银屑病的可靠性明显差些,且完全治愈需要更多的治疗次数。此外,炎症后色素沉着的存在带来长时间的美观问题。Gonzalez 等[35]同时观察到在 50% 只照射半身的患者其未照射部位也得到改善,提示 PUVA 可能除了局部效应,还可发挥系统性作用。PUVA 浴的疗效于 1980 年由 Vaatainen 等提出[148]。他们认为尽管两者都存在早期复发率,该疗法优于口服疗法[48]。在大部分的 PUVA 浴研究中使用的是 3-甲氧补骨脂素,尽管 Kerscher 等[70]在 4 例患者中成功使用 8-甲氧补骨脂素(8-methoxypsoralen, 8-MOP),他们只需低累积 UVA 剂量($7.2 \sim 11.2 J/cm^2$)就可缓解症状。而 3 例患者的非治疗区域黏膜皮损得到改善再一次提示 PUVA 的系统效应。同一研究小组后来在另 12 例患者证实了 PUVA 浴的疗效[154],除 1 例患者外,所有患者在 6 周内完全缓解,但累积剂量相对高($10.1 \sim 23.8 J/cm^2$)。

黏膜 LP 的治疗尤其困难,建议口服 PUVA。Jansen 等[59]在口服补骨脂素同时使用通常被用于牙科填充硬化的一种滤光照射装置,8 例患者中有 7 例明显改善。该作用在其他研究中也得到证实[83,86,102]。然而,要对口腔进行均匀照射足够时间存在较大技术问题,因此对患者来说较为困难。而且要是不谨慎可能导致潜在严重的热烧伤。因此,该技术尚未广泛使用。有报道使用 308nm 准分子光[72],8 例患者有 6 例临床改善,2 例完全缓解。

播散性和尤其是角化过度型 LP 可能对 PUVA 和维 A 酸联合治疗反应好。维 A 酸一般先使用 2~3 周,与银屑病的使用推荐一样[31]。

因此,PUVA 对于泛发性 LP 可能也是一有效的治疗选择。但比银屑病需要更长疗程和更高的累积剂量,并且可能早期复发。此外,可能致罕见的光化性 LP[151]恶化[35]。

近年来,NB-UVB 在 LP 以及其他疾病的治疗中,与 PUVA 比较其优势逐步显露。对患者而言,NB-UVB 更方便以及更轻的慢性副反应。一项回顾性分析显示,20 例患者使用 NB-UVB 治疗,有 11 例完全缓解,4 例部分缓解[42],与患者皮肤光类型、性别、年龄以及病程无关。Turkey[127]对 10 例患者的观察可得出类似结果。复发的时间虽没有记录,但由于 NB-UVB 的优势大于 PUVA, NB-UVB 目前可能成为 LP 光疗的选择,而 PUVA 仍然保留作为难治性病例的选择。

苔藓样糠疹和淋巴瘤样丘疹病

急性苔藓样糠疹(pityriasis lichenoides acuta, PLA)以及慢性苔藓样糠疹(chronic pityriasismosssamples, PLC)病程较长且对治疗抵抗。然而,日光对后者的显著疗效使得广谱 UVB 成功地作为传统使用[85]。随后,PUVA 也被注意到其类似作用[11,51,122]。最近在 3 例患者中 PUVA 与阿维 A 联合使用同样有疗效[110]。然而,考虑到广谱或窄谱 UVB(尚未有报道用于该病)相对安全,故应该首先考虑使用,而 PUVA 则作为难治性病例的选择[52]。Brenner 等[12]也证明了

PUVA 对 PLA 的疗效,并在后来为 Powell 等证实。因为 PLA 与 PLC 比更顽固且损伤性更大,Honiny 等[52]认为尽管可能复发,仍推荐 PUVA 作为 PLA 的治疗选择。

上述提到 Bremer 等在 PLA 的 PUVA 研究中[12],使用 PUVA 成功治疗一个可能淋巴瘤样丘疹病(lymphomatoid papulosis,LyP)相关的患者,随后逐渐减量治疗 3.5 个月以上,但在 4 个月后仍然复发了。尽管该疗效明显有限,Lange-Wantzin 和 Thomsen[77]在另外 5 例患者的研究中也显示出 PUVA 的疗效。其中,只有 1 例患者完全缓解,其余 4 例患者小部分缓解,当 PUVA 治疗停止后均出现复发,因此提示需要维持治疗。基于 PUVA 的长期副反应,并不推荐这种方法。因此,Willemze 和 Beljaards[159]认为 LyP 只是作为该疗法的相关适应证。近来一患有 LyP 的 6 岁儿童用可能相对安全的沐浴方式成功治疗的报道[153],经过 30 次治疗累积剂量达 28.5J/cm^2 时完全缓解。任何病例都建议对患者进行定期随访,确保发现早期恶性淋巴瘤的任何表现。

玫瑰糠疹

一般来说,玫瑰糠疹(pityriasis rosea,PR)是较轻的皮肤病,不需任何治疗通常可在数月内自行缓解。然而,Arndt 等[5]在一对照研究中对 BB-UVB 治疗 PR 进行评估,观察 20 例患者 5 次照射,初始剂量为 80% MED,结果 50% 患者只需 9 天就可以得到明显改善,包括治疗部位的瘙痒也明显减轻。因此,作者推荐对大部分 PR 早期使用 BB-UVB。另一对 17 例患者的对照研究再次证实其疗效[81]。安慰剂组使用 1J/cm^2 UVA 每周 5 次,超过两周。只有 UVB 组在 3 次照射后得到改善。但后来的研究未能证实该优势,且瘙痒无改善。因此考虑到本身的自限性及良性过程,BB-UVB 对 PR 可能只是一个可疑适应证,而可能会致炎症性 PR 加重[17]。

脂溢性皮炎

对脂溢性皮炎(seborrheic dermatitis,SD)患者而言,尽管存在极少数加剧的情况,大部份患者在夏天以及阳光灿烂的假期后改善,提示紫外线照射对 SD 似乎有效。无论如何,使用人工 UVB 可以达到良好疗效。PUVA 也已成功治疗 3 例在停止长期的局部类固醇治疗后出现的红斑性皮肤病[21]。然而,在一项 PUVA 治疗的研究中,有 8% 患者出面部脂溢性症状恶化[146]。不管怎样,Pirkhammer 等[119]对 18 例严重 SD 的开放性前瞻性研究中,发现他们对每周三次的 NB-UVB 治疗反应良好,其中 6 例完全缓解,12 例明显改善,尽管 3 周后全部复发。

掌跖皮肤病

　　手部慢性过敏性接触性皮炎有时十分困扰,特别当接触的致敏原未能证实或无法避免时。间断局部使用强效类固醇,通常联合使用渗透剂如丙二醇可以作为很好的治疗选择,但其潜在副反应需要我们寻求其他疗法。Mork 和 Austad[98]基于照射所致免疫抑制效应假设[1,7],在 1983 年使用 BB-UVB 治疗该病。尽管需要坚持至少每周一次来维持,10 例患者中有 7 例反应非常好。Sjovall 和 Christensen[133]通过对镍过敏患者斑贴试验反应观察比较 UVB 和 UVA 的局部和系统性效应,UVA 无明显作用而 UVB 可以明显减轻反应。当其余部位暴露而斑贴部位未暴露时斑贴试验活性会减轻,提示 UVB 的系统性效应,同时也提示近期暴露于 UVB 的患者不应进行斑贴试验。

　　作者进一步对手部湿疹进行 UVB 局部和系统性效应的评估[134],18 例各种致敏原所致的接触性皮炎患者分为安慰剂暴露、手部 UVB 暴露以及手和身体 UVB 暴露。安慰剂组未观察到任何改变,但手部照射明显改善且大于全身照射。然而,治疗停止后通常会复发。Mork 和 Austad 的研究也是一样[98]。另一开放性前瞻性研究对 30 例手部银屑病、湿疹或脓疱病评估 NB-UVB 的疗法[105]中发现,银屑病反应最好,在 20～38 次治疗后 11 例患者有 9 例明显改善;而湿疹在 11～31 次治疗后 16 例患者有 11 例改善。因此,NB-UVB 似乎对手部慢性炎症性疾病有效,尽管以后的进一步研究应该考虑最佳暴露剂量和疗程会更好。

　　Bruynzeel 等[15]对 9 例过敏接触性皮炎患者进行系统性 PUVA 治疗中有 6 例成功。平均 23 次治疗后完全缓解,尽管需要持续治疗来维持。尽管 PUVA 对严重病例无效,也存在复发现象,Hawk 和 leGrice[46]仍进一步报道了慢性掌跖湿疹使用外用 PUVA 以及系统性 PUVA 的良好效果。掌跖银屑病对其反应也不错,但脓疱型反应相对较差。掌跖脓疱病使用局部以及系统性 PUVA 的疗效也受到其他研究者的关注[96,99,111],而 Levine 等[84]用系统性 PUVA 成功治疗了出汗障碍性湿疹。

　　对慢性掌跖湿疹进行手掌和足底进行 PUVA 浴的疗效似乎比之前的外涂 PUVA 要好,通常可以避免光敏以及色素沉着。Schemp 等[129]认为对出汗障碍性湿疹比角化型湿疹的治疗更好,有效率分别达 93% 和 86%。外用 PUVA 乳霜是另一种可选择的疗法[140]。在 UVA 照射 2 小时前外用 8-MOP 乳膏,30% 油包水乳膏含 0.0006% 8-MOP。使用 PUVA 浴治疗手部皮肤病的进一步研究提示反应最好的是掌跖银屑病,接着是特应性湿疹[10],角化型皮炎反应最差。

　　一双盲、安慰剂对照试验显示中等剂量($40J/cm^2$)UVA-1 每周 3 次治疗出汗障碍性湿疹有效[129]，而对慢性水疱性出汗障碍湿疹进行局部、高剂量 UVA-1 照射治疗以及外用乳膏 PUVA 进行对比，结果显示 UVA-1 与 PUVA 效果和安全性相当，但 UVA-1 容易操作[118]。因此，UVB、PUVA 以及高剂量 UVA-1 看起来都可以作为掌跖湿疹不错的治疗选择，我们的经验可以证实其疗效。然而我们的经验同时提示治疗失败率可能高于报道的。原因可能是研究者倾向于报道成功例子而不是失败例子[58]。此外，患者吸烟可能是治疗失败的原因[58]，特别在出汗障碍性湿疹[23]。最后，目前有报道 308nm 氙光治疗掌跖脓疱性银屑病和手部异位性皮炎有效[6]，但需进一步研究来证实。

慢性苔藓样角化病

慢性苔藓样角化病是一泛发且经常致残的疾病。尤其是面部特征为线状、网状角化过度，伴有甲周肿胀、角化过度。然而，Lang[76]等报道 PUVA 成功治疗一例对任何治疗抵抗的患者。Ryatt 等也指出该疗法的疗效[126]，认为当 PUVA 与系统应用维 A 酸联合治疗可能更有效[24,26]。

色素性紫癜

色素性紫癜损伤性较小但经常影响外观，且常对传统治疗抵抗。不管怎样，Simon 和 Hunyadi[132]报道用 PUVA 成功治疗该病。Wong 和 Ratham 相互支持的研究对 UVB 抵抗的患者也取得一样疗效[161]。同样，Krisza 等[75]在另 7 例患者证实，祛除如药物诱发等原因后，PUVA 似乎可以作为色素性紫癜的治疗选择。

硬皮病

局限性硬皮病（硬斑病）通常较轻，对治疗抵抗。但一旦广泛播散，可以导致关节以及胸腔活动受限。好发于青年人，女性多于男性。其发病机制未明，基因、免疫、毒性、病毒、激素以及血管等因素均被认为与之有关。某些病例存在伯氏疏螺旋体感染可以解释有时抗生素治疗有效。

外用类固醇对轻症患者有效，但对于重症患者需要其他治疗。尽管口服免疫抑制剂如环磷酰胺比较可靠，系统性药物如苯妥英、氯喹、灰黄霉素、青霉胺以及维 A 酸在少数病例中同样有效。另一有效的治疗方法为 PUVA。Kerscher 等[71]在 1994 年报道用 PUVA 浴成功治疗 2 例患者，初始剂量为 0.2J/cm^2，每周 4 次治疗 20 次，并在 5 周后逐渐减至每周 2 次，30 次后所有患者的硬斑完全缓解或大部分缓解，所有皮损临床上变软且组织学改善。尽管至少需要 6～8 周的疗程,复发率也有待评估,该疗法仍被其他学者所证实[43,68]。尽管只限于极少数患者,如 1 例 8 岁急进性进展为严重的全硬化性硬皮病伴有关节挛缩的女孩患者,口服 PUVA 也被证明有效[128]。类固醇和 α-干扰素系统性治疗该患者,不管是单一使用还是与己酮可可碱联用均无效,而使用系统性 PUVA,起始剂量 UVA 为 $0.5J/cm^2$,每周 4 次,2 个月后加到最大剂量 $1.8J/cm^2$,该剂量每周 2 次保持 6 个月后,患者硬皮病明显减轻,所有的溃疡愈合且关节活动性改善。但患者在 14 个月后病情复发。

近来,Kerscher 等报道 UVA-1 光疗成功治疗了 10 例局限性硬斑病[67]。患者接受 $20J/cm^2$,每周 4 次,照射 6 周,所有病例在最多 15 次照射后硬皮病皮损明显改善,24 次治疗后,80% 以上的皮损改善。在另外 30 例患者使用 $20J/cm^2$ UVA-1 超过 12 周(总治疗次数为 30,累积剂量为 $600J/cm^2$)也得到成功结果[69]。该治疗方式用于 1 例 16 岁有严重致残性全硬化性硬斑病的男性患者同样有效[40]。Stege 等也用 $130J/cm^2$ 或者 $20J/cm^2$ 高剂量 UVA-1,治疗次数大于 30 次,成果治疗 17 例局限性硬斑病[139]。研究提示,高剂量疗法优于低剂量,UVA-1 疗法对叠加的硬化萎缩性苔藓(LSA)[41]和生殖器外的 LSA[73] 后期皮损也有效。

欧洲进行了大量关于 UVA-1 疗法应用的研究,尽管来自美国的首次报道支持这些结果[57]。最后,近来一项来自 Pubmed 数据库引擎的研究也证明 UVA-1 光疗可作为各种结缔组织及相关疾病的有效治疗选择[14]。

PUVA 和 UVA-1 疗法对硬皮病的作用方式尚有待研究,但体外和体内研究均显示,紫外线照射诱导胶原合成,从而增加胶原分解[139,160]。因此,硬斑病与胶原合成增加有关,紫外线照射对该病可能就是通过此机制起作用的。此外,UVA 和 PUVA 可诱导细胞因子释放,尤其是 α-TNF 和 IL-6,它们也可诱导胶原酶生成并抑制胶原合成从而产生治疗效果。最后,光疗的免疫抑制效应可能也参与其中。

环状肉芽肿

撇开偶尔不美观的外表以及罕见的瘙痒来说,环状肉芽肿(granuloma annulare,GA)一般属于良性疾病。此外,它通常呈自限性。因此,很少需要激进治疗,外用、皮损内注射、短期口服类固醇或冷冻疗法通常已经足够了。然而,该病偶尔会泛发并且治疗抵抗,为了美观要求,有必要寻求其他治疗。该病病因尚未清楚,各种方法尝试用于其治疗,包括砜、碘化钾、氯喹、维 A 酸、烟酰胺和金,都未见明显疗效。尽管免疫抑制剂环孢素似乎有效。在 1981 年,PUVA 增加为其中一个疗法[88],使用 0.15% 8-MOP 外用疗法证明有用。此后,其他研究同样证实 PUVA 的疗效，UVA 累积剂量从 10.5J/cm² 到 110J/cm² 甚至 400J/cm² 均有报道[50,66,164]。一更近的报道[78]以及我们几例的治疗经验表明，沐浴以及系统性 PUVA 同样有效。而对于局部病例还有一个选择就是乳膏 PUVA 疗法，已在 5 例局限性 GA 患者取得明显疗效[39]。PUVA 在 GA 治疗中的作用仍有待研究，尽管可能主要是免疫抑制。尝试的各种疗法表明，目前尚无统一清晰的治疗方案。潜在的副作用在治疗前也应考虑。尤其是儿童和年轻患者特发型进展，当其他可以考虑的方法都无效且患者坚持寻求其他疗法时才应考虑该疗法。

肥大细胞增多症

肥大细胞增多症是一疾病谱，特征为肥大细胞的异常增生，可累及多个器官，特别是皮肤，但因为它既可以为良性也可以为恶性，如肥大细胞瘤和肥大细胞白血病，因此需要采取不同的治疗方法，年轻患者局部淋巴瘤以及散在的肥大细胞增生症一般呈特发型进展，不需要任何处理，而系统性肥大细胞增生症累及内脏可能需要系统性应用 α-TNF 或其他化学疗法如苯丁酸氮芥。某些病例伴有系统性潮红、腹泻、心动过速可能需要 H_1 和 H_2 抗组胺剂。最后，经典的色素性荨麻疹(urticaria pigmentosa, UP)伴有广泛的斑疹，尽管无主观症状或内脏受累，可能患者为了单纯美观上的原因寻求治疗，不过有时可以出现严重的瘙痒，经常与机械刺激后的风团有关，就是所谓的 Darier 征。

经典 UP 经常对传统疗法抵抗，尽管外用类固醇或皮损内封闭有时对局部的皮损有效。目前 PUVA 可作为一种更有用的治疗方法。Christophers 等[18]首次报道 PUVA 对 10 例患者的疗效。尽管皮损的色素沉着并无改善，所有这些患者瘙痒和 Darier 征均有明显改善。Vella Briffa 等[152]则治疗了另 8 例患者，其中一个伴有系统性受累，除了此患者，其余患者再次证明瘙痒和风团均明显改善。此外，PUVA 也可改善典型斑疹，甚至可致部分完全消退。尽管最初治疗时可出现瘙痒加重，但随着治疗的继续，会逐渐改善。在儿童 PUVA 也可能有效，尤其是泛发的、致残性肥大细胞增多症[135]。对任何其他疗法无效的 4 例患者，在应用系统性 PUVA 治疗后，戏剧性地出现改善，而且观察 6 年未出现复发。然而经验提示，对于成人在数月内至多 1 年或 2 年经常出现复发。

为了避免 UP 患者在治疗过程中肥大细胞突然释放介质，PUVA 治疗原则为逐步增加剂量，尤其是初始剂量。治疗应该根据常规指南进行，8-MOP 0.6mg/kg，每周 2 次、3 次或 4 次。治疗反应也应该在疗程中根据瘙痒、潮红或 Darier 征改善评分来进行评估。然而，在一项研究中 PUVA 治疗前后病理活检并无显示任何肥大细胞的改善。不管是受累或非受累皮肤，皮肤组胺浓度也无改变[152]。另一方面，在另一研究显示，PUVA 治疗后肥大细胞数量减少以及尿液组胺代谢产物 1-甲基-4 乙咪唑乙酸水平下降。这些发现与瘙痒和典型斑疹改善有关[38]。Väätäinen 等[148]也把 PUVA 浴应用在 UP 上,三甲补骨脂内酯沐浴后 UVA 照射,有 5 例患者反应良好。相反地,Godt 等发现沐浴方式无效而系统性 PUVA 有效[37],可能是因为外用 8-MOP 主要集中在表皮而系统应用更容易达到真皮肥大细胞。因此,皮肤 UP 似乎对 PUVA 反应也可以,但经常较慢且部分无效,治疗停止后很容易复发。另一方面,有报道 4 例患者使用高剂量 UVA-1(130J/cm^2,每周 5 次,治疗 2 周)可相对延长缓解时间[141]。在该患者,只在 3 次治疗后瘙痒即消失,同时,腹泻和头痛也改善,尿组胺代谢物水平下降,缓解持续 10~23 个月。但只是 10 次只看便达到如此好的反应且缓解期这么长是没有预料到的,这些令人鼓舞的观察结果有待证实。

硬化性黏液性水肿

硬化性黏液性水肿是一种广泛的慢性进展性疾病,主要累及皮肤,但后期可以为系统性,预后不理想,且对治疗反应差。在进展期,内脏受累常需要环磷酰胺化学疗法,此为目前的治疗选择。然而,系统性 PUVA 可能对皮肤表现有改善。Farr 和 Zve[28]首次治疗了一例患者,该患者只对联合应用环磷酰胺和类固醇有一点反应,进行 PUVA 治疗 2 月后皮损明显改善。Schirren 等[130]也报道一例进展期患者联合马法兰和 PUVA 取得较好的皮肤反应。从我们的经验,早期应用 PUVA 更合适。举例来说,一 30 岁女性患者,联合应用 PUVA 和系统性类固醇反应非常满意[138],而单独使用 PUVA 也可有效[2]。

以上这些报道清晰地提示 PUVA 可能经常能改变硬化性黏液性水肿的皮损但无系统效应,循环异常蛋白水平无改变。然而,尽管 PUVA 治疗后皮损消失,仍建议规则随诊以提高内脏进展的早期发现。对于苔藓样黏液性水肿,UVB 治疗似乎无效,且有报道加重的情况[162]。

组织细胞增多症 X

组织细胞增多症 X 类似于硬化性黏液性水肿,因此光疗也可以考虑使用,伴有内脏受累是化学疗法的适应证。但 PUVA 倾向于对皮损有效,特别对于成人。因此,Iwatsuki 等[56]用 UVB 和 PUVA 治疗 2 例患者,PUVA 更有效,然而 PUVA 治疗停止后很快复发,而复发后 PUVA 治疗仍有效。这些观察结果由 Neumann[103]以及 Kaudenitz 等[65]证实。进一步,组织细胞增生症 X 的源头表皮朗格汉细胞对 UV 特别敏感,但这么满意的反应是没有预料到的。

嗜酸性粒细胞增多性皮肤病

嗜酸性粒细胞增多综合征的特征为外周血嗜酸性粒细胞增多,广泛器官受累以及系统性症状,为确证,需排除其他原因的嗜酸性粒细胞增多,如寄生虫感染需要排除,该综合征为嗜酸性粒细胞增多性皮肤病的病谱性疾病,从一边的Nir-Westfried 嗜酸性粒细胞增多性皮炎到另一边嗜酸性粒细胞白血病[107],伴有明显瘙痒且对传统治疗抵抗。然而,Vander Hoogenband 等报道 PUVA 成功治疗系统性类固醇以及砜无效的病例[149]。而 Wenmer 等[158]也报道了 PUVA 对一仅有皮肤受累的患者反应极佳。因此,PUVA 似乎可作为高嗜酸性粒细胞综合征的皮肤表现的治疗选择,即使在 HIV 感染患者[89]。当系统性受累时,它可与类固醇以及抑制细胞生长的药物一起使用。PUVA 浴似乎也有效[25]。此外,Ofuji 嗜酸性脓疱性毛囊炎,可能作为角层下脓疱病毛囊变异型,特征为面部和躯干不对称分布环状疹和脓疱,对系统性 PUVA[15]以及 UVB[27]也可能有一定疗效。

瘙痒症

UVB 光疗对各种类型的瘙痒症有效,特别与糖尿病、肝炎相关的以及某些特发型,然而部分对照研究也证实对尿毒症性瘙痒症有效[34,49]。奇怪的是,一尿毒症性瘙痒症患者 BB-UVB 反应很好却对 NB-UVB 无效[54],不过这只是个例报道。尽管 Person 观察到一胆汁淤积性瘙痒症患者有明显反应[117],然而对肝炎相关瘙痒症的缓解是很短暂的[45]。沐浴和系统性 PUVA 也证实对水源性瘙痒有明显疗效[91,136],甚至在一例与真性红细胞增多症(polycythemia rubra vera,PRV)或骨髓增生异常综合征相关的患者也有效[91]。不过 PUVA 对 PRV 瘙痒的疗效已经由 Swerlick[144]和 Jeanmougin[60]等报道过。这些血液疾病引起的瘙痒症通常较严重,此疗法清楚地被证明是有道理的[97],尽管经常需要维持治疗[60]。NB-UVB 似乎也有作用,这在 10 例 PRV 相关的瘙痒症研究中得到证明[8]。光疗明显可作为瘙痒症治疗的一个有价值的选择[124]。

PUVA 对瘙痒症的明确作用机制有待研究,然而,疗效可能与肥大细胞脱颗粒、皮肤组胺活性以及神经敏感阈值有关[97]。Fjellner 和 Hägermark 在 1982 年证明了 BB-UVB、UVA 以及 PUVA 均可以明显降低皮肤对组胺释放剂 40/80 的反应性,尽管 UVB 仅在直接注射组胺后有效。虽然长期反复 UV 照射可导致干燥以及相关瘙痒,但还是值得的。因此建议对光疗患者常规使用乳剂。

人类免疫缺陷病毒(HIV)相关性皮肤病

光疗对 HIV 感染患者的安全性仍不确定[3]。因此,尽管很多皮肤问题会在该病发生,如银屑病、瘙痒症、瘙痒性丘疹以及毛囊炎,对光疗反应不错,但是该疗法有免疫抑制效应[7,74],可能会潜在有助于HIV复制[131,156,165]。UVB光疗对HIV相关的瘙痒性丘疹有效,Pardo等[113]已治疗8例患者,每周3次,初始为60% MED,然后以10%的增幅,如果瘙痒消失在一个月后停止光疗,如果未消失则继续治疗。7个患者有改善,主要以 CD4$^+$、CD8$^+$以及 CD2$^+$为主的炎症浸润也减轻,尽管8周左右经常复发。UVB对HIV患者的嗜酸性脓疱性毛囊炎也有效[16,94],而Weiss和Taylor[157]也报道HIV相关的瘙痒症有效,尽管治疗停止后多迅速复发。Gorin等[36]用PUVA治疗严重的HIV瘙痒症,观察4周取得明显改善,同时存在的毛囊炎也有改善。在另4个患者,单独使用UVA治疗对HIV性瘙痒症也有效。May等[89]报道2例高嗜酸性粒细胞综合征相关的HIV性瘙痒症基本完全缓解。因此,总之,UVB光疗和PUVA对HIV相关的瘙痒症有效[53]。

光疗是否可以加快HIV的病程进展尚不清楚。Ranki等[123]用系统性PUVA治疗了5例HIV阳性的患者,数周后除了2例患者,其余患者的银屑病、脂溢性皮炎、毛囊炎以及瘙痒症都得到改善,CD4$^+$淋巴细胞数量减少,尽管他们血清和尿 β_2-微球蛋白、新蝶呤以及血清HIV抗原水平无影响。有趣的是,在进一步研究,其中2个患者,在光疗前结核菌素反应阴性而治疗后阳性。另一方面,Horn等[53]用PUVA治疗了一系列HIV阳性患者,CD4$^+$细胞数目以及病毒抗原水平并无改变。Meda等[92]治疗6例,5例伴有银屑病,再次用UVB治疗数周,发现血清 CD4$^+$或 CD8$^+$细胞数目或 β_2-微球蛋白浓度无改变,尽管有1例患者治疗开始时P24-抗原阴性而治疗后变为阳性。不管怎样,没有任何一个研究观察到机会性感染的增加。然而,一项访问调查以及文献检索提示,与正常患者对比,HIV阳性患者较倾向于使用UVB而不是PUVA,更倾向于用于治疗瘙痒而不是银屑病[142]。而且,UVB光疗被作为HIV相关的嗜酸性脓疱性毛囊炎的金标准治疗[27]。

总之,综合各种体外研究[131,156,165],很明显是长期治疗前关于确定HIV阳性患者考虑治疗的最后决定需根据监测医生的个人意见倾向[3]。增加光敏感的可能风险也应该考虑到[112]。最后,HIV患者总的来说应该建议尽可能地避免日光UV照射环境来保护他们自己。

斑秃

斑秃(AA)治疗抵抗仍然是皮肤科中的一个治疗难题,所以除了其他各种疗法用于该病,光疗也有相关的研究并不奇怪。在1974年Rolliver和Warcewski[125]报道给AA患者系统应用8-MOP后日光暴露很快出现头发生长。在1980年,Lassus

等[79]对41例各种类型AA进行局部PUVA和系统性PUVA的疗效,局限型效果最好,全秃和普秃型成功率较低,患者具有异位性体质以及病程较长的反应也较差。如果病程超过8年无任何反应。然而,总的来说,PUVA对其他治疗抵抗的AA似乎是个适当的治疗选择。

在1983年,Claudy等[20]再次提出PUVA对23例患者有效,17例患者有多处皮损,或全秃或普秃中的11例在系统性PUVA治疗后完全缓解或者改善接近90%,平均UVA累积剂量为505J/cm^2,治疗后有3例复发。这些发现与Vander Schar和Sillevis Swit[150]的结果形成鲜明对比,他们的治疗结果很差,30例患者进行系统性全身PUVA治疗,只有9例出现各种程度的头发生长,在8个月内有6例复发。Mitchell和Douglass[95]也复制出同样的结果,他们用局部PUVA治疗22例患者,只有45%出现不同程度的头发生长,且长期效果不佳。因此,Mitcheu和Douglass不建议将PUVA用于AA,除非对于特别严重的病例作为最后的方法。1993年的另一项目前最大的由Healy和Rogers对102例患者的研究乐观地显示出在治疗中,53%的患者有90%的头发再生长,但超过10年以上的随访发现高复发率使得作者总结出PUVA不应常规用于AA。Taylor和Hark研究PUVA对70例局部性AA、全秃型AA及普秃型AA患者的疗效进行研究,观察到长期反应不佳,局部型AA患者6%反应,全秃型AA患者为12.5%,普秃型AA为13.3%。最后,Alabdulkareem等进一步对25例患者进行研究得出类似结论[4]。尽管目前有首次报道308nm氙光治疗AA有效[163],但这只限于局限型AA,并且同样可能达不到长期疗效。

寻常痤疮

因为如今对痤疮有各种有效药物,如口服抗生素和维A酸,光疗对痤疮的作用可能更主要的是历史价值。然而,很多患者可以观察到症状在夏天可以改善[93],而更多针对性的研究显示目前已经基本过时的UVB选择性紫外线光疗(selective ultraviolet phototherapy,SUP)[80]以及UVA[90]有效。另一方面,一项对126例患者的研究并未证明UVB或PUVA有任何疗效[93],与Parrish等[114]发现一致,Nielsen和Thormann[104]甚至观察到PUVA治疗过程中诱导痤疮样皮疹,而长期UVB暴露的致粉刺反应也有提出。因此,UVB和PUVA显示并不适应用于痤疮的治疗,除了患者要参加重大活动需要紧急短期治疗或作为一个少见的方法使用。也有研究报道蓝光(415nm)和红光(660nm)光疗以及来自激光的该段波长对痤疮有效[64,111]。尽管这些疗效基本被否定[108],被认定的模式为作用于细菌卟啉的光动力疗法,使用该疗法需进一步的认真研究。

红斑狼疮

在红斑狼疮(lupus erythematosus,LE)中,光疗和光化学疗法长期被认为是禁忌证,因为该病的严重性以及临床上观察而且有实验证据证实 UV 暴露后会恶化。然而,一位 71 岁患有亚急性皮肤 LE 的患者因为禁忌使用类固醇以及其他免疫抑制疗法,实验性地考虑使用 UVA-1(340~400nm),9 周以上总剂量为 $186J/cm^2$ [137]。6 周以上皮损改善,并且几个月内继续保持缓解。因此,尽管皮肤狼疮确定是潜在 UV 介导或 UV 加重,诱导的作用光谱主要为 UVB[382],使得 UVA-1 理论上安全,但目前要证实其疗效需要大样本。因此,在得到这样的数据以前,UVA-1 治疗皮肤狼疮仍需谨慎。

在一双盲、交叉研究[121],11 例系统性 LE 患者也使用 UVA-1 冷光或安慰剂光源治疗。长达 2 个以上连续 12 周的治疗,头 3 周用 UVA-1 或安慰剂治疗,反之亦然。只需 3 周 UVA-1 治疗后,平均系统性 LE 疾病活动次数和系统性 LE 活性测量均显示明显下降。因此,低剂量 UVA-1 冷光显示可以降低系统性 LE 疾病活动性,且无副反应,与传统免疫抑制疗法相比,可作为一种选择方案之一。

其他皮肤病

短暂性棘层松解性皮炎(Grover 病)为一间断性、瘙痒性疾病,表现为躯干皮疹,通常累及有毛皮肤、光老化的老年男性。一般 UV 暴露后加重或诱导。然而,Paul 和 Arndt[115]观察到一例患者在系统性 PUVA 后明显改善,其改善不像是自然发生的,因为非暴露部位并无反应,尽管该病本来就加重。

Ofuji 丘疹性红皮病特征为持续瘙痒,皱褶部位泛发棕红色扁平丘疹(所谓的 deckchair 征)以及循环嗜酸性颗粒细胞增多,而且治疗不理想。然而,Wakeel 等[155]报道予以系统性 PUVA 后一患者缓解达 9 个月,该结果也被另一使用系统性维 A 酸化合物的研究指出。

2 例回旋形线状鱼鳞病对系统性 PUVA 也有效[87,101],而联合盐水浴和 UVB 照射(联合紫外线照射的浴光疗法)也似乎有效[32]。然而,在该不稳定性疾病,即使很少的照射或盐的浓度超量容易导致严重恶化。

30 例类脂质渐进性坏死(其中 13 例有胰岛素依赖性糖尿病),每周 2 次,使用 0.005% 补骨脂水凝胶,然后 UVA 照射[22],5 例症状完全好转,11 例改善,10 例无反应,4 例加重,是否伴有糖尿病结果无明显不同。因此,PUVA 对这难治性疾病似乎为一合适的选择。

结节性痒疹也是众所周知的难治性疾病,包括使用系统性 PUVA 和 UVB。

然而，Väätäinen 等[147]和 Karvonen 等[63]报道，用三甲补骨脂内酯的 PUVA 浴有较好的疗效。然而尚待进一步研究证实。

亚急性单纯性痒疹对 PUVA 浴[143]反应较好，正如 Clark 等在一项关于光疗对该病疗效的一项回顾性分析中所显示[19]，尽管所有患者在一定时间内复发，PUVA 患者反应率最好且之后保持症状清除的几率最大。

使用 BB-UVB 和 NB-UVB 治疗穿通性皮肤病也有有效的报道[29]，5 例对 NB-UVB 疗效很好[106]，治疗后缓解期可达 8 个月。

苔藓样淀粉样变性为一瘙痒特别明显疾病，经常对治疗抵抗。基于对一例患者的一项研究[55]，Jin 等[61]用 BB-UVB 或 PUVA 浴治疗 20 例患者，每周 3 次，与未治疗区域比，所有光疗部位均有改善，尽管区别并无明显意义，可能是样本量太小，PUVA 显示出疗效稍优于 UVB。

持续性虫咬反应也对系统性 PUVA 有效[9]，当然尽管他们对更简单的治疗如外用或注射皮质类固醇也有效，偶尔可使用 PUVA。

Halkier-sørensen 等[44]用局部 PUVA 成功治疗 20 例甲萎缩，在甲上皮部位外用 0.15% 8-MOP 溶液，45 分钟后 UVA 照射，只有治疗的甲有改善，尽管只基于一个报道，该疗法可作为一个新的方法。

最后，Kalimo 等[62]用 PUVA 成功治疗 5 例对无谷蛋白饮食也无改善的疱疹样皮炎患者。该病除去谷蛋白饮食或者使用氨苯砜一般即可取得较好疗效，因此 PUVA 治疗机会罕见。

总结

光疗还是一种重要的皮肤科疗法，过去十年大量的研究（随机、安慰剂对照、双盲）已经毫无疑问地证实其主要适应证为银屑病、特应性皮炎和皮肤 T 细胞淋巴瘤。然而，该疗法可能因为其抗炎和免疫抑制特性，对少见的适应证也有疗效。很多这些适应证是基于个例报道或小型研究，并无统计学标准，也不可能进行大量研究。因为很多疾病罕见，其他治疗也经常可以选择，新 UV 设备的发展使得治疗多样化。目前光疗有时被认为是过时的，特别是考虑到使用了数十年之久，治疗花费时间且不便利，比起新开发的药物如生物制剂，又无特别的治疗靶点。无论如何，它仍然是一种非常有用的治疗方法，考虑到它的有效性，无较大的短期副作用，并且容易施用，因此仍然适用于比较棘手的皮肤病。

（梁碧华 译，张倩雯　陈荃 校，朱慧兰 审）

参考文献

1. Aberer W, Schuler G, Stingl G, Hönigsmann H, Wolff K (1981) Ultraviolet light depletes surface markers of Langerhans cells. J Invest Dermatol 76:202–210
2. Adachi Y, Iba S, Horio T (2000) Successful treatment of lichen myxoedematosus with PUVA photochemotherapy. Photodermatol Photoimmunol Photomed 16:229–231
3. Adams ML, Houpt KR, Cruz PD (1996) Is phototherapy safe for HIV-infected individuals? Photochem Photobiol 64:234–237
4. Alabdulkareem AS, Abahussein AA, Okoro A (1996) Minimal benefit from photochemotherapy for alopecia areata. Int J Dermatol 35:890–891
5. Arndt KA, Paul BS, Stern RS, Parrish JA (1983) Treatment of pityriasis rosea with UV radiation. Arch Dermatol 119:381–382
6. Aubin F, Vigan M, Puzenat E, Blanc D, Drobacheff C, Deprez P, Humbert P, Laurent R (2005) Evaluation of a novel 308-nm monochromatic excimer light delivery system in dermatology: a pilot study in different chronic localized dermatoses. Br J Dermatol 152:99–103
7. Baadsgaard O (1991) In vivo ultraviolet irradiation of human skin results in profound perturbation of the immune system. Arch Dermatol 127:99–109
8. Baldo A, Sammarco E, Plaitano R, Martinelli V, Monfrecola G (2002) Narrowband (TL-01) ultraviolet B phototherapy for pruritus in polycythaemia vera. Br J Dermatol 147:979–981
9. Beacham BE, Kurgansky D (1990) Persistent bite reactions responsive to photochemotherapy. Br J Dermatol 123:693–694
10. Behrens S, von Kobyletzki G, Gruss C, Reuther T, Altmeyer P, Kerscher M (1999) PUVA-bath photochemotherapy (PUVA-soak therapy) of recalcitrant dermatoses of the palms and soles. Photodermatol Photoimmunol Photomed 15:47–51
11. Boelen RE, Faber WR, Lambers JCCA, Cormane RH (1982) Long-term follow-up of photochemotherapy in pityriasis lichenoides. Acta Derm Venereol 62:442–444
12. Brenner W, Gschnait F, Hönigsmann H, Fritsch P (1978) Erprobung von PUVA bei verschiedenen Dermatosen. Hautarzt 29:541–544
13. Breit R, Röcken M (1991) Klassische Form einer eosinophilen pustulösen Follikulitis—erfolgreiche Therapie mit PUVA. Hautarzt 42:247–250
14. Breuckmann F, Gambichler T, Altmeyer P, Kreuter A (2004) UVA/UVA1 phototherapy and PUVA photochemotherapy in connective tissue diseases and related disorders: a research based review. BMC Dermatol 20:4–11
15. Bruynzeel DP, Boonk WJ, van Ketel WG (1982) Oral psoralen photochemotherapy of allergic contact dermatitis of the hands. Dermatosen 30:16–20
16. Buchness MR, Lim HW, Hatcher VA, Sanchez M, Soter NA (1988) Eosinophilic pustular folliculitis in the acquired immunodeficiency syndrome. Treatment with ultraviolet B phototherapy. N Engl J Med 318:1183–1186
17. Castanedo-Cazares JP, Lepe V, Moncada B (2003) Should we still use phototherapy for pityriasis rosea? Photodermatol Photoimmunol Photomed 19:160–161
18. Christophers E, Hönigsmann H, Wolff K, Langner A (1978) PUVA-treatment of urticaria pigmentosa. Br J Dermatol 98:701–702
19. Clark AR, Jorizzo JL, Fleischer AB (1998) Papular dermatitis (subacute prurigo, "itchy red bump" disease): pilot study of phototherapy. J Am Acad Dermatol 38:929–933
20. Claudy AL, Gagnaire D (1983) PUVA treatment of alopecia areata. Arch Dermatol 119:975–978
21. Dahl KB, Reymann F (1977) Photochemotherapy of erythrodermic seborrheic dermatitis. Arch Dermatol 113:1295–1296
22. De Rie MA, Sommer A, Hoekzema R, Neumann HA (2002) Treatment of necrobiosis lipoidica with topical psoralen plus ultraviolet A. Br J Dermatol 147:743–747
23. Douwes KE, Karrer S, Abels C, Landthaler M, Szeimies RM (2000) Does smoking influence

the efficacy of bath-PUVA therapy in chronic palmoplantar eczema? Photodermatol Photoimmunol Photomed 16:25–29
24. Duschet P, Schwarz T, Gschnait F (1987) Keratosis lichenoides chronica. Hautarzt 38:678–682
25. Eberlein A, von Kobyletzki G, Gruss C, Dirschka T, Kerscher M, Altmeyer P (1997) Erfolgreiche Monotherapie der hypereosinophilen Dermatitis mit PUVA-Bad-Photochemotherapie. Hautarzt 48:820–823
26. Elbracht C, Wolf AF, Landes E (1983) Keratosis lichenoides chronica. Z Hautkr 58:701–708
27. Ellis E, Scheinfeld N (2004) Eosinophilic pustular folliculitis: a comprehensive review of treatment options. Am J Clin Dermatol 5:189–197
28. Farr PM, Ive FA (1984) PUVA treatment of scleromyxoedema. Br J Dermatol 110:347–350
29. Faver IR, Daoud MS, Su WP (1994) Acquired reactive perforating collagenosis. Report of six cases and review of the literature. J Am Acad Dermatol 30:575–580
30. Fjellner B, Hägermark Ö (1982) Influence of ultraviolet light on itch and flare reactions in human skin induced by histamine and the histamine liberator compound 48/80. Acta Derm Venereol 62:137–140
31. Fritsch PO, Hönigsmann H, Jaschke E, Wolff K (1978) Augmentation of oral methoxsalen-photochemotherapy with an oral retinoic acid derivative. J Invest Dermatol 70:178–182
32. Gambichler T, Senger E, Altmeyer P, Hoffmann K (2000) Clearance of ichthyosis linearis circumflexa with balneophototherapy. J Eur Acad Dermatol Venereol 14:397–399
33. Gambichler T, Breuckmann F, Boms S, Altmeyer P, Kreuter A (2005) Narrowband UVB phototherapy in skin conditions beyond psoriasis. J Am Acad Dermatol 52:660–670
34. Gilchrest BA (1979) Ultraviolet phototherapy of uremic pruritus. Int J Dermatol 18:741–748
35. Gonzalez E, Momtaz K, Freedman ST (1984) Bilateral comparison of generalized lichen planus treated with psoralens and ultraviolet A. J Am Acad Dermatol 10:958–961
36. Gorin I, Lessana-Leibowitch M, Fortier P, Leibowitch J, Escande JP (1989) Successful treatment of the pruritus of human immunodeficiency virus infection and acquired immunodeficiency syndrome with psoralen plus ultraviolet A therapy. J Am Acad Dermatol 20:511–513
37. Godt O, Proksch E, Streit V, Christophers E (1997) Short- and long-term effectiveness of oral and bath PUVA therapy in urticaria pigmentosa and systemic mastocytosis. Dermatology 195:35–39
38. Granerus G, Roupe G, Swanbeck G (1981) Decreased urinary histamine metabolite after successful PUVA treatment of urticaria pigmentosa. J Invest Dermatol 76:1–3
39. Grundmann-Kollmann M, Ochsendorf FR, Zollner TM, Tegeder I, Kaufmann R, Podda M (2001) Cream psoralen plus ultraviolet A therapy for granuloma annulare. Br J Dermatol 144:996–999
40. Gruss C, Stücker M, von Kobyletzki G, Schreiber D, Altmeyer P, Kerscher M (1997) Low dose UVA1 photochemotherapy in disabling pansclerotic morphoea of childhood. Br J Dermatol 136:293–294
41. Gruss CJ, Von Kobyletzki G, Behrens-Williams SC, Lininger J, Reuther T, Kerscher M, Altmeyer P (2001) Effects of low dose ultraviolet A-1 phototherapy on morphea. Photodermatol Photoimmunol Photomed 17:149–155
42. Habib F, Stoebner PE, Picot E, Peyron JL, Meynadier J, Meunier L (2005) Narrow band UVB phototherapy in the treatment of widespread lichen planus. Ann Dermatol Venereol 132:17–20
43. Hager CM, Sobhi HA, Hunzelmann, N, Wickenhauser C, Scharenberg R, Krieg T, Scharffetter-Kochanek K (1998) Bath PUVA therapy in three patients with scleroderma adultorum. J Am Acad Dermatol 38:240–242
44. Halkier-Sørensen L, Cramers M, Kragballe K (1990) Twenty-nail dystrophy treated with topical PUVA. Acta Derm Venereol 70:510–511
45. Hanid MA, Levi AJ (1980) Phototherapy for pruritus in primary biliary cirrhosis. Lancet ii:530

46. Hawk JLM, Le Grice P (1994) The efficacy of localized PUVA therapy for chronic hand and foot dermatoses. Clin Exp Dermatol 19:479–482
47. Healy E, Rogers S (1993) PUVA treatment for alopecia areata—does it work? A retrospective review of 102 cases. Br J Dermatol 129:42–44
48. Helander I, Jansén CT, Meurman L (1987) Long-term efficacy of PUVA treatment in lichen planus: comparison of oral and external methoxsalen regimens. Photodermatology 4:265–268
49. Hindson C, Taylor A, Martin A, Downey A (1981) UVA light for relief of uraemic pruritus. Lancet i:215
50. Hindson TC, Spiro JG, Cochrane H (1987) PUVA therapy of diffuse granuloma annulare. Clin Exp Dermatol 13:26–27
51. Hofmann C, Weissmann I, Plewig G (1979) Pityriasis lichenoides chronica—eine neue Indikation zur PUVA-Therapie? Dermatologica 159:451–460
52. Honig B, Morison WL, Karp D (1994) Photochemotherapy beyond psoriasis. J Am Acad Dermatol 31:775–790
53. Horn TD, Morison WL, Frazadegan H, Zmudzka BZ, Beer JZ (1994) Effects of psoralen plus UVA radiation (PUVA) on HIV-1 in human beings: a pilot study. J Am Acad Dermatol 31:735–740
54. Hsu MM, Yang CC (2003) Uraemic pruritus responsive to broadband ultraviolet (UV) B therapy does not readily respond to narrowband UVB therapy. Br J Dermatol 149:888–889
55. Hudson LD (1986) Macular amyloidosis: treatment with ultraviolet B. Cutis 38:61–62
56. Iwatsuki K, Tsugiki M, Yoshizawa N, Takigawa M, Yamada M, Shamoto M (1985) The effect of phototherapies on cutaneous lesions of histiocytosis X in the elderly. Cancer 57:1931–1936
57. Janiga JJ, Ward DH, Lim HW (2004) UVA-1 as a treatment for scleredema. Photodermatol Photoimmunol Photomed 20:210–211
58. Jansén CT, Malmiharju T (1981) Inefficacy of topical methoxsalen plus UVA for palmoplantar pustulosis. Acta Derm Venereol 61:354–356
59. Jansén CT, Lehtinen R, Happonen RP, Lehtinen A, Söderlund K (1987) Mouth PUVA: a new treatment for recalcitrant oral lichen planus. Photodermatology 4:165–166
60. Jeanmougin M, Rain D, Najean Y (1996) Efficacy of photochemotherapy on severe pruritus in polycythemia vera. Ann Hematol 73:91–93
61. Jin AG, Por A, Wee LK, Kai CK, Leok GC (2001) Comparative study of phototherapy (UVB) vs. photochemotherapy (PUVA) vs. topical steroids in the treatment of primary cutaneous lichen amyloidosis. Photodermatol Photoimmunol Photomed 17:42–43
62. Kalimo K, Lammintausta K, Viander M, Jansén CT (1986) PUVA treatment of dermatitis herpetiformis. Photodermatology 3:54–55
63. Karvonen J, Hannuksela M (1982) Long term results of topical trioxsalen PUVA in lichen planus and nodular prurigo. Acta Derm Venereol [Suppl] 120:53–55
64. Kawada A, Aragane Y, Kameyama H, Sangen Y, Tezuka T (2002) Acne phototherapy with a high-intensity, enhanced, narrow-band, blue light source: an open study and in vitro investigation. J Dermatol Sci 30:129–135
65. Kaudewitz P, Przybilla B, Schmoeckel C, Gollhausen R (1986) Cutaneous lesions in histiocytosis X: successful treatment with PUVA. J Invest Dermatol 86:324–325
66. Kerker B, Huang CP, Morison WL (1990) Photochemotherapy of generalized granuloma annulare. Arch Dermatol 126:359–361
67. Kerscher M, Dirschka T, Volkenandt M (1995) Treatment of localised scleroderma by UVA1 phototherapy. Lancet 346:1166
68. Kerscher M, Meurer M, Sander C, Volkenandt M, Lehmann P, Plewig G, Röcken M (1996) PUVA bath photochemotherapy for localized scleroderma. Arch Dermatol 132:1280–1282
69. Kerscher M, Volkenandt M, Gruss C, Reuther T, von Kobylletzki G, Freitag M, Dirschka T, Altmeyer P (1998) Low-dose UVA1 phototherapy for treatment of localized scleroderma.

J Am Acad Dermatol 38:21–26
70. Kerscher M, Volkenandt M, Lehmann P, Plewig G, Röcken M (1995) PUVA-bath photochemotherapy of lichen planus. Arch Dermatol 131:1210–1211
71. Kerscher M, Volkenandt M, Meurer M, Lehmann P, Plewig G, Röcken M (1994) Treatment of localised scleroderma with PUVA bath photochemotherapy. Lancet 343:1233
72. Kollner K, Wimmershoff M, Landthaler M, Hohenleutner U (2003) Treatment of oral lichen planus with the 308-nm UVB excimer laser—early preliminary results in eight patients. Lasers Surg Med 33:158–160
73. Kreuter A, Jansen T, Stucker M, Herde M, Hoffmann K, Altmeyer P, Von Kobyletzki G (2001) Low-dose ultraviolet-A1 phototherapy for lichen sclerosus et atrophicus. Clin Exp Dermatol 26:30–32
74. Kripke ML (1990) Photoimmunology. Photochem Photobiol 52:919–924
75. Krizsa J, Hunyadi J, Dobozy A (1992) PUVA treatment of pigmented purpuric lichenoid dermatitis (Gougerot-Blum). J Am Acad Dermatol 27:778–780
76. Lang PG (1981) Keratosis lichenoides chronica. Successful treatment with psoralen-ultraviolet-A therapy. Arch Dermatol 117:105–108
77. Lange-Wantzin G, Thomsen K (1982) PUVA-treatment in lymphomatoid papulosis. Br J Dermatol 107:687–690
78. Langrock A, Weyers W, Schill WB (1998) Balneophotochemotherapie bei disseminiertem Granuloma anulare. Hautarzt 49:303–306
79. Lassus A, Kianto U, Johansson E, Juvakoski T (1980) PUVA treatment for alopecia areata. Dermatologica 161:298–304
80. Lassus A, Salo O, Förström L, Lauharnta J, Kanerva L, Juvakoski T (1983) Behandlung der Akne mit selektiver Ultraviolettphototherapie (SUP). Dermatol Monatsschr 169:376–379
81. Leenutaphong V, Jiamton S (1995) UVB phototherapy for pityriasis rosea: a bilateral comparison study. Arch Dermatol 33:996–999
82. Lehmann P, Hölzle E, Kind P, Goerz G, Plewig G (1990) Experimental reproduction of skin lesions in lupus erythematosus by UVA and UVB radiation. J Am Acad Dermatol 22:181–187
83. Lehtinen R, Happonen RP, Kuusilehto A, Jansén CT (1989) A clinical trial of PUVA treatment in oral lichen planus. Proc Finn Dent Soc 85:29–33
84. LeVine MJ, Parrish JA, Fitzpatrick TB (1981) Oral methoxsalen photochemotherapy (PUVA) of dyshidrotic eczema. Acta Derm Venereol 61:570–571
85. LeVine MJ (1983) Phototherapy of pityriasis lichenoides. Arch Dermatol 119:378–380
86. Lundquist G, Forsgren H, Gajecki M, Emtestam L (1995) Photochemotherapy of oral lichen planus. Oral Surg Oral Med Oral Pathol Oral Radiol Endod 79:554–558
87. Manabe M, Yoshiike T, Negi M, Ogawa H (1983) Successful therapy of ichthyosis linearis circumflexa with PUVA. J Am Acad Dermatol 8:905–906
88. Marsch WCH, Stüttgen G (1981) Granuloma anulare—eine Indikation für die Photochemotherapie? Z Hautkr 56:44–49
89. May LP, Kelly J, Sanchez M (1990) Hypereosinophilic syndrome with unusual cutaneous manifestations in two men with HIV infection. J Am Acad Dermatol 23:202–204
90. Meffert H, Kölzsch J, Laubstein B, Sönnichsen N (1986) Phototherapie bei Akne vulgaris mit dem Teilkörperbestrahlungsgerät "TuR" UV10. Dermatol Monatsschr 172:9–13
91. Menagé HduP, Norris PG, Hawk JLM, Greaves MW (1993) The efficacy of psoralen photochemotherapy in the treatment of aquagenic pruritus. Br J Dermatol 129:163–165
92. Meola T, Soter NA, Ostreicher R, Sanchez M, Moy JA (1993) The safety of UVB phototherapy in patients with HIV infection. J Am Acad Dermatol 29:216–220
93. Mills OH, Kligman AM (1978) Ultraviolet phototherapy and photochemotherapy of acne vulgaris. Arch Dermatol 114:221–223
94. Misago N, Narisawa Y, Matsubara S, Hayashi S (1998) HIV-associated eosinophilic pustular folliculitis: successful treatment of a Japanese patient with UVB phototherapy. J Dermatol 25:178–184

95. Mitchell AJ, Douglass MC (1985) Topical photochemotherapy for alopecia areata. J Am Acad Dermatol 12:644–649
96. Morison WL, Parrish JA, Fitzpatrick TB (1978) Oral methoxsalen photochemotherapy of recalcitrant dermatoses of the palms and soles. Br J Dermatol 99:297–302
97. Morison WL, Nesbitt JA (1983) Oral psoralen photochemotherapy (PUVA) for pruritus associated with polycythemia vera and myelofibrosis. Am J Hematol 42:409–410
98. Mørk NJ, Austad J (1983) Short-wave ultraviolet light (UVB) treatment of allergic contact dermatitis of the hands. Acta Derm Venereol 63:87–89
99. Murray D, Corbett MF, Warin AP (1980) A controlled trial of photochemotherapy for persistent palmoplantar pustulosis. Br J Dermatol 102:659–663
100. Mutluer S, Yerebakan O, Alpsoy E, Ciftcioglu MA, Yilmaz E (2004) Treatment of papuloerythroderma of Ofuji with Re-PUVA: a case report and review of the therapy. J Eur Acad Dermatol Venereol 18:480–483
101. Nagata T (1980) Netherton's syndrome which responded to photochemotherapy. Dermatologica 161:51–56
102. Narwutsch M, Narwutsch M, Dietz H (1990) Erste Ergebnisse zum Langzeiteffekt des PUVA-therapierten Lichen ruber oralis. Dermatol Monatsschr 176:349–355
103. Neumann C, Kolde G, Bonsmann G (1988) Histiocytosis X in an elderly patient. Ultrastructure and immunocytochemistry after PUVA photochemotherapy. Br J Dermatol 119:385–391
104. Nielsen EB, Thormann J (1978) Acne-like eruptions induced by PUVA-treatment. Acta Derm Venereol 58:374–375
105. Nordal EJ, Christensen OB (2004) Treatment of chronic hand dermatoses with UVB-TL01. Acta Derm Venereol 84:302–304
106. Ohe S, Danno K, Sasaki H, Isei T, Okamoto H, Horio T (2004) Treatment of acquired perforating dermatosis with narrowband ultraviolet B. J Am Acad Dermatol 50:892–894
107. Oppolzer G, Duschet P, Schwarz T, Hutterer J, Gschnait F (1988) Die Hypereosinophile Dermatitis (Nir-Westfried). Eine Variante im Spektrum des Hypereosinophiliesyndroms. Z Hautkr 63:123–125
108. Orringer JS, Kang S, Hamilton T, Schumacher W, Cho S, Hammerberg C, Fisher GJ, Karimipour DJ, Johnson TM, Voorhees JJ (2004) Treatment of acne vulgaris with a pulsed dye laser: a randomized controlled trial. JAMA 291:2834–2839
109. Ortonne JP, Thivolet J, Sannwald C (1978) Oral photochemotherapy in the treatment of lichen planus (LP). Br J Dermatol 99:77–87
110. Panse I, Bourrat E, Rybojad M, Morel P (2004) Photochemotherapy for pityriasis lichenoides: 3 cases. Ann Dermatol Venereol 131:201–203
111. Papageorgiou P, Katsambas A, Chu A (2000) Phototherapy with blue (415nm) and red (660nm) light in the treatment of acne vulgaris. Br J Dermatol 142:973–978
112. Pappert A, Grossman M, DeLeo V (1994) Photosensitivity as the presenting illness in four patients with human immunodeficiency viral infection. Arch Dermatol 130:618–623
113. Pardo RJ, Bogaert MA, Penneys NS, Byrne GE, Ruiz P (1992) UVB phototherapy of the pruritic papular eruption of the acquired immunodeficiency syndrome. J Am Acad Dermatol 26:423–428
114. Parrish JA, Strauss JS, Fleming TS, Fitzpatrick TB (1978) Oral methoxsalen photochemotherapy for acne vulgaris. Arch Dermatol 114:1241–1242
115. Paul BS, Arndt KA (1984) Response of transient acantholytic dermatosis to photochemotherapy. Arch Dermatol 120:121–122
116. Paul R, Jansén CT (1983) Suppression of palmoplantar pustulosis symptoms with oral 8-methoxypsoralen and high-intensity UVA irradiation. Dermatologica 167:283–285
117. Person JR (1981) Ultraviolet A (UV-A) and cholestatic pruritus. Arch Dermatol 117:684
118. Petering H, Breuer C, Herbst R, Kapp A, Werfel T (2004) Comparison of localized high-dose UVA1 irradiation versus topical cream psoralen-UVA for treatment of chronic vesicular dyshidrotic eczema. J Am Acad Dermatol 50:68–72

119. Pirkhammer D, Seeber A, Hönigsmann H, Tanew A (2000) Narrow-band ultraviolet B (ATL-01) phototherapy is an effective and safe treatment option for patients with severe seborrhoeic dermatitis. Br J Dermatol 143:964–968
120. Polderman MC, Govaert JC, le Cessie S, Pavel S (2003) A double-blind placebo-controlled trial of UVA-1 in the treatment of dyshidrotic eczema. Clin Exp Dermatol 28:584–587
121. Polderman MC, le Cessie S, Huizinga TW, Pavel S (2004) Efficacy of UVA-1 cold light as an adjuvant therapy for systemic lupus erythematosus. Rheumatology 43:1402–1404
122. Powell FC, Muller SA (1984) Psoralens and ultraviolet A therapy of pityriasis lichenoides. J Am Acad Dermatol 10:59–64
123. Ranki A, Puska P, Mattinen S, Lagerstedt A, Krohn K (1991) Effect of PUVA on immunologic and virologic findings in HIV-infected patients. J Am Acad Dermatol 24:404–410
124. Rivard J, Lim HW (2005) Ultraviolet phototherapy for pruritus. Dermatol Ther 18:344–354
125. Rollier R, Warcewski Z (1974) Le traitement de la pelade par la méladinine. Bull Soc Fr Dermatol Syph 81:97
126. Ryatt KS, Greenwood R, Cotterill JA (1982) Keratosis lichenoides chronica. Br J Dermatol 106:223–225
127. Saricaoglu H, Karadogan SK, Baskan EB, Tunali S (2003) Narrowband UVB therapy in the treatment of lichen planus. Photodermatol Photoimmunol Photomed 19:265–267
128. Scharffetter-Kochanek K, Goldermann R, Lehmann P, Hölzle E, Goerz G (1995) PUVA therapy in disabling pansclerotic morphea of children. Br J Dermatol 132:830–831
129. Schempp CM, Müller H, Czech W, Schöpf E, Simon JC (1997) Treatment of chronic palmoplantar eczema with local bath PUVA therapy. J Am Acad Dermatol 36:733–737
130. Schirren CG, Bethe M, Eckert F, Przybilla B (1992) Skleromyxödem Arndt-Gottron. Fallbericht und Übersicht über die therapeutischen Möglichkeiten. Hautarzt 43:152–157
131. Schreck S, Panozzo J, Milton J, Libertin CR, Woloschak GE (1995) The effects of multiple UV exposures on HIV-LTR expression. Photochem Photobiol 61:378–382
132. Simon M Jr, Hunyadi J (1986) PUVA-Therapie der Ekzematid-artigen Purpura. Aktuel Dermatol 12:100–102
133. Sjövall P, Christensen OB (1986) Local and systemic effect of ultraviolet irradiation (UVB and UVA) on human allergic contact dermatitis. Acta Derm Venereol 66:290–294
134. Sjövall P, Christensen OB (1987) Local and systemic effect of UVB irradiation in patients with chronic hand eczema. Acta Derm Venereol 67:538–541
135. Smith ML, Orton PW, Chu H, Weston WL (1990) Photochemotherapy of dominant, diffuse, cutaneous mastocytosis. Pediatr Dermatol 7:251–255
136. Smith RA, Ross JS, Staughton RCD (1994) Bath PUVA as a treatment for aquagenic pruritus. Br J Dermatol 131:584
137. Sönnichsen N, Meffert H, Kunzelmann V, Audring H (1993) UV-A-1-Therapie bei subakutkutanem Lupus erythematodes. Hautarzt 44:723–725
138. Ständer H, Nashan D, Schwarz T (1997) Skleromyxödem Arndt-Gottron: erfolgreiche Behandlung mit einer kombinierten Steroid-PUVA-Therapie. Z Hautkr 72:365–370
139. Stege H, Berneburg M, Humke S, Klammer M, Grewe M, Grether-Beck S, Boedeker R, Diepgen T, Dierks K, Goerz G, Ruzicka T, Krutmann J (1997) High-dose UVA1 radiation therapy for localized scleroderma. J Am Acad Dermatol 36:938–944
140. Stege H, Berneburg M, Ruzicka T, Krutmann J (1997) Creme-PUVA-Photochemotherapie. Hautarzt 48:89–93
141. Stege H, Schöpf E, Ruzicka T, Krutmann J (1996) High dose UVA1 for urticaria pigmentosa. Lancet 347:64
142. Stern RS, Mills DK, Krell K, Zmudzka BZ, Beer JZ (1998) HIV-positive patients differ from HIV-negative patients in indications for and type of UV therapy used. J Am Acad Dermatol 39:48–55
143. Streit V, Thiede R, Wiedow O, Christophers E (1996) Foil bath PUVA in the treatment of prurigo simplex subacuta. Acta Derm Venereol (Stockh) 76:319–320

144. Swerlick RA (1985) Photochemotherapy treatment of pruritus associated with polycythemia vera. J Am Acad Dermatol 4:675–677
145. Taylor CR, Hawk JLM (1995) PUVA treatment of alopecia areata partialis, totalis and universalis: Audit of 10 years' experience at St John's Institute of Dermatology. Br J Dermatol 133:914–918
146. Tegner E (1983) Seborrheic dermatitis of the face induced by PUVA treatment. Acta Derm Venereol 63:335–339
147. Väätäinen N, Hannuksela M, Karvonen J (1979) Local photochemotherapy in nodular prurigo. Acta Derm Venereol 59:544–547
148. Väätäinen N, Hannuksela M, Karvonen J (1981) Trioxsalen baths plus UV-A in the treatment of lichen planus and urticaria pigmentosa. Clin Exp Dermatol 6:133–138
149. van den Hoogenband HM, van den Berg WHHW, van Diggelen MW (1985) PUVA therapy in the treatment of skin lesions of the hypereosinophilic syndrome. Arch Dermatol 121:450
150. van der Schaar WW, Sillevis Smitt JH (1984) An evaluation of PUVA therapy for alopecia areata. Dermatologica 168:250–252
151. van der Schroeff JG, Schothorst AA, Kanaar P (1983) Induction of actinic lichen planus with artificial UV sources. Arch Dermatol 119:498–500
152. Vella Briffa D, Eady RAJ, James MP, Gatti S, Bleehen SS (1983) Photochemotherapy (PUVA) in the treatment of urticaria pigmentosa. Br J Dermatol 109:67–75
153. Volkenandt M, Kerscher M, Sander C, Meurer M, Röcken M (1995) PUVA-bath photochemotherapy resulting in rapid clearance of lymphomatoid papulosis in a child. Arch Dermatol 131:1094
154. von Kobyletzki G, Gruss C, Altmeyer P, Kerscher M (1997) Balneophotochemotherapie des Lichen ruber. Hautarzt 48:323–327
155. Wakeel RA, Keefe M, Chapman RS (1991) Papuloerythroderma. Another case of a new disease. Arch Dermatol 127:96–98
156. Wallace BM, Lasker JS (1992) Awakenings... UV light and HIV gene activation. Science 257:1211–1212
157. Weiss DS, Taylor JR (1990) Treatment of generalized pruritus in an HIV-positive patient with UVB phototherapy. Clin Exp Dermatol 15:316–317
158. Wemmer U, Thiele B, Steigleder GK (1988) Hypereosinophilie-Syndrom (HES)—erfolgreiche PUVA-Therapie. Hautarzt 39:42–44
159. Willemze R, Beljaards RC (1993) Spectrum of primary cutaneous CD30 (Ki-1)-positive lymphoproliferative disorders. J Am Acad Dermatol 28:973–980
160. Wlaschek M, Heinen G, Poswig A, Schwarz A, Krieg T, Scharffetter-Kochanek K (1994) UVA-induced autocrine stimulation of fibroblast-derived collagenase/MMP-1 by interrelated loops of interleukin-1 and interleukin-6. Photochem Photobiol 59:550–556
161. Wong K, Ratnam KV (1990) A report of two cases of pigmented purpuric dermatoses treated with PUVA therapy. Acta Derm Venereol 71:68–70
162. Yamazaki S, Fujisawa T, Yanatori A, Yamakage A (1995) A case of lichen myxedematosus with clearly exacerbated skin eruptions after UVB irradiation. J Dermatol 22:590–593
163. Zakaria W, Passeron T, Ostovari N, Lacour JP, Ortonne JP (2004) 308-nm excimer laser therapy in alopecia areata. J Am Acad Dermatol 51:837–838
164. Ziemer A, Göring HD (1989) Disseminiertes Granuloma anulare—Rückbildung unter PUVA-Therapie. Z Hautkr 64:1095–1097
165. Zmudzka BZ, Beer JZ (1990) Activation of human immunodeficiency virus by ultraviolet radiation. Photochem Photobiol 52:1153–1162

第 10 章 光疗与 HIV 感染

H. McDonald, P. D. Cruz, Jr.

内容

引言 ·· 198
紫外线辐射安全性的证据 ··· 198
紫外线辐射诱发 HIV 活动的机制 ······························· 199
光疗副作用的潜在机制 ··· 200
光疗安全性的临床研究 ··· 201
指南 ·· 203

要点

- 体外研究表明,紫外线辐射可激活 HIV 基因表达。
- 为了修复紫外线造成的 DNA 损伤,细胞启动基因,包括 HIV 基因;然而对皮肤病毒载量增加的整体影响很小。
- 紫外线可能通过抑制 Th1 免疫反应和促进 Th2 免疫耐受免疫反应产生副作用。
- 光疗可以改善 HIV 感染者的银屑病、嗜酸性毛囊炎、特应性皮炎和瘙痒症。
- 没有令人信服的证据证明 UVB 或 PUVA 治疗会引起 HIV 感染者出现有害的系统性作用。

引言

由于大多数医疗干预生物事件在完成有益任务的过程中,不可避免地会出现意想不到的副作用。以前关于感染人类免疫缺陷病毒(HIV)患者的光疗就说明了光疗带来的双刃剑情况。自西方世界艾滋病疫情爆发25年来,现在我们有更多的关于各种光疗治疗HIV感染患者各种相关性疾病的临床疗效以及安全性的信息,包括银屑病、嗜酸性毛囊炎、特应性皮炎、痒疹。

在这一章节中,我们总结了紫外线(UV)辐射对HIV感染的影响,回顾了近年来HIV感染患者相关光疗的经验。

紫外线辐射安全性的证据

体外研究第一次表明紫外线辐射可增加促进HIV感染的可能性(表10.1)[1-5]。转染了HIV病毒的长末端重复序列(long terminal repeat,LTR)(是病毒复制的"开关"序列)的HeLa细胞,与编码氯霉素乙酰转移酶(chloramphenicol acetyl transferase,CAT)的报告基因融合,这一酶活性可以检测。通过CAT活性的检测测定了HeLa细胞暴露于不同波长紫外线下的活性变化。结果显示UVC(小于290nm)能够刺激CAT活性至50~150倍[2];PUVA,UVB+UVA2(280~340nm),或太阳光也能增强CAT活性,但增加的幅度较小[5]。相比之下,小于100nm和UVA1(340~400nm)的辐射均不会增强CAT活性[5]。

Valerie以及他的同事、Stanley与他的同事均证明了紫外辐射对HIV活性有更加明确的刺激作用。他们通过体外培养潜伏感染HIV的细胞,发现UVC,UVB,或太阳光能激活HIV本身(不仅仅HIV LTR结构)。

类似的结果也出现在转基因小鼠实验中。三组独立的研究人员利用不同转基因小鼠进行实验,测试紫外线辐射对HIV基因表达的影响(表10.2)[6-8]。Cavard和同事用细菌β-半乳糖苷酶连接到HIV-LTR上[6];Morrey和同事用荧光素酶用荧光素酶连接到HIV-LTR上[7];Vogel和同事直接利用HIV-LTR与TAT基因[8]。三组体内研究表明各种波长的紫外线辐射均导致各自的转基因编码蛋白在皮肤上的表达。与以前的体外研究结果一样[2-5],UVC,UVB,太阳光,特别是PUVA,都激活HIV[6-8],然而UVA没有激活作用[7]。

我们采用定量聚合酶链反应(PCR)测量HIV病毒在皮肤上的载量[9]。在HIV阳性的银屑病,嗜酸性毛囊炎,或痒疹患者中,我们在皮损和非皮损处皮肤中均检测到HIV。我们还发现最小红斑剂量的UVB在体内或体外辐射均能激活病毒6~10倍,这种研究结果类似于前面提到的细胞培养和转基因小鼠的研究结果[9]。相比之下,高剂量UVA-1却未激活病毒(观察结果尚未发表)。

第10章 光疗与HIV感染

表 10.1 体外研究显示紫外线辐射可能会促进 HIV 感染的可能性

年, 第一作者	因素	细胞系	结果
1987 Folks	佛波醇酯 GM-CSF IL-1, IL-2, IFNα, TNFα	感染 HIV 的幼稚单核细胞(U1)	佛波醇酯和 GM-CSF 刺激 HIV 复制；IL-1, IL-2, IFN-γ 和 TNF-α 不能
1988 Valerie	丝裂霉素 UVC(254nm) 阳光	HIV-LTR 控制的有 CAT 基因的 Hela 细胞 感染 HIV 的 T 细胞	丝裂霉素, UVC, 和阳光能增强 HIV-CAT 的表达 紫外线和阳光能刺激感染 HIV 的 T 细胞的复制
1989 Stanley	UVC(254nm) UVB(312nm) UVA(320~380nm)	感染 HIV 的幼稚单核细胞(U1)	UVB 和 UVC 能增加逆转录酶的活性和 P24, UVA 不能
1993 Zmudzka	PUVA	连接到 HIV 启动子上的有 CAT 基因的 Hela 细胞	PUVA 能增强 CAT 基因的活性
1994 Beer	UVC(254nm) UVB+UVA2 (280~340nm) UVA1(340~400nm) 辐射波长<100nm	连接到 HIV 启动子上的有 CAT 基因的 Hela 细胞	UVC 和 UVB+UVA2 能增强 CAT 基因的活性；UVA1 和辐射波长<100nm 不能
2001 Breuer-McHam	UVB	收集 HIV 阳性患者和暴露于体外 UVB 个体的皮肤样本	UVB 能使 HIV 在皮肤上的表达增加 6~10 倍

紫外线辐射诱发 HIV 活动的机制

紫外辐射如何激活 HIV？紫外线会引起 DNA 损伤，正常细胞试图修复这些 DNA 损伤。在修复过程中，细胞启动病毒（包括艾滋病）基因整合到宿主 DNA 中[10]。从这一点来看，有趣且值得注意的是，不同药物和不同 UV 治疗所诱导的 DNA 损伤与其其所报道的激活 HIV 的能力相关。例如，丝裂霉素 C、顺铂和蒽环类抗生素是众所周知的细胞毒性药物；UVC、UVB 和 PUVA 也是如此。已证实所有这些均能激活 HIV[2,11,12]。相比之下，UVA 的基因毒性较小，不能激活病毒[3]。

在细胞修复转换成 HIV 基因过程中发生了什么？修复过程包括让 DNA 分子解螺旋，从染色体内的高度自然卷曲状态到展开状态。在这种展开状态下，裸露的 DNA 部件不仅让修复 DNA 损伤的酶容易发挥修复作用，而且也可通过与转录因子结合而成为激活目标[13]。

表 10.2　紫外辐射对 HIV 基因表达影响的三组测试结果

年，第一作者	因素	转基因	结果
1990 Cavard	UVC(254nm) UVB(280~300nm)	细菌 lac-2（β-半乳糖苷酶 β 编码）受 HIV-LTR 控制	UVC 和 UVB 刺激 β-半乳糖苷酶在皮肤上的表达
1991 Morrey	UVB UVA PUVA 日光 补骨脂素+日光	受 HIV-LTR 基因控制的萤火虫荧光素酶	UVB、PUVA、日光、补骨脂素+日光均能激活萤火虫荧光素酶在皮肤上的活性，而 UVA 没有激活作用
1992 Vogel	UVC(254nm) UVB(290~320nm) 日光	LTR 和 TAT 的 HIV 基因	UVC、UVB 和阳光能够刺激转基因在皮肤上的表达

光疗副作用的潜在机制

理论上，光疗能够通过两个途径对艾滋病感染者产生不良影响。如前所述，一个直接的途径就是光疗能够活化增殖暴露于紫外线辐射下的组织如皮肤中的 HIV[1-8]。

因为 HIV 可以潜伏在感染细胞内多年，一些能够触发激活的因素则视为危险因素。另一方面，皮肤或许不是 HIV 的重要储存库[14-21]。因此，如果皮肤中病毒载量很小或几乎为零，即使紫外线照射能够引起 HIV 复制，其整体作用也是微乎其微。

紫外辐射也会间接产生不利影响。已证明 UVB 和 PUVA 疗法能够通过几个机制抑制 T 细胞介导的免疫反应，包括诱导抑制性 T 细胞，扰乱抗原呈递、皮肤细胞分泌(尤其是角质形成细胞)的免疫抑制细胞因子如白细胞介素-10、α-肿瘤坏死因子和抗原递呈细胞和T细胞在紫外线照射部位的迁入迁出改变[20-24]。推测UVB照射能够抑制保护性免疫应答(Th1)而增强耐受性免疫应答(Th2)[25]。值得注意的是,已被证明在许多HIV感染者进展为艾滋病过程中,其免疫反应从Th1免疫应答转向Th2主导的免疫应答,独立于紫外线辐射之外[26-28]。

无论发生的细胞机制如何,在分子水平上,NF-κB的转录途径参与了UV诱导的HIV激活。这种间接的证据来自于NFκB寡核苷酸诱饵和水杨酸钠,它们都是已被人们认知的能够抑制NF-κB通路的因素。这两个因素都有部分阻挡紫外线诱导HIV感染者皮肤中HIV活化的作用[9]。

光疗安全性的临床研究

用细胞系和转基因小鼠做的研究均不能完全模仿出人类自然感染艾滋病病毒所发生的情况。从某种意义上说,对HIV感染者好发的适合光疗的皮肤病进行研究可体内评估紫外线辐射对HIV感染患者的影响(表10.3)[11-18]。

Ranki等人、Horn等人分析了PUVA治疗对HIV感染者的银屑病、嗜酸性毛囊炎或瘙痒的影响。这两人的研究均证明了PUVA可有效缓解皮肤病。尽管Ranki等人记载了8例患者中有2例于光化学疗法后出现了轻微病毒复制的增加,但是还没有研究证明患者的免疫或临床状况出现明显恶化[12]。

也有用UVB治疗患有类似皮肤病的HIV感染患者的报道。Meola等人观察到除1例患者经过42次治疗后其HIV p24抗原呈阳性,其他所有患者的皮肤病经治疗后均得到改善,而免疫和病毒指标均没有恶化[14]。Fotiades等人对比了UVB治疗HIV阳性和HIV阴性患者银屑病的效果[16]。该两组患者的皮肤病症状均有明显改善,而HIV感染患者的免疫状态也没有恶化[16,17]。

DUVic等人的研究也对比了UVB对HIV阳性和HIV阴性患者银屑病治疗的影响[18]。其对比的结果是,尽管照射后CD4细胞计数不变,但是HIV感染患者的p24抗原水平却出现了显著的增加[18]。

Gelfand等人评估了UVB对HIV阳性患者各种皮肤疾病的(24次)治疗情况。观察到CD4细胞计数没有显著变化。他们还报道尽管至少有四名患者血浆HIV计数增加但是血浆中HIV病毒载量没有显著增加(定义为三倍增量)[19]。最近,Breur-McHam等人计算了HIV阳性患者经UVB治疗前后其皮肤上的HIV载量,显示HIV在皮肤上的载量增加了6~10倍[9]。

最近的研究表明使用5-氨基酮戊酸光动力治疗可降低艾滋病病毒感染者传染性软疣的数量和严重程度[29,30]。

临床研究并无令人信服的证据证明 UVB 或 PUVA 治疗对 HIV 感染者会造成不利影响。此外，有报道显示联合光疗可增加病毒复制，例如几个患者血浆中 p24 或 HIV 的 RNA 水平有所升高[12,15,18,19]。目前尚无光疗引起的系统性副作用的报道，尤其自使用组合抗逆转录病毒治疗艾滋病病毒感染者成为普遍现象以来。

表 10.3　紫外线对 HIV 感染者的治疗作用

年份，第一作者	治疗(治疗时间)	患者(病例数)	结果
1988 Buchness	UVB(6~9)	HIV 阳性的嗜酸性毛囊炎的患者($n=6$)	所有患者的瘙痒症状消失
1991 Ranki	PUVA(12~24)	HIV 阳性的银屑病、脂溢性皮炎、毛囊炎或慢性荨麻疹($n=5$)	所有患者银屑病症状有所改善；血浆 HIV 浓度没有增加；有 3 例患者皮肤检测由阴性转为阳性
1992 Pardo	UVB(8)	HIV 阳性的瘙痒性丘疹患者($n=8$)	7 例患者的瘙痒症状减轻；6 例患者的皮肤活检显示炎症减轻；血浆免疫球蛋白没有变化
1993 Meola	UVB(21~57)	HIV 阳性的银屑病患者($n=5$) HIV 阳性的瘙痒症患者($n=1$)	所有患者的临床症状得以改善；CBC，CD4，或 CD8 的计数没有变化；血清 β2 微球蛋白的水平；HIV-1 或 p24 的水平。没有机会性感染或恶性肿瘤发生
1994 Horn	PUVA(24)	HIV 阳性的银屑病、嗜酸性毛囊炎、瘙痒症患者($n=10$)	CD4 和病毒载量计数没有变化；没有机会性感染的发生 8 名被评估的患者中有 2 名患者在 2 个月内病毒载量有所增加
1995 Fotiades	UVB(21)	HIV 阳性的银屑病患者($n=10$) HIV 阴性的银屑病患者($n=10$)	CBC，CD4，或 CD8 计数或血清 β2 微球蛋白的水平没有变化
1995 Fotiades	UVB(42)	HIV 阳性的银屑病患者($n=28$)	淋巴细胞计数没有变化；12 例患者的 β2 微球蛋白的水平；没有机会性感染或恶性肿瘤发生

续表

年份,第一作者	治疗(治疗时间)	患者(病例数)	结果
1995 Duvic	UVB(18)	HIV 阳性的银屑病患者($n=28$) 使用 AZT($n=10$)或者 UVB 或 PUVA($n=10$)	CD4 计数没有变化,但是 p24 水平升高
1998 Gelfand	UVB(24)	HIV 阳性的嗜酸性毛囊炎患者($n=3$),瘙痒症患者($n=3$),痒疹($n=3$),特应性皮炎($n=2$)	CD4 计数没有变化;4 例患者显示 HIV 病毒载量有增加
2001 Breuer-McHam	UVB(1) UVB(6)	HIV 阳性的银屑病($n=5$),嗜酸性毛囊炎($n=7$),瘙痒症($n=6$) HIV 阳性的银屑病,嗜酸性毛囊炎和瘙痒症患者($n=16$)	皮肤上的 HIV 表达增加 6~10 倍

指南

我们认为患有光敏感性皮肤病的血清学上诊断为 HIV 的患者,其 UVB 和 PUVA 治疗是可行的选择。决定是否采用光疗取决于对以下问题的回答:
1. 是否是光敏感性皮肤病? 若答案肯定,考虑光疗。
2. 替代疗法是否给患者带来的风险更少? 如果是,首先尝试替代治疗或许是明智的选择。
3. 是否光疗对疾病的治疗作用远大于其潜在的风险? 如果是,请继续光疗。
4. 病人能否保证可以做足够的治疗次数? 如果可以,请继续治疗。如果否,考虑其他治疗。
5. 有没有其他光疗的禁忌证(如光敏性药物)? 如果有,要衡量利弊。

目前,我们建议 HIV 阳性患者患有皮肤病(尤其是银屑病、嗜酸性毛囊炎或原因不明的瘙痒)可作为光疗的人选。对于 HIV 阳性的患者,尤其是那些接受组合抗逆转录病毒治疗的患者,不管他们是否光疗,都要监测 CD4 细胞计数和病毒载量。

(李振洁 译,周欣　陈荃 校,朱慧兰 审)

参考文献

1. Folks TM et al (1995) Cytokine-induced expression of HIV-1 in a chronically infected promonocyte cell line. Science 228:800–802
2. Valerie K et al (1988) Activation of human immunodeficiency virus type 1 by DNA damage in human cells. Nature 333:78–81
3. Stanley SK, Folks TM, Fauci AS (1989) Induction of expression of human immunodeficiency virus in a chronically infected promonocytic cell line by ultraviolet irradiation. AIDS Res Hum Retroviruses 5:375–384
4. Zmudzka BZ et al (1993) Activation of the human immunodeficiency virus promoter by UVA radiation in combination with psoralens or angelicins. Photochem Photobiol 58:226–232
5. Beer JZ et al (1994) Reassessment of the differential effects of ultraviolet and ionizing radiation on HIV promoter: the use of cell survival as the basis for comparisons. Photochem Photobiol 59:643–649
6. Cavard C et al (1990) In vivo activation by ultraviolet rays of the human immunodeficiency virus type 1 long terminal repeat. J Clin Invest 86:1369–1374
7. Morrey JD et al (1991) In vivo activation of human immunodeficiency virus type 1 long terminal repeat by UV type A (UV-A) light plus psoralen and UV-B light in the skin of transgenic mice. J Virol 65:5045–5051
8. Vogel J et al (1992) UV activation of human immunodeficiency virus gene expression in transgenic mice. J Virol 66:1–5
9. Breuer-McHam J et al (2001) Activation of HIV in human skin by ultraviolet B radiation and its inhibition by NFκB blocking agents. Photochem Photobiol 74:805–810
10. Stern RS et al (1998) HIV-positive patients differ from HIV-negative patients in indications for and type of UV therapy used. J Am Acad Dermatol 39:48–55
11. Buchness MR et al (1988) Eosinophilic pustular folliculitis in the acquired immunodeficiency syndrome. N Eng J Med 318:1183–1186
12. Ranki A et al (1991) Effect of PUVA on immunologic and virologic findings in HIV-infected patients. J Am Acad Dermatol 24:404–410
13. Pardo RJ et al (1992) UVB phototherapy of the pruritic papular eruption of the acquired immunodeficiency syndrome. J Am Acad Dermatol 26:423–428
14. Meola T et al (1993) The safety of UVB phototherapy in patients with HIV infection. J Am Acad Dermatol 29:216–220
15. Horn TD et al (1994) Effects of psoralen plus UVA radiation (PUVA) on HIV-1 in human beings: a pilot study. J Am Acad Dermatol 31:735–740
16. Fotiades J et al (1995) Efficacy of ultraviolet B phototherapy for psoriasis in patients infected with human immunodeficiency virus. Photodermatol Photoimmunol Photomed 11:107–111
17. Fotiades J et al (1995) A three-year follow-up evaluation on 28 HIV-positive patients treated with ultraviolet B (UVB) phototherapy. J Invest Dermatol 104:660a
18. Duvic M et al (1995) Treatment of HIV+ patients with UVB is associated with a significant increase in p24 antigen levels. J Invest Dermatol 104:581
19. Gelfand JM et al (1998) Effect of UV-B phototherapy on plasma HIV type 1 RNA viral level: a self-controlled prospective study. Arch Dermatol 134:940–945
20. Simpson E, Dawson B, Cruz PD Jr (1997) UVB radiation activates HIV in human skin. J Invest Dermatol 110:485a
21. Lauerma AI et al (1994) Topical FK506: suppression of allergic and irritant contact dermatitis in the guinea pig. Arch Dermatol Res 286:337–340
22. Cruz PD Jr et al (2000) Thymidine dinucleotides inhibit contact hypersensitivity and activate the gene for TNFα. J Invest Dermatol 114:253–258
23. Romerdahl CA, Okamoto H, Kripke ML (1989) Immune surveillance against cutaneous malignancies in experimental animals. Immunol Ser 46:749–769

24. Kripke ML, Morison WL (1986) Studies on the mechanism of systemic suppression of contact hypersensitivity by UVB radiation. II. Differences in the suppression of delayed and contact hypersensitivity in mice. J Invest Dermatol 86:787–790
25. Ullrich SE (1996) Does exposure to UV radiation induce a shift to a Th-2-like immune reaction? Photochem Photobiol 64:254–258
26. Clerici M et al (1989) Detection of three distinct patterns of T helper cell dysfunction in asymptomatic, human immunodeficiency virus-seropositive patients. J Clin Invest 84:1892–1899
27. Clerici M, Shearer GM (1993) A T_H1/T_H2 switch is a critical step in the etiology of HIV infection. Immunol Today 14:107–111
28. Mosmann TR (1994) Cytokine patterns during the progression to AIDS. Science 265:193–194
29. Moiin A (2003) Photodynamic therapy for molluscum contagiosum infection in HIV-coinfected patients: review of 6 patients. J Drugs Dermatol 2:637–639
30. Gold MH et al (2004) The successful use of ALA-PDT in the treatment of recalcitrant molluscum contagiosum. J Drugs Dermatol 3:187–190

第 3 篇

特殊光疗模式

第2編

林業水文模式

第11章 光动力疗法在皮肤科的应用

R-M. szeimies, S. Karrer, C. Abels, M. Landthaler, C. A. Elmets

内容

引言 ································· 209
光动力疗法的元素 ····················· 211
皮肤科光动力疗法 ····················· 221
展望 ································· 235

引言

光动力疗法(photodynamic therapy, PDT)是一种应用系统或局部非补脂骨素光敏剂于个体的新型治疗方法。单独使用光敏剂是无效的,但一旦被高强度的光(通常为激光)激活,光敏剂能有效抑制过度增生组织的生长。由于几种光敏剂优先定位于肿瘤的独特性质,PDT最初设计用于治疗恶性肿瘤。第一代PDT光敏剂,卟吩姆钠已经在美国、加拿大、日本和欧洲获得监管机构的批准,用于治疗膀胱癌、食管癌和肺癌。尽管光动力学疗法还没有被正式批准为皮肤恶性肿瘤的治疗方法,其疗效已在一些浅表皮肤癌治疗的临床研究中得到论证[23,38,43,85,103,125,151,163,185]。目前这种方法正在进行临床试验,这表明了光动力学疗法在未来几年内可能会得到批准。由于皮肤的易及性,越来越多的使用这种新兴形式治疗银屑病以及其他良性皮肤疾病。

光动力疗法的历史

大约在一百年前Oscar Raab发现了光敏剂的作用和光致光敏剂损伤细胞。作为他的博士论文的一部分,他发现草履虫暴露于玫瑰红和可见光中,可致其死亡[131]。临床上应用光动力学疗法治疗一位70岁的面部鳞状细胞癌的女性患者首次被报道[73,169]。反复多次涂以5%伊红溶液,随之暴露于阳光或碳弧灯光中两个月。肿瘤愈合迅速,且具有良好的美容效果。1905 年,Von Tappeiner 和 Jesionek 报道了 PDT 治疗 6 例面部皮肤肿瘤,其中主要为基底细胞癌。每天使用同样的方法进行治疗,持续 2~8 周,共治愈 4 例(图 11.1 示)。1937 年,Silver 报道了其应用 PDT 成功治疗慢性炎症性皮肤病[151]。27 岁的慢性银屑病患者肌内注射和口服应用血卟啉后照射紫外线灯。这种治疗方法可以使银屑病大斑块得到部分缓解,小斑块得以完全缓解。尽管取得令人鼓舞的结果,但直到 20 世纪 60 年代初,Lipson 和 Baldes 静脉注射血卟啉衍生物进行组织定位实验,很少进行 PDT 治疗[101]。他们试图通过血卟啉光暴露后发出的荧光以检测诊断肿瘤。1966 年,他们通过系统应用血卟啉 PDT 治疗复发性溃疡型乳腺癌患者。尽管肿瘤反复治疗后复发,仍能观察到显著的治疗效果[102]。

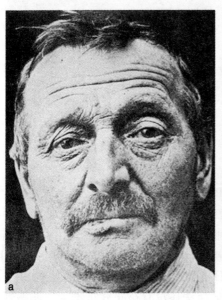 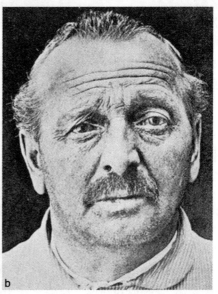

图 11.1 **a.** 55 岁男性患者,下唇溃疡型基底细胞癌。PDT 治疗:应用伊红溶液(浓度达到 5%)后,随之光曝露在 1904 年 3 月和 5 月份之间进行。**b.** 治疗结束时观察到患处完全再生上皮化,并且相隔一年后无复发[73]

20 世纪 70 年代中期,Thomas Dougherty 表明,在动物模型中应用血卟啉衍生物后照氙弧灯,多种不同类型的肿瘤能够得到治疗或完全缓解[37]。血卟啉衍生物(HpD)是一种从酯化和醚化血卟啉类而来的低聚混合物。三年后,他进行了第一次临床试验,全身应用 HpD-PDT 成功地治疗了 25 例皮肤及皮下恶性肿瘤患者。试验表明,在 113 个肿瘤中的 111 个得到完全或部分缓解[38]。在世界上的几个国家中,血卟啉衍生物(卟吩姆钠,商品名又称为光卟啉或 Photosan-3)-PDT 已被批准于临床使用。

氨基酮戊酸(aminolevulinic acid, ALA)是最新的获得监管部门批准的 PDT 药物。在这方面,它的主要适应证为光线性角化病。ALA 本身并不是一种光敏剂,但它可代谢转化成具有光敏能力的原卟啉 IX(PpIX)。ALA 的主要优势是它可外用于皮肤,因此与皮肤光敏性延长无关。

尽管卟吩姆钠(血卟啉)被用于临床治疗恶性肿瘤患者。但它不是一种纯化合物;用于治疗的光源波长渗入组织的深度通常不够;治疗常伴有严重的皮肤光敏性,这可能会持续长达 2 个月。由于这些缺陷,更少缺陷的二代光敏剂正处于研发和评估阶段。

光动力疗法的元素

光动力疗法需要同时存在的氧气、组织中可吸收光的光敏剂,以及适合波长的光(图 11.2)。

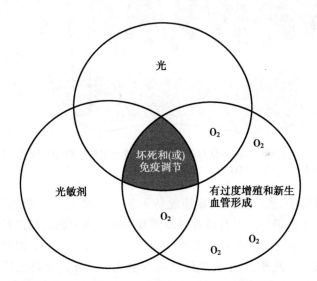

图 11.2 有效的 PDT 主要需要一个光敏剂、氧气及靶位点的光敏化光源的同时存在。如果其中缺失一个元素,PDT 不起作用

光源与剂量

尽管卟吩姆钠(光卟啉)与其他卟啉化合物一样,在较短的波长中具有较强的吸收峰,如在 630nm 处的吸收峰可最有效地利用光卟啉-PDT 实现光穿透组织的最大深度,以保证光敏剂能足够吸收光子。然而,即便在这个波长,渗透到皮肤的深度也小于 4mm。目前,常选择的光源为氩离子染料激光($\lambda=630$nm)和金

蒸气激光（λ=628nm），因为它们与光敏剂的吸收带630nm相适应（图11.3示）。对于大多数非皮肤恶性肿瘤的治疗，如膀胱、胃肠道及支气管，将光耦合到高功率密度的光纤系统中是非常必要的。使用这些激光系统的主要缺点是它们的成本高，并且需要持续更换和维护光学零件。在过去的几年里，因为半导体激光更便宜、更可靠，已发展成一个有前途的领域。此外，它们比染料激光器要小得多。

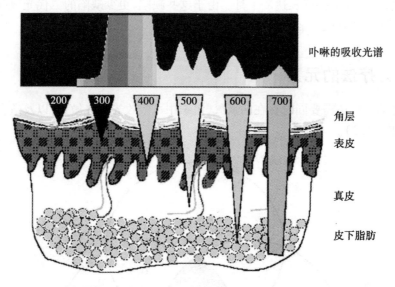

图11.3 波长越大（最多至1100nm），光渗透到组织中越深。因此，卟啉吸收峰630nm应用于PDT

在皮肤病学中，耦合光到内窥镜设备不是必须的。因此，在皮肤科PDT可以使用非相干光源进行。具有特殊过滤器和高功率密度的幻灯片投影仪已被用于照光[50,85,182]，并且市场上可以买到一些高性能的灯[159]。非相干光源的另一个优点是低成本。此外，一个更广泛的发射光谱的光源允许使用具体不同吸收峰的光敏剂（表11.1）[158]。

为了避免非特异性的热效应，在治疗区，光的强度不应超过$200mW/cm^2$。因为皮肤上的瘢痕、结痂、鳞屑和黑色素能影响光到达组织中的数量，所以，选择最适合的光能量密度时必须把它们带入考量。为了建立光照强度和光照密度的标准化方案，一个标准的PDT光剂量必须按不同的光敏剂去确定。实验和临床经验表明，在光卟啉PDT中，$100\sim150J/cm^2$的小剂量治疗肿瘤是必要的。应用这些参数的照射程序通常需要不到30分钟。用于治疗慢性炎症性皮肤病例如银屑病，需要不到一半的光剂量[23,100]。相关的亚致死损伤或PDT诱导的免疫调节作用是造成治疗反应的原因。此外，可以分级处理这些迹象。

表 11.1　不同 PDT 光源比较

光源	优点	缺点
阳光	免费	可用剂量测定
激光（金属蒸气、气体、染料激光）	可以连接到纤维 剂量可控	价格昂贵 需要维护 系统固定 常限制一个波长
二极管激光器	可以连接到光纤 剂量可控 相对便宜	目前只有较大的波长（630nm 及以上） 仅限于一个波长
宽光谱	价格低廉 可使用于几种光敏剂 照明范围大剂量	只可能照到表面

光敏剂

光卟啉是唯一得到监管部门批准的用于治疗肿瘤的光敏剂。尽管它被证实有效，但该药有几个特点，限制了其治疗应用：

1. 作为一个纯化合物，不能人工合成。

2. 与正常组织相比，它的选择性积累较差。

3. 大多数光卟啉 PDT 方案选择 625～630nm 之间的光源。这些光源穿透组织的最大深度约为 3mm。拥有更长波长的光可激活更好的光敏剂，因为光的长波具有更大的组织穿透深度。

4. 光卟啉只有通过静脉注射才有效。

5. 使用光敏剂后，在药物被光激活之前，有一个 24～27 小时的等待期。大多数治疗方案要求进行 2 次随访。

6. 光卟啉与严重而持久的皮肤光敏相关。这一问题已被归因于皮肤科长期保留这种光敏剂。（图 11.4）

用于理想的皮肤科药物应具有以下特点：

1. 纯化学物质。由于有关审批的法律要求和专利药物，只有化学物质纯净，才会被评估。

2. 高产量的单态氧。大多数光敏剂产生单线态氧产率为 5%～20%[144]。与低量子产率的物质相比，单态氧高产率的物质可以其较少的物质积累即引起

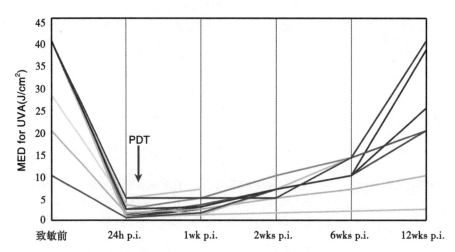

图 11.4 检测 HpD-PDT 治疗泌尿生殖系统和胃肠道肿瘤患者（$n=16$）随时间推移的 UVA 致其的最小红斑量（MED）

组织内的光动力学反应。然而,这样的考虑只具有理论价值,作为光敏剂还需取决于其染料的生物化学性质（例如,亲脂性或亲水性）,它可影响药物在亚细胞的分布[87,99,187]（表11.2）。

表 11.2 细胞吸收和不同光敏剂的定位

光敏剂	细胞的吸收机制	细胞内分布
亲水性（若丹明、菁、氯、光谱）	胞饮作用	胞内体 溶酶体
亲脂性（卟啉、酞菁）	扩散 低密度脂蛋白介导的内吞作用	膜（核膜、质膜和细胞器膜）

3. 渗透到组织的深度。正如已经提到的,光穿透到组织的深度相当有限。目前正在受评估的光敏剂有 600 到 700nm 之前的吸收峰。在这些波长下,病变只能是 3~4mm 厚度。在近红外区域吸收的合成物质,也产生了高量子产率的单态氧,利于较厚肿瘤的治疗。炎症性皮肤病如银屑病,光敏剂的渗透深度似乎是足够的。

4. 靶组织选择性的积累。光敏剂对病变组织的选择性高,则在 PDT 治疗中周围的组织损伤较少。多发性病变（如:光线性角化病）可达到极佳的美容效果[83,161]（图 11.5）。尽管组织靶向性是一个不错的特性,但应该指出的是,对于

第 11 章 光动力疗法在皮肤科的应用

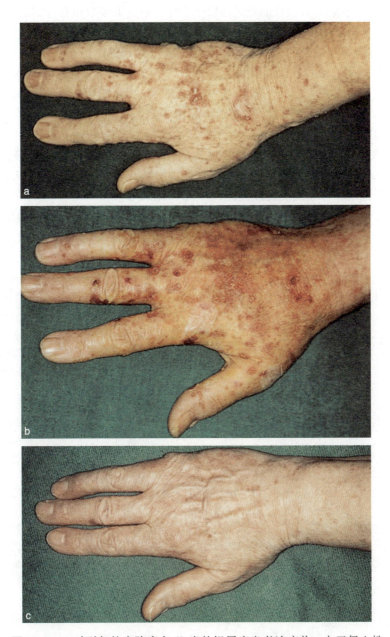

图 11.5 **a.** 砷引起的皮肤癌在 62 岁的银屑病患者治疗前。由于侵入性 Bowen 病,右手第 5 指已被截肢。**b.** 外用 ALA-PDT 治疗后 3 天:炎症和溃疡受限于受影响的组织。**c.** PDT 治疗后 6 个月:活组织检查证实完全缓解(许可转载自)[160]

大多数 PDT 光敏剂,其吸收的靶向性仅是中等。目前大多数正在评估的光敏剂被吸收到肿瘤和正常组织中的比例一般约为 3∶1。光源的限制和作用区域的给药方式,也有助于 PDT 的靶向选择性。已经尝试通过将其整合到脂质体中,增强光敏剂的选择性酯化,或将它们连接到抗体中[100,146]。总体来看,这些尝试收效不大。

目前正在临床使用的光敏剂在评估中显示,ALA 的组织靶向性最高[2,96]。外用 ALA 后病变部位(肿瘤)和周围组织中的药物比例大于 10∶1[93,162]。这种选择性的原因尚不清楚。

5. 缺乏皮肤光敏性。广义的皮肤光敏性,可能会持续一周,系统光动力治疗后对患者的生活质量会产生一个戏剧性的影响,最佳的光敏剂应该很少或没有这一副作用。它应该被迅速代谢,不应积累在皮肤。

目前一批二代光敏剂正处于评估阶段,它们有潜质可能作为光卟啉的补充或替代。表 11.3 显示了目前正在临床研究中的光敏剂其潜在的适应证和各自的性质。

表 11.3 光敏剂在皮肤病学中潜在的作用和发展现状

公司	光敏剂	波长	意义	使用途径	现状
QLT 光疗、Sanofi Winthrop,美国、欧洲	卟吩姆钠(光卟啉)	630nm	已批准用于治疗膀胱癌、食管癌和肺癌;尚在评估中的基底细胞癌和皮肤转移癌	静脉注射	批准用于加拿大、美国、日本、欧洲;皮肤肿瘤的Ⅱ/Ⅲ期
DUsA、Berlex,美国	5-氨基酮戊酸(ALA,Levulan)	635nm	日光性角化病、BCC、皮肤 T-cell 淋巴瘤、永久性头发脱失	局部	在美国批准用于光线性角化病(蓝光)
Medac,德国	ALA、spectrila	635nm	膀胱癌的诊断	膀胱内	预期德国在2001年批准
Photocure,挪威	ALA-methylester、Metvix	635nm	日光性角化病,基底细胞癌	局部	Ⅱ/Ⅲ期
Miravant,美国	Tin ethyl etiopurpurin(snET$_2$,purlytin)	660~665nm	卡波西肉瘤的皮肤转移,黄斑变性	静脉、液体扩散	Ⅱ/Ⅲ期
Pharmacyclics,美国	Lutetium texaphyrin PCI-0123(Lu-Tex)	720~760nm	皮肤肿瘤	静脉注射	Ⅱ/Ⅲ期
Cytopharm Inc.,美国	9-Acetoxy-2,7,12,17-tetrakis-(β-methoxyethyl)-porphycen(ATMPn)	640nm	银屑病	局部	Ⅱ期

续表

公司	光敏剂	波长	意义	使用途径	现状
QLT PhotoTherapeutics,加拿大	Benzoporphyrin derivative monoacid ring A (BPD-MA, Verteporfin)	690nm	基底细胞癌、银屑病、黄斑变性(MD)	静脉、脂质体配方	Ⅱ期、已批准用于MD
scotia Pharmaceuticals,英国	meso-tetra-hydroxy-phenyl-chlorin (mTHPC,Foscan)	650nm	基底细胞癌、头颈部肿瘤	静脉、局部	Ⅰ/Ⅱ期
Nippon Petrochemical,日本	Mono-L-aspartyl chlorin e6(NPe6)	660~665nm	皮肤肿瘤	静脉	Ⅰ/Ⅱ期

*作者不要求本表的完整性。因为他们已在文献或电子媒体中报道过这些商品名

最近,在美国 ALA 被批准用于治疗光线性角化病。ALA 的作用机制相当独特。ALA 不是一种光敏剂,而是血红素生物合成途径的代谢产物,其可诱导卟啉的合成,特别是原卟啉 IX[15,158]。其吸收增强,合成卟啉增强,或因病变导致细胞酶活性降低,血红素生成减少等可能是这种光敏剂的选择性积累的原因[84](图 11.6)。

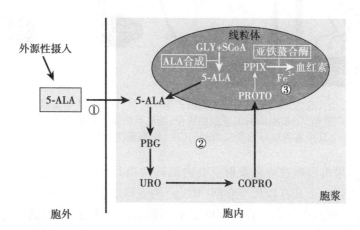

图 11.6 血红素的生物合成:当绕过负反馈机制(ALA 合成)时,卟啉代谢产物积累。合成卟啉的组织选择性基于吸收增强的 ALA(1),卟啉合成增强(2),或减低亚铁螯合酶的活性(3)。GLY,甘氨酸;SCoA,乙酰辅酶 A;5-ALA,5-氨基酮戊酸;PBG,胆色素原;URO,尿卟啉原;COPRO,粪卟啉原;PROTO,原卟啉原;PpIX,原卟啉 IX

作用机制

氧依赖

PDT诱导的作用是通过光氧化反应介导的(图11.7)。"光动力"一词是用于区分其他不需要氧气的反应过程。在治疗照射过程中,光敏剂吸收光,使其转化为能量较高的状态——单状态。经过一个短的半衰期(约10^{-9}秒),被激活的光敏剂返回激态。

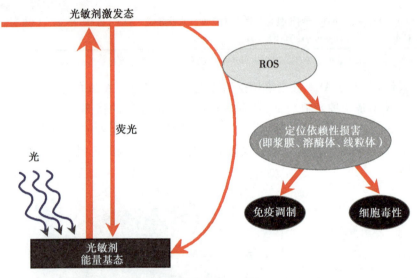

图11.7 处于激发态的光敏剂分子能够产生活性氧(ROS),主要是经光氧化的单态氧(反应Ⅱ型)。根据染料的亚细胞定位,细胞器的特发损害常发生。特定的损伤位点加上其损害程度导致免疫调制和(或)细胞毒性

这一结果可以通过荧光发射或其内部转换得到。另外,被激活的光敏剂从单重态变化到一个具有较长半衰期(10^{-3}s)的更稳定的三重态("窜跃")。在Ⅰ型光氧化反应中,有一个氢直接和电子从光敏剂的三重态转移到底物。底物反应生成自由基。这些自由基能与分子氧形成过氧化物,生成羟基自由基、超氧阴离子。这种类型的反应具有强烈的浓度依赖性。通过反应可对细胞产生直接损伤。尤其是容易被光敏剂氧化的分子。在Ⅱ型反应中,能量或电子被直接转移到分子氧的基态(三重态),形成单重态氧。单重态氧的高反应状态发生引起一种非常有效的生物底物氧化途径。这两种反应类型可以同时发生。需要注意的是,在何种程度上发生何种反应取决于光敏剂,染料的亚细胞定位,底物和氧气供应被激活的光敏剂,而不是其他条件。尽管有来自实验室的数据表明,超氧阴

离子可能参与皮肤光敏性的进展[11,12],但体外间接实验表明,单态氧是许多PDT诱导的生物学效应的主要中介[76,176]。

生物学机制

PDT 的生物学效应可分为直接作用和间接作用。直接作用指对肿瘤细胞的直接作用。间接作用是指 PDT 对免疫反应和炎症反应的作用,及对肿瘤血管的作用,其通过限制血液供应肿瘤,促进肿瘤消退。

直接作用

PDT 治疗后可以检测对细胞的直接损伤[97]。二磺化和硅酞菁光敏剂介导肿瘤破坏似乎是主要的机制[8,48]。除了光敏剂的类型,对细胞结构的影响取决于在光照处理时光敏剂的亚细胞定位。据报道,PDT 损伤细胞结构包括线粒体[87]、溶酶体[178]和内质网[113]。膜损伤引起一系列反应导致细胞凋亡,并可以影响细胞周期调节蛋白[4];可在体内和体外检测细胞凋亡。在分子水平上,PDT也可以诱导应激蛋白[57](图 11.8)。

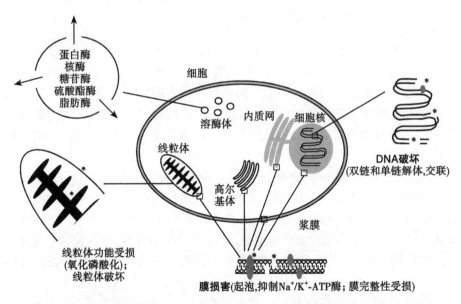

图 11.8 PDT 相关亚细胞损伤取决于光敏剂的定位应用。重大损害大多发生在细胞膜和线粒体、溶酶体。这将导致膜的完整性受损、溶酶体酶的释放和呼吸链受损。DNA 受损对细胞死亡的作用不显著

间接作用

当光敏剂应用于 PDT 中,间接效应占主导地位,最重要的生物效应是病理上对肿瘤血管产生不可逆性损害破坏[47,64](图 11.9)。

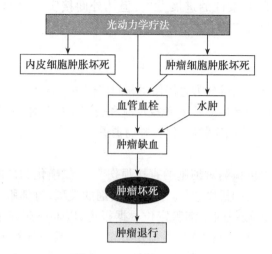

图11.9 在细胞水平上，PDT 导致内皮细胞和肿瘤细胞肿胀和/或坏死。血栓形成后，肿瘤细胞的高脆性导致血管闭塞。细胞肿胀和血管周围水肿，致组织间质压力增大，压迫血管，随后发生肿瘤缺血

光敏剂 PDT 可引起动脉瘤内血管收缩，及周围组织静脉的红细胞流速降低，肿瘤血管内血液淤滞及血栓形成，血管周围水肿[28,31,46,153]。当使用足量光敏剂和光时，影响是不可逆的。组织间隙压力增大同时压迫肿瘤血管[60,98]，随后肿瘤缺血，肿瘤细胞内高能磷酸盐累积[32]。组胺释放[86]，花生四烯酸的代谢产物诱导，如前列腺素 E2[65]，血栓烷 B2[46]，以及其他促凝物质，例如，血管性假血友病因子[51]，参与周围组织和肿瘤中的血管效应[92]。

除了对肿瘤血管的间接影响，还有许多免疫和炎症作用，至少部分造成 PDT 诱导的肿瘤消融。这些作用也被用于治疗一些良性病变[35,36,90]。PDT 治疗的组织中均可发现深部的炎症，并有令人信服的证据表明炎症细胞参与 PDT 诱导肿瘤衰退[29,31,47,91]。例如，在动物模型中，光敏剂 PDT 治疗后，中性粒细胞减少症可显著降低治愈率[29,89]。此外，PDT 通过共同作用于粒细胞集落刺激因子(G-CSF)及细胞因子增加中性粒细胞计数，实验性 PDT 的疗效可显著提高。

单核/巨噬细胞也有助于 PDT 诱导肿瘤转归。在小鼠实验中，低浓度的卟啉和光有免疫增强作用[189,190]。这可能是因为光敏剂 PDT 治疗后，巨噬细胞可优先针对 PDT 治疗癌细胞，释放肿瘤坏死因子(TNF-α)[41,88]。

T 细胞介导的免疫，也有助于 PDT 诱导的肿瘤治疗。肿瘤特异性 T 细胞可以消除恶性细胞的小病灶，这可能是肿瘤细胞直接受 PDT 的细胞毒性和血管效应影响而被消除的方式。一项强有力的证据表明，PDT 实际可诱导肿瘤特异性免疫；来自动物的研究模型表明，在免疫缺陷小鼠中不能实现长期的肿瘤治愈，

但可在免疫功能正常的动物中发生[89,90]。

炎症过程通常是由促炎症介质的合成与释放开始[9,41,56,119]。PDT 增加了几种介质的产生。组胺和其他血管活性胺[9]，细胞因子如 TNF-α[9,41,119]、白细胞介素-2(IL-2)[119]、IL-6[56]、IL-10[56]、IL-1[30]和粒细胞集落刺激因子[30]，急性期反应物[45,122]及补体成分均被报道在行 PDT 后有所增加。

相对于浅表皮肤癌或癌前病变的治疗，慢性炎症性皮肤病的治疗目标不是组织不可逆性损伤。对于 PDT 免疫抑制效应，文献中的证据显示，如减少接触性超敏反应，增加皮肤移植存活率及改善实验性自身免疫性疾病如胶原诱导性关节炎和实验性变态性脑脊髓炎[21,39,66,74,100,107,121,130,132,135,139]。PDT 诱导的免疫效应研究是今后研究的一个重要方向，将有助于确定 PDT 新适应证。

皮肤科光动力疗法

表 11.4 概述 PDT 在皮肤科的临床适应证。与其他器官相比，皮肤在静脉或直接外用或注射光敏剂致敏后，可更容易接触到光。

表 11.4　皮肤科中的 PDT 适应证

肿　瘤	非肿瘤
光化性角化病(也含砷角化病)	寻常型银屑病
Bowen 病	HPV 相关皮肤病
浅基底细胞癌	疣状表皮发育不良
Gorlin-Goltz 综合征	尖锐湿疣
角化棘皮瘤	
鳞状细胞癌初期	
卡波西肉瘤	
蕈样肉芽肿	
皮肤转移	

系统光动力疗法

卟啉混合物 HpD 和部分纯化及临床批准的形式——卟吩姆钠目前广泛应用于临床。系统疗法可用于治疗皮肤肿瘤。包括鲍温病、基底细胞癌、鳞状细胞癌和复发性转移性乳腺癌(表 11.5)。尽管大量光动力学系统疗法治疗非黑色素瘤皮肤癌的临床研究已经发表，但大部分是不受控制的开放性试验；试验中，小数目的患者使用多种药物浓度和光照剂量，随访时间、肿瘤类型及患者个体均有差异。

表 11.5　系统光动力治疗皮肤肿瘤的适应证治疗情况及疗效

适应证	著者	治疗的病变	敏化剂及治疗	波长、光及其剂量	完全缓解率
鲍温病	Waldow et al. 1987[171]	3	光卟啉 2.0mg/kg	630nm 40~60J/cm²	100%
	Robinson et al. 1988[140]	>500 90	光卟啉 2.0 vs 1.0mg/kg	628nm 25 vs 50J/cm²	100% 50%
	BucHAnan et al. 1989[24]	50	光卟啉 2.0mg/kg	630nm 50J/cm²	98%
	McCaughan et al. 1989[109]	2	HpD/光卟啉 3.0/2.0mg/kg	630nm 20~30J/cm²	50%
	Jones et al. 1992[75]	8	光卟啉 1.0mg/kg	630nm 185~250J/cm²	100%
鳞癌	Pennington et al. 1988[128]	32	HpD 5.0mg/kg	630nm 30J/cm²	<50%
	McCaughan et al. 1989[109]	5	HpD/光卟啉 3.0/2.0mg/kg	630nm 20~30J/cm²	40%
	Gross et al. 1990[58]	1	光卟啉 2.0mg/kg	630nm 150J/cm²	100%
	Feyh et al. 1993[42]	7	Photosan-3 2.0mg/kg	630nm 100J/cm²	86%
基底细胞癌	Tse et al. 1984[167]	40	HpD 3.0mg/kg	600~700nm 38~180J/cm²	83%
	Bandieramonte et al. 1984[14]	42	HpD 3.0mg/kg	480~515, 630nm 60~120J/cm²	60%
	Waldow et al. 1987[171]	6	光卟啉 1.5~2.0mg/kg	630nm 40~60J/cm²	100%
	Pennington et al. 1988[128]	21	HpD 5.0mg/kg	630nm 30J/cm²	0%
	Robinson et al. 1988[140]	15	光卟啉 2.0mg/kg	628nm 50J/cm²	93%
	Buchanan et al. 1989[24]	13	光卟啉 1.5~2.0mg/kg	630nm 50~100J/cm²	39%

续表

适应证	著者	治疗的病变	敏化剂及治疗	波长、光及其剂量	完全缓解率
乳癌的皮肤转移（最后一列为完全缓解率和部分缓解率）	McCaughan et al. 1989[109]	27	HpD/光卟啉 3.0/2.0mg/kg	630nm 20~30J/cm²	15%
	Feyh et al. 1993[42]	67	Photosan-3 2.0mg/kg	630nm 100J/cm²	97%
	Calzavara et al. 1991[26]	17	HpD/光卟啉 3.0/2.5~3.0mg/kg	600~700nm 25~225J/cm²	59%
	Wilson et al. 1992[180]	151	光卟啉 1.0mg/kg	630nm 72~288J/cm²	89%
	Hintschich et al. 1993[67]	27	Photosan-3 2.0mg/kg	630nm 100J/cm²	52%
	Dougherty 1981[34]	35	HpD 2.5~5.0mg/kg	? ?	97%
	schuh et al. 1987[147]	30	光卟啉 1.0~2.0mg/kg	630nm 36~288J/cm²	80%
	McCaughan et al. 1989[109]	29	HpD/光卟啉 3.0/2.0mg/kg	630nm 20~30J/cm²	100%
	Sperduto et al. 1991[152]	20	光卟啉 1.5mg/kg	630nm 20~359J/cm²	65%
	综述 schlag et al. 1992[145]	846	HpD/光卟啉 1.0~5.0mg/kg	- 8~300J/cm²	83%

系统 PDT 治疗肿瘤适应证

光卟啉和血卟啉衍生物

系统 PDT 疗法治疗鲍温病非常有效。联合卟吩姆钠（2mg/kg b. w.）和波长为 630nm 的光（20~50J/cm²）治疗治愈率可达 98%~100%[24,140,171]。低剂量的卟吩姆钠（1 毫克/公斤体重）用来减少皮肤光敏反应。完全缓解的鲍温病（$n=8$）也可使用高光剂量（630nm, 185~250J/cm²）[75]。然而，应用光剂量 50~100J/cm² 和卟吩姆钠 1mg/kg b. w. 却只有 50% 治愈率[24,140]。

系统 PDT 治疗皮肤鳞癌的疗效不及鲍温病。有报道随访用 HpD-PDT（HpD 剂量:5mg/kg b. w.）治疗后 6 个月的 32 例 SCC 患者复发率为 50%[128]。对于低反应率的一个合理解释可能是这项研究使用低剂量光（30J/cm²）。类似的结果也被McCaughan等报道,HpD(3mg/kg b. w.)和光卟啉(2mg/kg b. w.)也采用20~30J/cm²的低剂量光[109]。应用PDT治疗后1年的5例SCC患者缓解率却只有40%。只有一个案例报道显示随访系统应用PDT治疗后6个月的下唇大片鳞癌患者得到完全缓解(卟吩姆钠,2mg/kg b. w.,630nm,150J/cm²)[58]。

系统治疗基底细胞癌(BCC)有更多的经验报道。1981年,Dougherty第一次使用HpD(5mg/kg b. w.)治疗一位面部有3处基底细胞癌的72岁男患者。HpD给药4天和5天后分别照射氙气灯(600~700nm,100mW/cm²,120J/cm²)。Feyh等应用HpD(2mg/kg b. w.)联合氩离子泵浦染料激光(630nm,100J/cm²)治疗67例BCC患者。在4.5年的随访中,仅有3例复发[42]。另一项研究显示,同一组使用相同参数治疗位于眼睑的基底细胞癌皮损的反应性低[67]。Tse等使用HpD联合染料激光或氙气灯治疗3例有40处基底细胞癌皮损的痣样基底细胞癌综合征患者。所有肿瘤均在行治疗后4~6周内得到临床治愈。然而,治疗后的肿瘤组织学检查发现,17.5%患者中发现肿瘤细胞巢。在长达12~14个月的随访期中,复发率为10.8%。反复发作的、皮损较大的、溃疡样或结痂的肿瘤反应性较差[167]。

系统治疗的另一个适应证是乳腺癌皮肤转移的姑息治疗[145]。在所报道的病例中,PDT在常规疗法(放疗、化疗、激素治疗、常规手术)失效时实施。治疗目的是消除瘤体或减少瘤体体积,以避免发生溃疡或无法控制的出血(表11.5）。Dougherty对35例乳腺癌皮肤转移的患者行HpD-PDT治疗4~6周后,34例患者得到部分缓解(瘤体体积减少>50%)[34]。McCaughan在对乳腺癌皮肤转移的患者应用HpD(3mg/kg b. w.)或卟吩姆钠(2mg/kg b. w.),随后行光照射(60~120J/cm²)后,得到部分或完全缓解[109]。在对所有行系统PDT治疗的乳腺癌皮肤转移患者(n=118,病灶总数=846)的统计中,schlag等人发现得到治疗的病变中63%得到完全缓解,20%得到部分缓解,16%对治疗没有反应[145]。直径小于2cm的肿瘤可得到最好的治疗效果。

Boehncke等人发现在体外,使用不同的光敏剂浓度和光剂量(UVA 0.75J/cm²对630nm激光,1J/cm²)PDT治疗皮肤T淋巴细胞瘤可产生与补骨脂素联合紫外线A(即PUVA)类似效果[22]。1980年,Forbes等人成功地治疗1例斑块期蕈样肉芽肿患者,HpD(5mg/kg b. w.)和重复照射非相干光源(λ=620~640nm,40mW/cm²,48~96J/cm²,使用敏化剂后72小时及96小时照射)[50]。他使用同样的治疗方案治疗转移性卡波西肉瘤患者,实现部分缓解[50]。Dougherty[34]和Calzavara[26]应用2.5~3.0mg/kg b. w. HpD,分别使用光剂量120J/cm²、50~200J/cm²,治疗经典地中海卡波西肉瘤患者。PDT治疗的3例患者所有瘤体和4例患者85%瘤体显示完全缓解。

schweitzer 和 Visscher 应用卟吩姆钠 2mg/kg b. w. ,皮肤表面间歇性照射红光(50~200J/cm^2)治疗 5 例艾滋病相关卡波西肉瘤。观察 8 周后,其 92 个病变灶中的 54 个(58.7%)皮肤或黏膜结节性病变得到完全或部分缓解[150]。Hebeda 等人得出几乎相同的结果。其应用卟吩姆钠 2mg/kg b. w. 联合染料激光(630nm,70~120J/cm^2)照射治疗 8 例共有 83 处卡波西肉瘤病灶的 HIV 阳性患者。尽管缓解率达 60%~70%,但由于发生持久性色素沉着和瘢痕形成,美容效果不佳[63]。

第二代光敏剂

苯并卟啉衍生物单环(维替泊芬,BPD-MA)代表一系列的第一代光敏剂光卟啉和 HpD 的替代品。它有一个显著较短的组织半衰期。它是一种来自 PpIX 的半卟啉合成物。该药的一个主要优点是,给药时间和照射时间可以是同一天。不同于 HpD,BPD-MA 以惰性形式代谢和分泌[16,162]。其潜在的敏感性皮肤光敏性时间为小于 72 小时[103,186]。Ⅰ/Ⅱ期研究证实 BPD-MA 在治疗一些上皮性皮肤肿瘤的有效性,静脉注射 0.375~0.50mg/kg b. w. 脂质体配方药物,随之照射波长为 690nm(50~150J/cm^2)光 2 至 6 小时。达到约 100% 的缓解率[100]。

一种扩展的卟啉大环化合物 lutetium texaphyrin 的Ⅰ期研究,已经完成对 19 例基底细胞癌、卡波西肉瘤和转移性黑色素瘤患者的观察。这种药剂的吸收波长峰值是 732nm,这允许在组织内有更大的渗透深度。这种光敏剂似乎比正常皮肤对肿瘤有高度的选择性,当系统给药时没有明显的皮肤光毒性[136]。

SnET$_2$,是一种卟啉类光敏剂,目前正处于治疗皮肤转移性乳腺癌、卡波西肉瘤的Ⅱ期临床试验中[36]。有报道称在总共 121 处卡波息肉瘤病灶的患者中,整体有 75% 的完全缓解率并美容效果极佳[5]。有 8 例晚期乳腺癌转移(病灶数 86 个)的患者行单一 PDT 治疗,使用 SnET$_2$(1.2mg/kg b. w.)和激光(660±3nm,150mW/cm^2,200J/cm^2),完全有效率为 92%[6]。

另一种卟吩光敏剂——tetra(m-hydroxyphenyl) chlorin(mTHPC),含有间-羟基苯基,在欧洲和美国,正进行对头部和颈部癌症的临床试验;mTHPC 似乎是最有效的,且只需非常低的药物剂量和光剂量的光敏剂[33]。

另一种新的活性光敏剂,单-L-天冬酰胺二氢卟吩 E6(Npe6)在Ⅰ期临床研究中对 11 例有实体肿瘤(基底细胞癌、鳞癌、复发性乳腺癌)的患者进行评价[165]。Npe6 可迅速从组织中清除,从而减少皮肤光敏性的时间。应用 Npe6 2.5~3.5mg/kg b. w. 联合光能量密度 100J/cm^2 治疗后,随访 12 周,66% 的癌灶无复发。

系统 PDT 疗法治疗非肿瘤性皮肤病适应证

银屑病

早在 1937 年初,Silver 报道了应用血卟啉和紫外线光治疗银屑病的临床应用。6例银屑病患者接受肌肉注射和口服HpD连续数日后用UV光照射。治疗开始后2周,观察到银屑病斑块明显减少[151]。静脉注射低剂量血卟啉衍生物(1mg/kg b.w.)和紫外线照射,治疗15天可使90%的斑块型银屑病患者得到缓解,19例中15例患者没有明显副作用[18]。Emtestam等人对10例银屑病患者使用锡-原卟啉单一剂量(2.0μmol/kg b.w.)和UVA连续几天[40]。累积的UVA剂量产生光动力反应需要剂量为98.3J/cm^2,其中时间需超过21天。在所有患者中,银屑病斑块明显得到改善[40]。

Berg和Emtestam使用HpD和紫外线光治疗银屑病的研究显示要取得更好的疗效,更深地渗透到皮肤中的红光并非必要的。这将促进PDT的临床应用如紫外线光源一样广泛。Weinstein等人对8例银屑病患者使用单剂量卟吩姆钠(0.5mg/kg b.w.),随之使用波长405nm和630nm的UVA照射[175]。UVA或光在405nm处的光疗效明显比630nm处的疗效低[175]。目前,使用BPD-MA系统PDT治疗银屑病正处于研究阶段。在Ⅰ期研究中(0.2mg/kg b.w.,3小时后照射,690nm,75J/cm^2),单次治疗60天后银屑病斑块完全缓解[100]。目前,系统PDT BPD-MA正在研究银屑病。在Ⅰ期研究(0.2mg/kg体重,照射3h后,690nm,75J/cm^2),60天单次治疗后银屑病斑块完全缓解[100]。

鲜红斑痣

为评价PDT治疗鲜红斑痣的疗效,对15例患者使用卟吩姆钠(0.75和1mg/kg b.w.),在不同时间照射(15min、30min、60min、2h、4h、8h、24h)及使用不同的光照剂量(630nm,40~50mW/cm^2,25~100J/cm^2)。在这些患者中,使用光敏剂后,接受小剂量75~100J/cm^{2}的光能量密度,照射30min~2h的患者得到明显的改善。经过治疗后,鲜红斑痣的减轻持续长达6个月。治疗中并没有导致瘢痕形成或萎缩[117]。

Xiao-xi等人用一种卟啉分子的纯化混合物PsD-007,联合PDT治疗鲜红斑痣。相比于第一代卟啉光敏剂,PsD-007在系统用药后可被较长波长激活,并表现一定程度的皮肤光敏性。130例鲜红斑痣患者接受静脉注射4~7mg/kg b.w. PsD-007。不到半小时后,使用铜蒸气激光照射病灶(578nm,40~90mW/m^2)。对118例患者的临床资料进行回顾性分析,在一次治疗后,98.3%患者对PDT有不同程度的反应。治疗的副作用如增生性瘢痕和持久性色素沉着或减退没有发生。这对鲜红斑痣的作用被认为是基于PDT介导的内皮细胞损伤和表皮下异常毛细血管的死亡[188]。

外用光动力疗法

系统PDT疗法最常见的副作用是持久性皮肤光敏性。对于许多皮肤科疾病,可以通过外用局部光敏剂来避免这种副作用。然而,卟啉的分子量太高以至于足够的量无法渗透进肌肤[137]。相反,有分子量小的亲水性分子如 ALA 具有优异的皮肤渗透性,特别是上皮性角化不全肿瘤或银屑病[84]。

由于上皮性肿瘤表现出较高的卟啉选择性积累,所有它们可以被破坏而不损伤周围组织[2,84,158]。有几个可能的原因解释局部病变组织选择性吸收 ALA。正常皮肤角质层比受损皮肤的渗透性差。此外,异常的肿瘤间质结构间隙空间大和游离水含量高,可能允许亲水性 ALA 更快地扩散[120]。另外,ALA 诱导的卟啉选择性积累发生在细胞内[77]。其他有助于 ALA 诱导卟啉的组织选择性的因素有:表皮细胞和毛囊皮脂腺单位合成卟啉的数量高于成纤维细胞、心肌细胞及血管内皮细胞[84,124]。由于卟啉对肿瘤组织的选择性积累,应用 ALA 后基底细胞癌的荧光显微镜示在肿瘤内的荧光强度明显高于周围基质[106,164]。

一些研究证明,在人类志愿者和动物模型中,不管是口服、局部或静脉注射给药,ALA 诱导产生的 PpIX 在 24 小时内几乎被完全从体内清除[2,19,84]。这种快速清除的方式减少了 PpIX 积累导致长期光敏性的风险,即使是一次 PDT 治疗也常隔天进行。此外,局部应用 ALA 后,没有明显的系统性积累卟啉和卟啉前体[54]。

局部应用 ALA-PDT 促进内源性合成卟啉的积累的合理改进方法已经被提出。这包括添加亚铁螯合酶抑制剂[133,134],铁螯合剂[43,61,123]或使用酯化 ALA(如丙氨酸甲酯)。然而,目前还没有临床证据证明其比单独使用 ALA 的疗效更好。只有 EDTA 被证实对患有基底细胞癌(肿瘤厚度<2mm)患者在治疗中有增强的作用[126]。

局部外用 ALA 唯一相关的副作用是照射过程中产生的针刺样不适。当治疗较大面积皮损,如全头皮部光线性角化病,有些患者不能耐受这种疼痛,需使用镇痛药甚至必要时麻醉[157,160,161]。近日有报道一例 ALA 或其衍生物的接触性过敏性皮炎[55]。

ALA 较其他光敏剂是最常作为局部外用的。四苯基卟啉磺酸盐(Tetrasodium-meso-tetraphenylporphinesulfonate, $TPPS_4$)作为一种卟吩异构体,已经试用于 PDT。33 例复发性原发性皮肤肿瘤性病变(23 例基底细胞癌,8 例鲍温病,1 例鳞癌,1 例复发性乳腺癌)得到治疗。27 个病灶中的 25 个肿瘤组织厚度小于 1mm 的病变的到完全缓解[143]。Sacchini 等人使用一 2% $TPPS_4$ 的溶液和波长在 645nm 的染料激光($120\sim150J/cm^2$)治疗了 50 例共有 292 个瘤体厚度小于 2mm 的基底细胞癌。局部应用 $TPPS_4$ 后 3 小时、6 小时、24 小时进行照射。93.5% 肿瘤得到完全缓解。10.6% 给予治疗的肿瘤复发[143]。然而,由于可能的药物神经毒性[181]和广泛的组织损伤,导致周围正常组织非选择性吸收 $TPPS_4$ 并渗透到皮下脂肪组织,这些最初作为有前景的研究并没有继续进行[69]。

Porphycenes 是一组新的可用于局部 PDT 的有前景的化合物[79,137]。化学结构上,Porphycenes 由四个吡咯环组成的合成性卟啉异构体[168]。他们产生高量的单重态氧[10]和显示出良好的肿瘤靶向性[59]。Porphycene 9-acetoxy-2,7,12,17-tetrakis-(β-methoxyethyl)-porph-ycene(ATMPn)系统应用于脂质体内[1]以及局部作为乙醇凝胶制剂[78]。目前正在进行局部 ATMPn-PDT 治疗银屑病和浅表性基底细胞癌患者的有效性,安全性及耐受性。

外用 PDT 治疗肿瘤性疾病适应证

1990 年,Kennedy 等人首先报道了 ALA-PDT 的临床疗效。应用 20% ALA 水包油乳剂后,封包 3~6 小时,用 500 瓦的幻灯机照射病灶处($150 \sim 300 mW/cm^2$,$15 \sim 150 J/cm^2$)。80 例基底细胞癌患者在治疗后 2~3 个月后,完全缓解率达 90%(表 11.6)。同时,PDT 治疗后每 6 个原位或早期浸润性鳞癌表现出完全缓解。在单一 ALA-PDT 治疗中,10 例中的 9 例光线性角化病同样对治疗反应良好。然而,转移性乳腺癌对 ALA-PDT 不敏感[85]。2 年后,这一团队报道了 ALA-PDT 治疗超过 300 例浅表性基底细胞癌患者,治疗 3 个月后完全缓解率为 79%[84]。Warloe 等人使用 20% ALA 溶液治疗 11 例有 96 个基底细胞癌病灶的患者。用药 3 小时后,光照射病灶。大多数病灶接受一次光动力治疗;11 处病灶接受 2 次治疗及 2 处病灶被治疗 3 次。治疗 3 个月后,96% 的病灶被治愈,并取得良好的美容效果[173]。

表 11.6 局部 PDT ALA 在皮肤肿瘤的适应证及疗效

适应证	著者	治疗的病变	ALA 剂量	波长和光剂量	完全缓解率
基底细胞癌	Kennedy et al. 1990[85]	80[a]	20% 3~6h	$150 \sim 300 mW/cm^2$ $15 \sim 150 J/cm^2$	90%
	Kennedy 和 Pottier 1992[84]	300[a]	20% 3~6h	$150 \sim 300 mW/cm^2$ $15 \sim 150 J/cm^2$	79%
	Warloe et al. 1992[173]	96	20% >3h	$100 \sim 150 mW/cm^2$ $50 \sim 100 J/cm^2$	96%
	Wolf et al. 1993[185]	37[a] 10[b]	20% 4h	$50 \sim 100 mW/cm^2$ —	97%[a] 10%[b]
	Hürlimann et al. 1994[71]	72a 15b	20% —	— —	94%[a] 33%[b]
	Cairnduff et al. 1994[25]	16	20% 3~6h	$150 mW/cm^2$ $125 \sim 250 J/cm^2$	50%
	Svanberg et al. 1994[157]	55[a] 25[b]	2% 4~6h	$110 mW/cm^2$ $60 J/cm^2$	100%[a] 64%[b]

续表

适应证	著者	治疗的病变	ALA 剂量	波长和光剂量	完全缓解率
	Lang et al. 1995[95]	12	10% 6h	– 100J/cm^2	83%
	Lui et al. 1995[106]	8[a]	20% 3h	19~44mW/cm^2 100J/cm^2	50%
	Calzavara-Pinton 1995[27]	23[a] 30[b]	20% 6~8h	100mW/cm^2 60~80J/cm^2	87%[a] 50%[b]
	Fijan et al. 1995[43]	34[a] 22[b]	20% +3% desferrioxamine 20h	150~250mW/cm^2 >300J/cm^2	88%[a] 32%[b]
	Fink-Puches et al. 1998[49]	95[a]	20% 4h	– 18~131J/cm^2	56%
	Hürlimann et al. 1998[70]	81[a]	10% (nanocolloidal) 6h	– 240J/cm^2	84%
	szeimies et al. unpublished	149[a]	10%~20% 5~6h	120~150J/cm^2 120~180J/cm^2	77%
鳞状细胞癌	Kennedy et al. 1990[85]	6	20% 3~6h	150~30mW/cm^2 15~150J/cm^2	100%
	Wolf et al. 1993[185]	6[a]	20% 4h	50mW/cm^2 –	83%
	Hürlimann et al. 1994[71]	4[a]	20% –	– –	100%
	Lui et al. 1995[106]	3[a] 2[b]	20% 3h	19~44mW/cm^2 100J/cm^2	67%[a] 0%[b]
	Calzavara-Pinton 1995[27]	12[a] 6[b]	20% 6~8h	100mW/cm^2 60~80J/cm^2	83%[a] 33%[b]
光线性角化病	Kennedy et al. 1990[85]	10	20% 3~6h	150~300mW/c^2 15~150J/cm^2	90%
	Wolf et al. 1993[185]	9	20% 4h	50~100mW/cm^2 –	100%
	Calzavara-Pin-ton 1995[27]	50	20% 6~8h	100mW/cm^2 60~80J/cm^2	84%
	Fijan et al. 1995[43]	43	20% +3% Desferrioxamine 20h	150~250mW/cm^2 >300J/cm^2	81%

续表

适应证	著者	治疗的病变	ALA 剂量	波长和光剂量	完全缓解率
	szeimies et al. 1996[161]	17 头部 19 手部和手臂	10% 5~6h	160mW/cm^2 150J/cm^2	71% 头部 0% 手部和手臂
	Jeffes et al. 1997[72]	55 头部 112 手部和手臂	10/20/30% 3h	- 10~150J/cm^2	76% 头部 38% 手部和手臂
	Karrer et al. 1999[80]	200 头部	20% 6h	60~160J/cm^2（灯） 16J/cm^2（激光585nm）	84%（灯） 79%（激光）
鲍温病	Hürlimann et al. 1994[71]	6	20% -	- -	100%
	Cairnduff et al. 1994[25]	36	20% 3~6h	150mW/cm^2 125~250J/cm^2	89%
	Svanberg et al. 1994[157]	10	20% 4~6h	110mW/cm^2 60J/cm^2	90%
	Calzavara-Pinton 1995[27]	6	20% 6~8h	100mW/cm^2 60~80J/cm^2	100%
	Fijan et al. 1995[43]	10	20% +3% desfer-rioxamine 20h	150~250W/cm^2 >300J/cm^2	30%
	Morton et al. 1996[116]	20	20% 4h	- 125J/cm^2	100%
	Wennberg et al. 1996[177]	11	20% 3h	- 100J/cm^2	100%
	szeimies et al. unpublished	10	10% 6h	150mW/cm^2 150~180J/cm^2	80%

[a] 浅表性肿瘤
[b] 结节性肿瘤

Hürlimann 等人使用 20% ALA 配方的 ALA-PDT 疗法得到非常好的疗效。接受治疗的 72 例浅表性基底细胞癌患者有 68 例达到完全缓解，接受治疗的 6 例鲍温病患者和 4 例鳞癌患者均得到完全缓解。结节性基底细胞癌患者的治愈率仅为 33%。同时，9 例皮肤淋巴瘤患者对 ALA-PDT 治疗反应差[71]。Hürlimann 等人同时对 19 例共有 55 处浅表性基底细胞癌病灶的患者进行治疗，局部应用一种含 10% ALA 的新型纳米乳胶溶液后，使用传统幻灯机光源照射[70]。由于ALA在高pH水平的水溶液中的化学性质不稳定,这种新兴ALA配方正在不断被研究开发。随访6个月后发现85%的肿瘤均对治疗有反应。Harth等人把一种改良的局部渗透促进剂(2% EDTA和2% DMsO)加入到20% ALA底霜中。经过12小时的孵育,肿瘤被暴露于高输出源发射的红光和红外光中,达到热疗的目的[62]。31例中26例浅表性或小的基底细胞癌患者(84%)或5例中4例浅表性鳞状细胞癌患者(80%)在1~3次ALA-PDT治疗后,完全缓解得以实现。Wennberg等人应用20% ALA乳剂联合过滤的氙气灯治疗157例浅表性基底细胞癌患者,取得92%的治愈率[177]。

Wolf等人应用局部ALA-PDT(20% ALA溶液,幻灯机照射)治疗13例共70个皮肤瘤体的患者。6例中5例早期鳞状细胞癌患者,治疗的9例光线性角化病患者及37例中有36例浅表性基底细胞癌患者治疗后完全缓解。皮肤转移性恶性黑色素瘤对治疗无应答[185]。色素性基底细胞癌($n=4$)也没有应答[27]。这些黑色素瘤和其他色素性肿瘤因其黑色素含量,可能不允许足够的量渗透到肿瘤组织中。因此,色素性病变是各种PDT疗法的禁忌证。svanberg等人报道了一个很好的疗效,他们应用局部ALA-PDT(波长630nm激光来源的光,110W/cm^2,60J/cm^2),治疗55例浅表细胞癌患者得到100%的治愈率,治疗10例鲍温病患者得到90%的治愈率。结节性基底细胞癌($n=25$)没有表现出其他疾病对PDT一样的应答(仅有64%缓解)[157]。Calzavara-Pinton反复应用ALA-PDT治疗取得很好的疗效,治疗中局部应用20% ALA溶液,氩离子泵浦染料激光照光(100mW/cm^2,60~80J/cm^2)[27]。每隔一天重复治疗,直到临床上检测不到明显的肿瘤(通常是1~3个月)。48%50例光线性角化病患者,87%23例浅表性基底细胞癌患者,100%6例鲍温病患者,84%12例浅表性鳞状细胞癌患者,50%30例结节性基底细胞癌患者,33%6例结节性鳞状细胞癌患者治疗后显示出临床完全缓解[27]。目前为止,只有在鲍温病治疗的Ⅲ期研究报告显示,ALA-PDT使用非激光光源,不良反应较少,似乎与冷冻疗法有类似疗效。

在一项Ⅱ期研究中,szeimies等人根据GCP指南调查了ALA-PDT局部治疗光线性角化病的有效性和耐受性[161]。10例共有36处光线性角化病病灶的患者得到治疗。病变处应用10% ALA溶液5~6个小时,结合非相干光源照射(Waldmann PDT 1200,160mW/cm^2,150J/cm^2)。治疗后3个月,71%位于头部的光线性角化病病灶得到完全缓解。较远端臂部和手部的病变仅表现出部分缓解,很可能是由于此处角化过度覆盖的病变范围更大[161]。Jeffes等人按照类似的治疗方案(0%、10%、20%及30% ALA,3小时孵育,用氩辐射泵浦染料激光器照光,630nm,10~150J/cm^2)治疗40例光线性角化病患者。单一30% ALA治疗8周后,91%的面部和头皮的病变及45%躯干和四肢的病变表现为完全清除。对ALA的不同浓度(10~30%)的临床反应并无显著差异[72]。最近,DUSA

制药(加拿大多伦多)报道了应用局部 ALA-PDT 治疗面部和头部光线性角化病的 2 个Ⅲ期临床试验结果。共有 240 例患者接受 20% ALA 或安慰剂,隔天用光能量密度 10J/cm² 的蓝光照射。在这 2 项研究中,86% 和 81% 的病灶在单一治疗后得到清除。与安慰剂组相比,32% 和 20% 的清除率有统计学意义[36]。

为了进一步减少照光时间和降低目前为止 ALA-PDT 唯一的副作用——照光引起的疼痛,Karrer 等人对 24 例患者进行了对比研究[80]。对头部光线性角化病患者($n = 200$)进行局部 ALA-PDT 治疗,应用 20% ALA 溶液 6 小时照光,使用非相干光源(160mW/cm²,60 ~ 160J/cm²)或长脉冲氪灯泵浦染料激光(LPDL)($t = 1.5ms; \lambda = 585nm; 16J/cm²$)。治疗后 28 天,100 例光线性角化病患者使用 LPDL 照光得到 79% 的完全缓解率;100 例光线性角化病患者使用非相干光源照光得到 84% 的完全缓解率。使用 LPDL 光疗过程产生的疼痛明显减少。对照组的病变应用 LPDL 照光而无 ALA 治疗疗效不确切。

一个局部 ALA-PDT 重要可能适应证是 Gorlin-Goltz 综合征(痣样基底细胞癌综合征),可在临床上和表现上有效控制其多发性肿瘤[83,112]。由于肾移植术后发生免疫抑制,ALA-PDT 同样适用于砷所致的皮肤癌或上皮性皮肤肿瘤[44,160,172]。

为探讨肿瘤厚度对 PDT 疗效的影响,Thiele 等人对 11 例共 19 处基底细胞癌癌灶患者进行治疗,应用 20% ALA 溶液,50 ~ 100J/cm² 的光能量密度。治疗后的组织学检查显示部分肿瘤表明破坏。然而,更深层的真皮结节病变在治疗后仍保持不变[166]。Fink-Puches 等人研究 ALA 联合多色光治疗后,对浅表性基底细胞癌和浅表性鳞状细胞癌患者组织学改变的长期影响[49]。他们的研究表明,治疗后 36 个月长期治愈率较低,BCC 为 50%,sCC 为 8%。组织病理学研究显示行 ALA-PDT 治疗后,发生真皮层纤维化,这比非侵袭性肿瘤的初始深度更深,表明 ALA-PDT 的疗效差,不能够用治疗渗透不足来解释。通过 PpIX 检测肿瘤标记物不足的假设来研究低应答的可能原因[49]。Hoerauf 报道了应用 20% ALA 局部 PDT 治疗眼睑基底细胞癌后,肿瘤对治疗反应性较低[68]。PDT 治疗 4 ~ 8 周后,10 例患者通过手术切除原肿瘤瘤体。组织学检查发现残留肿瘤[67]。在一个Ⅰ期研究中,Cairnduff 等人应用 20% ALA 软膏联合波长为 630nm 的染料激光照射治疗 36 例鲍温病患者,89% 得到完全缓解。然而,16 例基底细胞癌患者使用此种治疗方式,仅有 50% 患者表现完全缓解。在这个研究中,最有可能复发的病灶是应用 ALA 只有 3 ~ 4 个小时孵育时间[25]。

Szeimies 等人对基底细胞癌患者进行荧光显微镜检查,这些患者行术式切除前已应用 10% ALA 软膏。应用 ALA 4 小时后行切除术,只在毛囊皮脂腺单位可检测到荧光卟啉。只有在一个更长的封包时间至少 6 个小时,在浅表性或结节性基底细胞癌中方可检测出荧光卟啉[164]。然而,在一个长达 12 小时的孵育时间后,硬化性基底细胞癌表现出一个异构的荧光体[164]。这可能是这种亚型基底细胞癌中卟啉的合成减少[164,179]。一项渗透性研究对16例共有18处基底细胞癌癌灶的患者(7处浅表性、10处结节性、1处浸润性)应用20% ALA溶液,平均封包时间为6.9个小时,只有6处浅表性肿瘤和4处结节性肿瘤的荧光检查示全肿瘤厚度示PpIX荧光[108]。这些结果接近于不同工作组的临床经验,ALA-PDT对于肿瘤厚度超过3～4mm的基底细胞癌并不是一个有效的治疗方案,所以一些标准的治疗方法非常有必要,如切除术、莫氏显微外科手术或冷冻疗法[27,43,71,156,157,185]。

根据以上数据,目前局部ALA-PDT治疗(应用20% ALA油水相乳液封包4～6小时,$100～150mW/cm^2$;$100～150J/cm^2$照光)上皮性癌前病变或癌性病变适应证有光线性角化病、鲍温病和浅表性基底细胞癌(肿瘤厚度小于3mm)。对于照光来说,没有失去功效的非相干光是合适的[43,161]。回顾这些适应证和遵循治疗参数,光动力疗法提供了一个具有更好美容效果及可同时治疗多个病灶的能力的替代疗法。然而,直到Ⅲ期研究的长期随访期完成前,判断局部ALA-PDT治疗疗效均不确切。

除了皮肤上皮性肿瘤,光动力疗法也被成功地用于治疗蕈样肉芽肿。应用20% ALA乳剂4～6小时,然后用幻灯机照光($44mW/cm^2$,$40J/cm^2$)治疗2例斑块期蕈样肉芽肿患者。1例患者在18周内治疗了5次,另1例患者在7周治疗了4次,均在临床上和组织学上得到了一个完全缓解[182]。这个团队已对另外4例有超过60处蕈样肉芽肿病灶的患者进行治疗。在这项研究中,治疗参数如光源波长(UVA和可见光)、光能量密度($0.5～60J/cm^2$)和治疗次数(10～25天内达到3次)差异显著。只有反复治疗,才有病变的临床缓解[183]。在单一的ALA-PDT治疗后。尽管观察到病变达到临床上缓解,但病理检查显示真皮层内持久的非典型淋巴细胞[7]。美国布法罗罗斯威尔公园癌症研究所的Oseroff等人收治8例有超过50处孤立癌灶的不同阶段蕈样肉芽肿,包括瘤体厚度达1.5cm的溃疡型肿瘤。应用2%～20% ALA软膏于病变处12小时,然后用染料激光照射($30～150mW/cm^2$,$50～150J/cm^2$)。为了进行比较,2例患者使用了氮芥进行局部治疗。每2～4周进行治疗。斑块和较薄的斑片在2个治疗周期后得到解决;较厚的治疗则需5～7个治疗周期,直到组织学证实其完全缓解。溃疡型肿瘤在单次治疗后呈再上皮化。重叠感染的溃疡性皮肤T细胞淋巴瘤其治疗区域细菌浓度减少,可导致快速肉芽化和更好的愈合。ALA-PDT比氮芥能更快的治疗肿瘤。这两种治疗方法最终的疗效相近。因此,组织学证实治疗病变有61%得到缓解;39%得到部分缓解[13]。然而,还未有ALA-PDT治疗蕈样肉芽肿相关的前瞻性随机性临床研究。

外用 PDT 治疗非肿瘤性疾病的适应证

外用 PDT 非常有前景的适应证是良性皮肤疾病,如寻常型银屑病。相比于光动力疗法治疗肿瘤,大多数慢性疾病的单次治疗并不足以达到理想的临床效果[23,174]。Hürlimann 等人应用 ALA-PDT 治疗 15 例斑块型银屑病患者,治疗 1~5 次后部分得到缓解[71]。Weinstein 等人治疗银屑病患者的斑块,分别使用 10%、20% 及 30% ALA 溶液,染料激光($10~150J/cm^2$)照射。他观察到的最好疗效是应用 30% ALA 反复治疗[174]。McCullough and Weinstein 进行了一个应用 UVA 和光动力治疗银屑病的试验药物和光能量密度范围的研究[110]。14 例斑块型银屑病使用 ALA(2%、10%、20%)水包油型乳剂 3 小时,然后暴露于 UVA 递增剂量($2.5~30J/cm^2$)。这项研究的初步结果表明,治疗 4 周后,应用 10% ALA 组(UVA $80~120J/cm^2$)和 20% ALA 组(UVA $1~39J/cm^2$)有约 50% 患者得到改善。2% ALA 治疗患者无明显疗效。为了比较 ALA-PD 和蒽三酚的疗效,Boehncke 对 3 例慢性斑块型银屑病进行了治疗,应用 10% ALA 软膏 5 小时,以及非相干光源($70mW/cm^2$,$25J/cm^2$)照射病变区,每周 3 次。在 1 例病人上,PDT 治疗区域的皮损比蒽三酚治疗区域的消退早约 1 周[23]。一项早期的 II 期临床研究对局部 PDT 治疗 29 例慢性斑块型银屑病的疗效进行了评估[78]。用 0.1% 乙醇 ATMPn 配方和照射非相干光源单次治疗后,银屑病斑块明显改善。进一步的研究正在进行,研究重复使用这种新型光敏剂是否能够有效维持银屑病斑块的完全和长期缓解。

相比于已知的致癌物质 PUVA 或 UVB 辐射[142,155],PDT 细胞毒性的杀伤目标不是 DNA。文献中没有记录红血球生成素原卟啉症患者在长期随访中发生皮肤肿瘤的风险增加(Goerz,个人通信)。此外,相对于 PUVA,PDT 治疗成功所需要的治疗总数可能降低。然而,我们需要一个更好地了解相关 PDT 治疗银屑病患者的基本机制,这机制与皮肤恶性肿瘤的 PDT 治疗明显不同。

上个世纪 30 年代,我们已经知道光敏剂灭活病毒或噬菌体的能力[141,148]。在体外单纯疱疹病毒的这种能力已被证实(综述中可见[20])。作为一个结果,这种疗法在生殖器单纯疱疹感染的患者身上进行调查。中性红(1.0% 水溶液)作为光敏剂,随后用荧光灯照射。在 30 例患者中观察到了皮损症状显著减轻,复发频率降低[53]。吖啶黄和亚甲基蓝作为光敏剂治疗本病也显示出疗效(综述可见[20])。然而,在其他四项双盲、安慰剂对照治疗的研究中,PDT 被发现是无效的(综述可见[20])。因吖啶黄和亚甲基蓝的潜在致癌性及抗病毒化学治疗的开展,然而,PDT 已被评估于血液制品的病毒灭活中(如艾滋病毒)[17,118]。

另一个外用 PDT 治疗的潜在适应证是人乳头状瘤病毒(HPV)相关皮肤病。在这些条件下对 PDT 疗法的优势是随 CO_2 和可调节脉冲染料激光器产生的病毒相关激光束的缺失以及由于亚临床病灶清除，其可能的复发率较低。Frank 等人应用外用 ALA-PDT（20% ALA 凝胶，封包 14 小时，75-氩染料激光，75～100mW/cm^2，100J/cm^2）治疗 7 例生殖器尖锐湿疣患者得到完全缓解[52]。ALA-PDT 也被证明对顽固性手足病毒疣有效。Stender 等人对 45 例手足病毒寻常疣患者行 ALA-PDT 疗法（20% ALA 乳霜；4 小时封包；红光 70J/cm^2）或安慰剂 PDT 治疗。经过超过 18 周的 6 次治疗后，ALA-PDT 治疗组疣面积减少 100%，而安慰剂 PDT 治疗组则减少 71%。然而，一些研究对 6 例手足寻常疣患者行 ALA-PDT 治疗，应用 20% ALA 乳液 6 小时，随后非相干光源照光（50～150mW/cm^2，100J/cm^2），尽管之前使用了足够角质溶解剂，却显示没有任何疗效。疣状表皮发育不良的 HPV 相关疣患者对 ALA-PDT 反应非常好[81,184]。

研究证实光动力抗菌化学疗法对体外细菌有效，如耐药菌株、酵母菌和寄生虫[82,170]。因此，光动力抗菌化学疗法被推荐作为消毒血液制品和治疗局部感染的一个潜行方式。

一些除了 ALA 的外用光敏剂已进入临床评价阶段，以治疗良性疾病。Monfrecola 等人应用局部 HpD-PDT 治疗 2 例斑秃患者。应用 0.5% HpD 于无毛发区，然后照射无毛区（360～365nm），每周 3 次。治疗 8～10 周后，在处理区域发现细毳毛生长；再经过 4～8 周，毳毛被终毛取代[115]。1989 年，Meffert and Prěs 对 29 例寻常型银屑病患者行 HpD-PDT 疗法。其中，17 例患者合并掌跖银屑病[111,129]。Meffert 应用 0.0001% HpD 软膏和 5% DMsO 治疗 12 例斑片型银屑病。PDT 在可见光或紫外线光（2,4,6J/cm^2）下连续 3 天进行。斑块对治疗反应良好，部分表现出完全缓解[111]。Prěs 使用相同的 HpD 配方对 17 例掌跖银屑病行 20 次治疗。使用可见光照光（17J/cm^2）。治疗结果显示 PDT 几乎完全清除病灶[129]。

因为外用局部 ALA，皮肤附属器结构中可检测到 PpIX，外用 ALA-PDT 被推荐用于痤疮、多毛症及斑秃的治疗管理[104,127]。在这一方面，临床上却很少有证据确认或否认 ALA-PDT 对这些疾病的疗效。

展望

PDT 被证明其对皮肤浅表性瘤性肿瘤治疗有效，特别是光线性角化病、鲍温病、浅表基底细胞癌，以及慢性炎症性皮肤病如银屑病的治疗。

由于卟吩姆钠引起皮肤光敏性的延长，目前系统光动力治疗限制于治疗老年人多种肿瘤或巨大肿瘤。然而，一旦副作用极少的第二代光敏剂被认可，系统光动力疗法即表现出其巨大的治疗潜能。目前临床上众所周知的局部光敏剂是 ALA，且其最近已经在美国被批准用于治疗光线性角化病。

局部光动力疗法的优点之一是，它是一种可重复治疗的且具有极佳美容效果的非侵入性程序。此外,相比于其他形式的光疗,PDT 介导其作用造成的膜损伤,从而大大降低了可能造成 DNA 损伤、基因突变与肿瘤的发生[114]。尽管如此,光动力疗法的局限性是必须考虑的。光的穿透深度以及光敏剂渗透到皮肤的深度是一个极具关键的要点,应为每个患者制定个体化方案。此外,我们在选择患者时,应充分考虑皮肤癌是否有转移的潜在风险。组织学确认和肿瘤厚度测定是一个先决条件。

未来的研究目标是确定此种治疗方法的其他适应证和规范治疗参数,以及在皮肤肿瘤患者的长期临床试验中比较光动力疗法、手术或放射治疗的疗效。

(罗权　林玲　译,黄茂芳　陈荃　校,朱慧兰　审)

参考文献

1. Abels C, Dellian M, Szeimies RM, Steinbach P, Richert C, Goetz AE (1996) Targeting of the tumor microcirculation with a new photosensitizer. In: Ehrenberg B, Jori G, Moan J (eds) Photochemotherapy: photodynamic therapy and other modalities. Proc SPIE 2625:164–169
2. Abels C, Heil P, Dellian M, Kuhnle GEH, Baumgartner R, Goetz AE (1994) In vivo kinetics and spectra of 5-aminolevulinic acid-induced fluorescence in an amelanotic melanoma of the hamster. Br J Cancer 70:826–833
3. Agarwal R, Korman NJ, Mohan RR, Feyes DK, Jawed S, Zaim MT, Mukhtar H (1996) Apoptosis is an early event during phthalocyanine photodynamic therapy-induced ablation of chemically induced squamous papillomas in mouse skin. Photochem Photobiol 63:547–552
4. Ahmad N, Feyes DK, Agarwal R, Mukhtar H (1998) Photodynamic therapy results in induction of WAF1/CIP1/P21 leading to cell cycle arrest and apoptosis. Proc Natl Acad Sci USA 95:6977–6982
5. Allison RR, Mang TS (1997) A phase II/III clinical study for the treatment of HIV-associated cutaneous Kaposi's sarcoma with tin ethyl etiopurpurin (SnET2)-induced photodynamic therapy. Presented at the European Cancer Conference (ECC09), Hamburg, Germany
6. Allison RR, Mang TS, Wilson BD (1998) Photodynamic therapy for the treatment of non-melanomatous cutaneous malignancies. Semin Cut Med Surg 17:153–163
7. Ammann R, Hunziker T (1995) Photodynamic therapy for mycosis fungoides after topical photosensitization with 5-aminolevulinic acid. J Am Acad Dermatol 33:541
8. Anderson CY, Elmets CA (manuscript in preparation)
9. Anderson C, Hrabovsky S, McKinley Y, Tubesing K, Tang HP, Mukhtar H, Elmets CA (1997) Phthalocyanine (Pc) photodynamic therapy: disparate effects of pharmacologic inhibitors on cutaneous photosensitivity and on tumor regression. Photochem Photobiol 65:895–901
10. Aramendia PF, Redmond RW, Nonell S, Schuster W, Braslavsky SE, Schaffner K, Vogel E (1986) The photophysical properties of porphycenes: potential photodynamic therapy agents. Photochem Photobiol 44:555–559
11. Athar M, Mukhtar H, Elmets CA, Zaim MT, Lloyd JR, Bickers DR (1988) In situ evidence for the involvement of superoxide anions in cutaneous porphyrin photosensitization. Biochem Biophys Res Commun 151:1054–1059
12. Athar M, Elmets CA, Bickers DR, Mukhtar H (1989) A novel mechanism for the generation of superoxide anions in porphyrin mediated cutaneous photosensitization: Activation of the xanthine oxidase pathway. J Clin Invest 83:1137–1143
13. Babich D, Whitaker J, Conti C, Blaird-Wagner D, Stoll HL, Dozier S, Oseroff AR (1996) Treatment of all stages of cutaneous T-cell lymphomas with fractionated photodynamic ther-

apy using topical δ-aminolevulinic acid. J Invest Dermatol 106:840
14. Bandieramonte G, Marchesini R, Melloni E, Andreoli C, Di pietro D, Spinelli P, Pava G, Zunino F, Emanuelli H (1984) Laser phototherapy following HpD administration in superficial neoplastic lesions. Tumori 70:327–334
15. Batlle AM del C (1993) Porphyrins, porphyrias, cancer and photodynamic therapy—a model for carcinogenesis. J Photochem Photobiol B: Biol 20:5–22
16. Bellnier DA, Ho YK, Pandey RK, Missert JR, Dougherty TJ (1989) Distribution and elimination of Photofrin II in mice. Photochem Photobiol 50:221–228
17. Ben-Hur E, Horowitz B (1995) Advances in photochemical approaches for blood sterilization. Photochem Photobiol 62:383–388
18. Berg H, Bauer E, Gollmick FA, Diezel W, Böhm F, Meffert H, Sönnichsen N (1985) Photodynamic hematoporphyrin therapy of psoriasis. In: Jori G, Perria C (eds) Photodynamic therapy of tumors and other diseases. Progetto Editore, Padova, pp 337–343
19. Berlin NI, Neuberger A, Scott JJ (1956) The metabolism of δ-aminolevulinic acid. 1. Normal pathways, studied with the aid of [15]N. Biochem J 64:80–90
20. Bockstahler LE, Coohill TP, Hellman KB, Lytle CD, Roberts JE (1979) Photodynamic therapy for herpes simplex: a critical review. Pharmacol Ther 4:473–499
21. Boehncke WH, König K, Kaufmann R, Scheffold W, Prümmer O, Sterry W (1994) Photodynamic therapy in psoriasis: suppression of cytokine production in vitro and recording of fluorescence modification during treatment in vivo. Arch Dermatol Res 286:300–303
22. Boehncke WH, König K, Rück A, Kaufmann R, Sterry W (1994) In vitro and in vivo effects of photodynamic therapy in cutaneous T cell lymphoma. Acta Derm Venereol (Stockh) 74:201–205
23. Boehncke WH, Sterry W, Kaufmann R (1994) Treatment of psoriasis by topical photodynamic therapy with polychromatic light. Lancet 343:801
24. Buchanan RB, Carruth JAS, McKenzie AL, Williams SR (1989) Photodynamic therapy in the treatment of malignant tumours of the skin and head and neck. Eur J Surg Oncol 15:400–406
25. Cairnduff F, Stringer MR, Hudson EJ, Ash DV, Brown SB (1994) Superficial photodynamic therapy with topical 5-aminolevulinic acid for superficial primary and secondary skin cancer. Br J Cancer 69:605–608
26. Calzavara F, Tomio L (1991) Photodynamic therapy: clinical experience at the department of radiotherapy at Padova general hospital. J Photochem Photobiol B Biol 11:91–95
27. Calzavara-Pinton PG (1995) Repetitive photodynamic therapy with topical δ-aminolevulinic acid as an appropriate approach to the routine treatment of superficial non-melanoma skin tumours. J Photochem Photobiol B Biol 29:53–57
28. Castellani A, Page GP, Concioli M (1963) Photodynamic effect of hematoporphyrin on blood microcirculation. J Pathol Bacteriol 86:99–102
29. de Vree WJ, Essers MC, de Bruijn HS, Star WM, Koster JF, Sluiter W (1996) Evidence for an important role of neutrophils in the efficacy of photodynamic therapy *in vivo*. Cancer Res 56:2908–2911
30. de Vree WJ, Essers MC, Koster JF, Sluiter W (1997) Role of interleukin 1 and granulocyte colony-stimulating factor in photofrin-based photodynamic therapy of rat rhabdomyosarcoma tumors. Cancer Res 57:2555–2558
31. Dellian M, Abels C, Kuhnle GE, Goetz AE (1995) Effects of photodynamic therapy on leukocyte-endothelium interaction: differences between normal and tumour tissue. Br J Cancer 72:1125–1130
32. Dellian M, Walenta S, Gamarra F, Kuhnle GE, Mueller-Klieser W, Goetz AE (1994) High-energy shock waves enhance hyperthermic response of tumors: effects on blood flow, energy metabolism, and tumor growth. J Natl Cancer Inst 86:287–293
33. Dilkes MG, De Jode ML, Rowntree-Taylor A (1997) m-THPC photodynamic therapy for head and neck cancer. Lasers Med Sci 11:23–30

34. Dougherty TJ (1981) Photoradiation therapy for cutaneous and subcutaneous malignancies. J Invest Dermatol 77:122–124
35. Dougherty TJ (1996) A brief history of clinical photodynamic therapy development at Roswell Park Cancer Institute. J Clin Laser Med Surg 14:219–221
36. Dougherty TJ, Gomer CJ, Henderson BW, Jori G, Kessel D, Korbelik M, Moan J, Peng Q (1998) Photodynamic therapy. J Natl Cancer Inst 90:889–905
37. Dougherty TJ, Grindey GB, Fiel R, Weishaupt KR, Boyle DG (1975) Photoradiation therapy. II. Cure of animal tumors with hematoporphyrin and light. J Natl Cancer Inst 55:115–121
38. Dougherty TJ, Kaufman JE, Goldfarb A, Weishaupt KR, Boyle D, Mittleman A (1978) Photoradiation therapy for the treatment of malignant tumors. Cancer Res 38:2628–2635
39. Elmets CA, Bowen KD (1986) Immunological suppression in mice treated with hematoporphyrin derivative photoradiation. Cancer Res 46:1608–1611
40. Emtestam L, Berglund L, Angelin B, Drummond GS, Kappas A (1989) Tin-protoporphyrin and long wavelength ultraviolet light in treatment of psoriasis. Lancet 1:1231–1233
41. Evans S, Matthews W, Perry R, Fraker D, Norton J, Pass HI (1990) Effect of photodynamic therapy on tumor necrosis factor production by murine macrophages. J Natl Cancer Inst 82:34–39
42. Feyh J, Gutmann R, Leunig A (1993) Die photodynamische Lasertherapie im Bereich der Hals-, Nasen-, Ohrenheilkunde. Laryngo Rhino Otol 72:273–278
43. Fijan S, Hönigsmann H, Ortel B (1995) Photodynamic therapy of epithelial skin tumours using delta-aminolevulinic acid and desferrioxamine. Br J Dermatol 133:282–288
44. Fijan S, Hönigsmann H, Tanew A (1996) Photodynamic therapy of keratoacanthoma using topical delta-aminolevulinic acid. J Invest Dermatol 106:945 (abstract)
45. Fingar VH (1996) Vascular effects of photodynamic therapy. J Clin Laser Med Surg 14:323–328
46. Fingar VH, Wieman TJ, Doak KW (1990) Role of thromboxane and prostacyclin release on photodynamic therapy-induced tumor destruction. Cancer Res 50:2599–2603
47. Fingar VH, Wieman TJ, Wiehle SA, Cerrito PB (1992) The role of microvascular damage in photodynamic therapy: the effect of treatment on vessel constriction, permeability, and leukocyte adhesion. Cancer Res 52:4914–4921
48. Fingar VH, Wieman TJ, Karavolos PS, Doak KW, Ouellet R, van Lier JE (1993) The effects of photodynamic therapy using differently substituted zinc phthalocyanines on vessel constriction, vessel leakage and tumor response. Photochem Photobiol 58:251–258
49. Fink-Puches R, Soyer HP, Hofer A, Kerl H, Wolf P (1998) Long-term follow-up and histological changes of superficial nonmelanoma skin cancers treated with topical δ-aminolevulinic acid photodynamic therapy. Arch Dermatol 134:821–826
50. Forbes IJ, Cowled PA, Leong ASY, Ward AD, Black RB, Blake AJ, Jacka FJ (1980) Phototherapy of human tumours using hematoporphyrin derivative. Med J Aust 2:489–493
51. Foster TH, Primavera MC, Marder VJ, Hilf R, Sporn LA (1991) Photosensitized release of von Willebrand factor from cultured human endothelial cells. Cancer Res 51:3261–3266
52. Frank RGJ, Bos JD, Vandermeulen FW, Sterenborg HJCM (1996) Photodynamic therapy for condylomata acuminata with local application of 5-aminolevulinic acid. Genitourin Med 72:70–71
53. Friedrich EG (1973) Relief for herpes vulvitis. Obstet Gynecol 41:74–77
54. Fritsch C, Verwohlt B, Bolsen K, Ruzicka T, Goerz G (1996) Influence of topical photodynamic therapy with 5-aminolevulinic acid on porphyrin metabolism. Arch Dermatol Res 288:517–521
55. Gniazdowska B, Rueff F, Hillemann P, Przybilla B (1998) Allergic contact dermatitis from δ-aminolevulinic acid used for photodynamic therapy. Contact Derm 38:348–349
56. Gollnick SO, Liu X, Owczarczak B, Musser DA, Henderson BW (1997) Altered expression of interleukin 6 and interleukin 10 as a result of photodynamic therapy in vivo. Cancer Res 57:3904–3909

第 11 章 光动力疗法在皮肤科的应用

57. Gomer CJ, Ferrario A, Rucker N, Wong S, Lee AS (1991) Glucose regulated protein induction and cellular resistance to oxidative stress mediated by porphyrin photosensitization. Cancer Res 51:6574–6579
58. Gross DJ, Waner M, Schosser RH, Dinehart SM (1990) Squamous cell carcinoma of the lower lip involving a large cutaneous surface. Photodynamic therapy as an alternative therapy. Arch Dermatol 126:1148–1150
59. Guardiano M, Biolo R, Jori G, Schaffner K (1989) Tetra-*n*-propylporphycene as a tumour localizer: pharmacokinetic and phototherapeutic studies in mice. Cancer Lett 44:1–6
60. Gutmann R, Leunig M, Feyh J, Goetz AE, Messmer K, Kastenbauer E, Jain RK (1992) Interstitial hypertension in head and neck tumors in patients: correlation with tumor size. Cancer Res 52:1993–1995
61. Hanania J, Malik Z (1992) The effect of EDTA and serum on endogenous porphyrin accumulation and photodynamic sensitization of human K562 leukemic cells. Cancer Lett 65:127–131
62. Harth Y, Hirshowitz B, Kaplan B (1998) Modified topical photodynamic therapy of superficial skin tumors, utilizing aminolevulinic acid, penetration enhancers, red light, and hyperthermia. Dermatol Surg 24:723–726
63. Hebeda KM, Huizing MT, Brouwer PA, van der Meulen FW, Hulsebosch HJ, Reiss P, Oosting JH, Veenhof CHN, Bakker PJM (1995) Photodynamic therapy in AIDS-related cutaneous Kaposi's sarcoma. J Acquir Immune Defic Syndr Hum Retrovirol 10:61–70
64. Henderson BW, Waldow SM, Mang TS, Potter WR, Malone PB, Dougherty TJ (1985) Tumor destruction and kinetics of tumor cell death in two experimental mouse tumors following photodynamic therapy. Cancer Res 45:572–576
65. Henderson BW, Donovan JM (1989) Release of prostaglandin E_2 from cells by photodynamic treatment in vitro. Cancer Res 49:6896–6900
66. Hendrich C, Hüttmann G, Diddens H, Seara J, Siebert WE (1996) Experimentelle Grundlagen einer photodynamischen Lasertherapie für die chronische Polyarthritis. Orthopäde 25:30–36
67. Hintschich C, Feyh J, Beyer-Machule C, Riedel K, Ludwig K (1993) Photodynamic laser therapy of basal-cell carcinoma of the lid. Ger J Ophthalmol 2:212–217
68. Hoerauf H, Hüttmann G, Diddens H, Thiele B, Laqua H (1994) Die Photodynamische Therapie (PDT) des Lidbasalioms nach topischer Applikation von δ-Aminolävulinsäure (ALA). Ophthalmologe 91:824–829
69. Hohenleutner U, Szeimies RM, Landthaler M (1993) Photodynamische Therapie zur Behandlung oberflächlicher Basaliome. In: Braun-Falco O, Plewig G, Meurer M (eds) Fortschritte der praktischen Dermatologie und Venerologie, vol 13. Springer, Berlin, pp 472–474
70. Hürlimann AF, Hänggi G, Panizzon RG (1998) Photodynamic therapy of superficial basal cell carcinomas using topical 5-aminolevulinic acid in a nanocolloid lotion. Dermatology 197:248–254
71. Hürlimann AF, Panizzon RA, Burg G (1994) Topical photodynamic treatment of skin tumors and dermatoses. Dermatology 3:327 (abstract)
72. Jeffes EW, McCullough JL, Weinstein GD, Fergin PD, Nelson JS, Shull TF, Simpson KR, Bukaly LM, Hoffmann WL, Fong NL (1997) Photodynamic therapy of actinic keratosis with topical 5-aminolevulinic acid. A pilot dose-ranging study. Arch Dermatol 133:727–732
73. Jesionek A, von Tappeiner H (1905) Zur Behandlung der Hautcarcinome mit fluorescierenden Stoffen. Dtsch Arch Klin Med 85:223–239
74. Jolles CJ, Ott MJ, Straight RC, Lynch DH (1988) Systemic immunosuppression induced by peritoneal photodynamic therapy. Am J Obstet Gynecol 158:1446–1453
75. Jones CM, Mang T, Cooper M, Wilson DB, Stoll HL (1992) Photodynamic therapy in the treatment of Bowen's disease. J Am Acad Dermatol 27:979–982
76. Jones LR, Grossweiner LI (1994) Singlet oxygen generation by Photofrin in homogeneous and light-scattering media. J Photochem Photobiol B Biol 26:249–256

77. Kappas A, Sassa S, Galbraith RA, Nordmann Y (1989) The porphyrias. In: Scriver CR, Beaudet AL, Sly WS, Valle D (eds) The metabolic basis of inherited disease, 6th edn. McGraw-Hill, New York, pp 1305–1366
78. Karrer S, Abels C, Bäumler W, Ebert A, Landthaler M, Szeimies RM (1996) Topical photodynamic therapy of psoriasis using a novel porphycene dye. J Invest Dermatol 107:466
79. Karrer S, Abels C, Szeimies RM, Bäumler W, Dellian M, Hohenleutner U, Goetz AE, Landthaler M (1997) Topical application of a first porphycene dye for photodynamic therapy—penetration studies in human perilesional skin and basal cell carcinoma. Arch Dermatol Res 289:132–137
80. Karrer S, Bäumler W, Abels C, Hohenleutner U, Landthaler M, Szeimies RM (1999) Long pulse dye laser for photodynamic therapy—investigations in vitro and in vivo. Lasers Surg Med 25(1):51–59
81. Karrer S, Szeimies RM, Abels C, Wlotzke U, Stolz W, Landthaler M (1999) Epidermodysplasia verruciformis: topical 5-aminolevulinic acid photodynamic therapy. Br J Dermatol 140:935–938
82. Karrer S, Szeimies RM, Ernst S, Abels C, Bäumler W, Landthaler M (1999) Photodynamic inactivation of staphylococci with 5-aminolevulinic acid or photofrin. Lasers Med Sci 14:54–61
83. Karrer S, Szeimies RM, Hohenleutner U, Heine A, Landthaler M (1995) Unilateral localized basaliomatosis: treatment with topical photodynamic therapy after application of 5-aminolevulinic acid. Dermatology 190:218–222
84. Kennedy JC, Pottier RH (1992) Endogenous protoporphyrin IX, a clinically useful photosensitizer for photodynamic therapy. J Photochem Photobiol B Biol 14:275–292
85. Kennedy JC, Pottier RH, Pross DC (1990) Photodynamic therapy with endogenous protoporphyrin IX: basic principles and present clinical experience. J Photochem Photobiol B Biol 6:143–148
86. Kerdel FA, Soter NA, Lim HW (1987) In vivo mediator release and degranulation of mast cells in hematoporphyrin derivative-induced phototoxicity in mice. J Invest Dermatol 88:277–280
87. Kessel D (1986) Sites of photosensitization by derivatives of hematoporphyrin. Photochem Photobiol 44:489–493
88. Korbelik M, Krosl G (1994) Enhanced macrophage cytotoxicity against tumor cells treated with photodynamic therapy. Photochem Photobiol 60:497–502
89. Korbelik MJ (1996) Induction of tumor immunity by photodynamic therapy. J Clin Laser Med Surg 14:329–334
90. Korbelik M, Krosl G, Krosl J, Dougherty GJ (1996) The role of host lymphoid populations in the response of mouse EMT6 tumor to photodynamic therapy. Cancer Res 56:5647–5652
91. Krosl G, Korbelik M, Dougherty GJ (1995) Induction of immune cell infiltration into murine SCCVII tumor by Photofrin-based photodynamic therapy. Br J Cancer 71:549–555
92. Krosl G, Korbelik M, Krosl J, Dougherty GJ (1996) Potentiation of photodynamic therapy-elicited antitumor response by localized treatment with granulocyte-macrophage colony-stimulating factor. Cancer Res 56:3281–3286
93. Korell M, Untch M, Abels C, Dellian M, Kirschstein M, Baumgartner R, Beyer W, Goetz AE (1995) Einsatz der photodynamischen Lasertherapie in der Gynäkologie. Gynäkol Geburtshilfl Rundsch 35:90–97
94. Landthaler M (1992) Premalignant and malignant skin lesions. In: Achauer BM, Vander Kam VM, Berns MW (eds) Lasers in plastic surgery and dermatology. Thieme, New York, pp 34–44
95. Lang S, Baumgartner R, Struck R, Leunig A, Gutmann R, Feyh J (1995) Photodynamische Diagnostik und Therapie von Neoplasien der Gesichtshaut nach topischer Applikation von 5-Aminolävulinsäure. Laryngo Rhino Otol 74:85–89
96. Langer S, Abels C, Szeimies RM, Goetz AE (1995) Photodynamic diagnosis and therapy of

tumors with topically applied 5-aminolevulinic acid. J Invest Dermatol 105:511 (abstract)
97. Leunig A, Staub F, Peters J, Leiderer R, Feyh J, Goetz AE (1994) Die Schädigung von Tumorzellen durch die photodynamische Therapie. Laryngo Rhino Otol 73:102–107
98. Leunig M, Goetz AE, Gamarra F, Zetterer G, Messmer K, Jain RK (1994) Photodynamic therapy-induced alterations in interstitial fluid pressure, volume and water content of an amelanotic melanoma in the hamster. Br J Cancer 69:101–103
99. Leunig M, Richert C, Gamarra F, Lumper W, Vogel E, Jocham D, Goetz AE (1993) Tumour localisation kinetics of photofrin and three synthetic porphyrinoids in an amelanotic melanoma of the hamster. Br J Cancer 68:225–234
100. Levy JG, Jones CA, Pilson LA (1994) The preclinical and clinical development and potential application of benzoporphyrin derivative. Int Photodynam 1:3–5
101. Lipson RL, Baldes EJ (1960) The photodynamic properties of a particular haematoporphyrin derivative. Arch Dermatol 82:508–516
102. Lipson RL, Gray MJ, Baldes EJ (1966) Haematoporphyrin derivative for detection and management of cancer. Proc IX Internat Cancer Congr 393
103. Lui H, Anderson RR (1992) Photodynamic therapy in dermatology. Arch Dermatol 128:1631–1636
104. Lui H, Anderson RR (1993) Photodynamic therapy in dermatology: recent developments. Dermatol Clin 11:1–13
105. Lui H, Kollias N, Wimberly J, Anderson RR (1992) Photosensitizing potential of benzoporphyrin derivative-monoacid ring A (BPD-MA) in patients undergoing photodynamic therapy. Photochem Photobiol 55 [Suppl]:30S (abstract)
106. Lui H, Salasche S, Kollias N, Wimberly J, Flotte T, McLean D, Anderson RR (1995) Photodynamic therapy of nonmelanoma skin cancer with topical aminolevulinic acid: a clinical and histologic study. Arch Dermatol 131:737–738
107. Lynch DH, Haddad S, King VJ, Ott MJ, Straight RC, Jolles CJ (1989) Systemic immunosuppression induced by photodynamic therapy (PDT) is adoptively transferred by macrophages. Photochem Photobiol 49:453–458
108. Martin A, Tope WD, Grevelink JM, Starr JC, Fewkes JL, Flotte TJ, Deutsch TF, Anderson RR (1995) Lack of selectivity of protoporphyrin IX fluorescence for basal cell carcinoma after topical application of 5-aminolevulinic acid: implications for photodynamic treatment. Arch Dermatol Res 287:665–674
109. McCaughan JS Jr, Guy JT, Hicks W, Laufman L, Nims TA, Walker J (1989) Photodynamic therapy for cutaneous and subcutaneous malignant neoplasms. Arch Surg 124:211–216
110. McCullough JL, Weinstein GD (1998) Photodynamic therapy of psoriasis. In: Roenigk HH Jr, Maibach HI (eds) Psoriasis, 3rd edn. Marcel Dekker, New York, pp 757–760
111. Meffert H, Preš H, Diezel W, Sönnichsen N (1989) Antipsoriatische und phototoxische Wirksamkeit von Hämatoporphyrin-Derivat nach topischer Applikation und Bestrahlung mit sichtbarem Licht. Dermatol Monatsschr 175:28–34
112. Meijnders PJN, Star WM, De Bruijn RS, Treurniet-Donker AD, Van Mierlo MJM, Wijthoff SJM, Naafs B, Beerman H, Levendag PC (1996) Clinical results of photodynamic therapy for superficial skin malignancies or actinic keratosis using topical 5-aminolevulinic acid. Las Med Sci 11:123–131
113. Milanesi C, Zhou C, Biolo R, Jori G (1990) Zn(II)-phthalocyanine as a photodynamic agent for tumours. II. Studies on the mechanism of photosensitised tumour necrosis. Br J Cancer 61:846–850
114. Moan J (1986) Porphyrin photosensitization and phototherapy. Photochem Photobiol 43:681–690
115. Monfrecola G, Dána F, Delfino M (1987) Topical hematoporphyrin plus UVA for treatment of alopecia areata. Photodermatol Photoimmunol Photomed 4:305–306
116. Morton CA, Whitehurst C, Moseley H, McColl JH, Moore JV, Mackie RM (1996) Comparison of photodynamic therapy with cryotherapy in the treatment of Bowen's disease. Br J

Dermatol 135:766–771
117. Nelson JS (1993) Photodynamic therapy of port wine stain: preliminary clinical studies. In: Shapshay SM, Anderson RR, White JV, White RA, Bass LR (eds) Lasers in otolaryngology, dermatology, and tissue welding. Proc SPIE 1876:142–146
118. North J, Coombs R, Levy JG (1994) Photodynamic inactivation of free and cell-associated HIV-1 using the photosensitizer, benzoporphyrin derivative. J Acquir Immune Defic Syndr 7:891–898
119. Nseyo UO, Whalen RK, Duncan MR, Berman B, Lundahl SL (1990) Urinary cytokines following photodynamic therapy for bladder cancer. A preliminary report. Urology 36:167–171
120. Nugent LJ, Jain RK (1984) Extravascular diffusion in normal and neoplastic tissues. Cancer Res 44:238–244
121. Obochi MO, Canaan AJ, Jain AK, Richter AM, Levy JG (1995) Targeting activated lymphocytes with photodynamic therapy: susceptibility of mitogen-stimulated splenic lymphocytes to benzoporphyrin derivative (BPD) photosensitization. Photochem Photobiol 62:169–175
122. Ochsner M (1997) Photophysical and photobiological processes in the photodynamic therapy of tumours. J Photochem Photobiol B 39:1–18
123. Ortel B, Tanew A, Hönigsmann H (1993) Lethal photosensitization by endogenous porphyrins of PAM cells—modification by desferrioxamine. J Photochem Photobiol B Biol 17:273–278
124. Oseroff AR (1993) Photodynamic therapy. In: Lim HW, Soter NA (eds) Clinical photomedicine. Dekker, New York, pp 387–402
125. Pass HI (1993) Photodynamic therapy in oncology: mechanisms and clinical use. J Natl Cancer Inst 85:443–456
126. Peng Q, Warloe T, Moan J (1995) Topically-applied ALA-based PDT for nodulo-ulcerative basal cell carcinoma. IPA News 7:2
127. Peng Q, Warloe T, Berg K, Moan J, Kongshaug M, Giercksky KE, Nesland JM (1997) 5-Aminolevulinic acid-based photodynamic therapy. Clinical research and future challenges. Cancer 79:2282–2308
128. Pennington DG, Waner M, Knox A (1988) Photodynamic therapy for multiple skin cancers. Plast Reconstr Surg 82:1067–1071
129. Preš H, Meffert H, Sönnichsen N (1989) Photodynamische Therapie der Psoriasis palmaris et plantaris mit topisch appliziertem Hämatoporphyrin-Derivat und sichtbarem Licht. Dermatol Monatsschr 175:745–750
130. Qin B, Selman SH, Payne KM, Keck RW, Metzger DW (1993) Enhanced skin allograft survival after photodynamic therapy. Association with lymphocyte inactivation and macrophage stimulation. Transplantation 56:1481–1486
131. Raab O (1900) Über die Wirkung fluorescierender Stoffe auf Infusoria. Z Biol 39:524
132. Ratkay LG, Chowdhary RK, Iamaroon A, Richter AM, Neyndorff HC, Keystone EC, Waterfield JD, Levy JG (1998) Amelioration of antigen-induced arthritis in rabbits by induction of apoptosis of inflammatory cells with local application of transdermal photodynamic therapy. Arthritis Rheum 41:525–534
133. Rebeiz N, Arkins S, Rebeiz CA, Simon J, Zachary JF, Kelley KW (1996) Induction of tumor necrosis by δ-aminolevulinic acid and 1,10-phenantroline photodynamic therapy. Cancer Res 56:339–344
134. Rebeiz N, Rebeiz CC, Arkins S, Kelley KW, Rebeiz CA (1992) Photodestruction of tumor cells by induction of endogenous accumulation of protoporphyrin IX: enhancement by 1,10-phenanthroline. Photochem Photobiol 55:431–435
135. Reddan J, Anderson CY, Xu H, Hrabovsky S, Freye K, Fairchild R, Tubesing KA, Elmets CA (1999) Immunosuppressive effects of silicon phthalocyanine photodynamic therapy. Photochem Photobiol 70:72–77
136. Renschler MF, Yuen A, Panella TJ, Wieman TJ, Julius C, Panjehpour M, Taber S, Fingar V, Horning S, Miller RA, Lowe E, Engel J, Woodburn K, Young SW (1997) Photodynamic therapy trials with lutetium texaphyrin PCI-0123 (Lu-Tex). Photochem Photobiol 65:47S

(Abstract)
137. Richert C, Wessels JM, Müller M, Kisters M, Benninghaus T, Goetz AE (1994) Photodynamic antitumor agents: beta-methoxyethyl groups give access to functionalized porphycenes and enhance cellular uptake and activity. J Med Chem 37:2797–2807
138. Richter AM, Jain AK, Canaan AJ, Waterfield E, Sternberg ED, Levy JG (1992) Photosensitizing efficiency of two regioisomers of the benzoporphyrin derivative monoacid ring A. Biochem Pharmacol 43:2349–2358
139. Rittenhouse-Diakun K, Van Leengoed H, Morgan J, Hryhorenko E, Paszkiewicz G, Whitaker JE, Oseroff AR (1995) The role of transferrin receptor (CD71) in photodynamic therapy of activated and malignant lymphocytes using the heme precursor delta-aminolevulinic acid (ALA). Photochem Photobiol 61:523–528
140. Robinson PJ, Carruth JAS, Fairris GM (1988) Photodynamic therapy: a better treatment for widespread Bowen's disease. Br J Dermatol 119:59–61
141. Rosenblum LA, Hoskwith B, Kramer SD (1937) Photodynamic action of methylene blue on poliomyelitis virus. Proc Soc Exp Biol Med 37:166–169
142. Rünger TM (1995) Genotoxizität, Mutagenität und Karzinogenität von UVA und UVB. Z Hautkr 70:877–881
143. Sacchini V, Melloni E, Marchesini R, Fabrizio T, Cascinelli N, Santoro O, Zunino F, Andreola S, Bandieramonte G (1987) Topical administration of tetrasodium-*meso*-tetraphenylporphinesulfonate (TPPS) and red light irradiation for the treatment of superficial neoplastic lesions. Tumori 73:19–23
144. Schaffner K, Vogel E, Jori G (1994) Porphycenes as photodynamic therapy agents. In: Jung EG, Holick MF (eds) Biologic effects of light 1993. De Gruyter, Berlin, pp 312–321
145. Schlag P, Hünerbein M, Stern J, Gahlen J, Graschew G (1992) Photodynamische Therapie—Alternative bei lokal reziviertem Mamma-Karzinom. Dt Ärztebl 89:680–687
146. Schmidt S, Wagner U, Oehr P, Krebs D (1992) Klinischer Einsatz der photodynamischen Therapie bei gynäkologischen Tumorpatienten—Antikörper-vermittelte photodynamische Lasertherapie als neues onkologisches Behandlungsverfahren. Zentralbl Gynäkol 114:307–311
147. Schuh M, Nseyo UO, Potter WR, Dao TL, Dougherty TJ (1987) Photodynamic therapy for palliation of locally recurrent breast carcinoma. J Clin Oncol 5:1766–1770
148. Schultz EW, Krueger AP (1930) Inactivation of staphylococcus bacteriophage by methylene blue. Proc Soc Exp Biol Med 26:100–101
149. Schwartz SK, Absolon K, Vermund H (1955) Some relationships of porphyrins, x-rays and tumours. Univ Minn Med Bull 27:7–8
150. Schweitzer VG, Visscher D (1990) Photodynamic therapy for treatment of AIDS-related oral Kaposi's sarcoma. Otolaryngol Head Neck Surg 102:639–649
151. Silver H (1937) Psoriasis vulgaris treated with hematoporphyrin. Arch Dermatol Syph 36:1118–1119
152. Sperduto PW, DeLaney TF, Thomas G, Smith P, Dachowski LJ, Russo A, Bonner R, Glatstein E (1991) Photodynamic therapy for chest wall recurrence in breast cancer. Int J Radiat Oncol Biol Phys 21:441–446
153. Star WM, Marijnissen HP, van den Berg Blok AE, Versteeg JA, Franken KA, Reinhold HS (1986) Destruction of rat mammary tumor and normal tissue microcirculation by hematoporphyrin derivative photoradiation observed in vivo in sandwich observation chambers. Cancer Res 46:2532–2540
154. Stender IM, Na R, Fogh H, Glaud C, Wulf HC (2000) Photodynamic therapy with 5-aminolaevulinic acid or placebo for recalcitrant foot and hand warts: randomized double-blind trial. Lancet 355:963–966
155. Stern R, Zierler S, Parrish JA (1982) Psoriasis and the risk of cancer. J Invest Dermatol 78:147–149
156. Svaasand LO, Tromberg BJ, Wyss P, Wyss-Desserich MT, Tadir Y, Berns MW (1996) Light

and drug distribution with topically administered photosensitizers. Las Med Sci 11:261–265
157. Svanberg K, Andersson T, Killander D, Wang I, Stenram U, Andersson-Engels S, Berg R, Johansson J, Svanberg S (1994) Photodynamic therapy of non-melanoma malignant tumours of the skin using topical δ-aminolevulinic acid sensitization and laser irradiation. Br J Dermatol 130:743–751
158. Szeimies RM, Abels C, Fritsch C, Karrer S, Steinbach P, Bäumler W, Goerz G, Goetz AE, Landthaler M (1995) Wavelength dependency of photodynamic effects after sensitization with 5-aminolevulinic acid in vitro and in vivo. J Invest Dermatol 105:672–677
159. Szeimies RM, Hein R, Bäumler W, Heine A, Landthaler M (1994) A possible new incoherent lamp for photodynamic treatment of superficial skin lesions. Acta Derm Venereol (Stockh) 74:117–119
160. Szeimies RM, Karrer S, Heine A, Hohenleutner U, Landthaler M (1995) Topical photodynamic therapy with 5-aminolevulinic acid in the treatment of arsenic-induced skin tumors. Eur J Dermatol 5:208–211
161. Szeimies RM, Karrer S, Sauerwald A, Landthaler M (1996b) Topical photodynamic therapy with 5-aminolevulinic acid in the treatment of actinic keratoses: a first clinical study. Dermatology 192:246–251
162. Szeimies RM, Landthaler M (1993) Treatment of Bowen's disease with topical photodynamic therapy. J Dermatol Treat 4:207–209
163. Szeimies RM, Landthaler M (1995) Topische photodynamische Therapie in der Behandlung oberflächlicher Hauttumoren. Hautarzt 46:315–318
164. Szeimies RM, Sassy T, Landthaler M (1994) Penetration potency of topical applied δ-aminolevulinic acid for photodynamic therapy of basal cell carcinoma. Photochem Photobiol 59:73–76
165. Taber SW, Fingar VH, Coots CT, Wieman TJ (1998) Photodynamic therapy using mono-l-aspartyl chlorin e_6 (Npe6) for the treatment of cutaneous disease: a phase I clinical study. Clin Cancer Res 4:2741–2746
166. Thiele B, Grotmann P, Hüttmann G, Diddens H, Hörauf H (1994) Topische photodynamische Therapie (TPDT) von Basaliomen: klinische, histologische und experimentelle Ergebnisse (erste Mitteilung). Z Hautkr 3:161–164
167. Tse DT, Kersten RD, Anderson RL (1984) Hematoporphyrin derivative photoradiation therapy in managing nevoid basal cell carcinoma syndrome. Arch Ophthalmol 102:990–994
168. Vogel E, Köcher M, Schmickler H, Lex J (1986) Porphycene—a novel porphin isomer. Angew Chem 98:262–264
169. von Tappeiner H, Jesionek A (1903) Therapeutische Versuche mit fluorescierenden Stoffen. Münch Med Wochenschr 47:2042–2044
170. Wainwright M (1998) Photodynamic antimicrobial chemotherapy (PACT). J Antimicrob Chemother 42:13–28
171. Waldow SM, Lobraico RV, Kohler IK, Wallk S, Fritts HT (1987) Photodynamic therapy for treatment of malignant cutaneous lesions. Lasers Surg Med 7:451–456
172. Walter AW, Pivnick EK, Bale AE, Kun LE (1997) Complications of the nevoid basal cell carcinoma syndrome: a case report. J Pediatr Hematol Oncol 19:258–262
173. Warloe T, Peng Q, Moan J, Qvist HL, Giercksky KE (1992) Photochemotherapy of multiple basal cell carcinoma with endogenous porphyrins induced by topical application of 5-aminolevulinic acid. In: Spinelli P, Dal Fante M, Marchesini R (eds) Photodynamic therapy and biomedical lasers. Elsevier Science, Amsterdam, pp 449–453
174. Weinstein GD, McCullough JL, Jeffes EW, Nelson JS, Fong NL, McCormick AJ (1994) Photodynamic therapy (PDT) of psoriasis with topical delta aminolevulinic acid (ALA): a pilot dose ranging study. Photodermatol Photoimmunol Photomed 10:92 (abstract)
175. Weinstein GD, McCullough JL, Nelson JS, Berns MW, McCormick AJ (1991) Low-dose photofrin II photodynamic therapy of psoriasis. Clin Res 39:509A (abstract)
176. Weishaupt KR, Gomer CJ, Dougherty TJ (1976) Identification of singlet oxygen as the cyto-

toxic agent in photo-inactivation of a murine tumor. Cancer Res 36:2326–2329
177. Wennberg AM, Lindholm LE, Alpsten M, Larkö O (1996) Treatment of superficial basal cell carcinomas using topically applied delta-aminolaevulinic acid and a filtered xenon lamp. Arch Dermatol Res 288:561–564
178. Wessels JM, Strauss W, Seidlitz HK, Rück A, Schneckenburger H (1992) Intracellular localization of meso-tetraphenylporphine tetrasulphonate probed by time-resolved and microscopic fluorescence spectroscopy. J Photochem Photobiol B Biol 12:275–284
179. Wilson BD, Mang TS, Cooper M, Stoll H (1989) Use of photodynamic therapy for the treatment of extensive basal cell carcinomas. Facial Plast Surg 6:185–189
180. Wilson BD, Mang TS, Stoll H, Jones C, Cooper M, Dougherty TJ (1992) Photodynamic therapy for the treatment of basal cell carcinoma. Arch Dermatol 128:1597–1601
181. Winkelman JW, Collins GH (1987) Neurotoxicity of tetraphenylporphinesulfonate $TPPS_4$ and its relation to photodynamic therapy. Photochem Photobiol 46:801–807
182. Wolf P, Fink-Puches R, Cerroni L, Kerl H (1994) Photodynamic therapy for mycosis fungoides after topical photosensitization with 5-aminolevulinic acid. J Am Acad Dermatol 31:678–680
183. Wolf P, Fink-Puches R, Kerl H (1995) Photodynamic therapy for mycosis fungoides after topical photosensitization with 5-aminolevulinic acid. J Am Acad Dermatol 33:541
184. Wolf P, Kerl H (1995) Photodynamic therapy with 5-aminolevulinic acid: a promising concept for the treatment of cutaneous tumors. Dermatology 190:183–185
185. Wolf P, Rieger E, Kerl H (1993) Topical photodynamic therapy with endogenous porphyrins after application of 5-aminolevulinic acid. J Am Acad Dermatol 28:17–21
186. Wolford ST, Novicki DL, Kelly B (1995) Comparative skin phototoxicity in mice with two photosensitizing drugs: benzoporphyrin derivative monoacid ring A and porfimer sodium (Photofrin). Fundam Appl Toxicol 24:52–56
187. Woodburn KW, Vardaxis NJ, Hill JS, Kaye AH, Phillips DR (1991) Subcellular localization of porphyrins using confocal laser scanning microscopy. Photochem Photobiol 54:725–732
188. Xiao-xi L, Wie W, Shuo-fan W, Chuan Y, Ti-Sheng C (1997) Treatment of capillary vascular malformation (port-wine stains) with photochemotherapy. Plast Reconstr Surg 99:1826–1830
189. Yamamoto N, Hoober JK, Yamamoto N, Yamamoto S (1992) Tumoricidal capacities of macrophages photodynamically activated with hematoporphyrin derivative. Photochem Photobiol 56:245–250
190. Yamamoto N, Sery TW, Hoober JK, Willett NP, Lindsay DD (1994) Effectiveness of photofrin II in activation of macrophages and in vitro killing of retinoblastoma cells. Photochem Photobiol 60:160–164
191. Zaidi SI, Oleinick NL, Zaim MT, Mukhtar H (1993) Apoptosis during photodynamic therapy-induced ablation of RIF-1 tumors in C3H mice: electron microscopic, histopathologic and biochemical evidence. Photochem Photobiol 58:771–776

第 12 章　体外光化学免疫疗法

R. Knobler

内容

引言	247
皮肤 T 细胞淋巴瘤	248
T 细胞介导疾病的体外光化学免疫疗法	248
寻常型天疱疮	249
进行性系统性硬化症	249
类风湿性关节炎	250
移植物抗宿主病	251
系统性红斑狼疮	252
口腔扁平苔藓	253
多发性硬化症	253
总结	253

要点

> 在跨学科背景下,有文献证明体外光化学免疫疗法似乎是一种有效且无显著相关副反应的免疫调节治疗方法。

> 已证实,体外光化学免疫疗法可有效治疗皮肤 T 细胞淋巴瘤、变异型 Sézary 综合征,且有相关资料显示治疗后患者将获得长期的缓解及长久的寿命。

> 在骨髓移植(急性、慢性 GvHD)、实体器官移植以及选择性 T 淋巴细胞所介导的疾病,如系统性硬化和肾源性纤维性皮病(NFD)中,体外光化学免疫疗法已成为一种可接受且行之有效的辅助性治疗措施。

第12章 体外光化学免疫疗法

引言

自1985年Edelson等人发明了体外光免疫化学疗法/光分离置换疗法(extracorporeal photoimmunotherapy, ECP, photopheresis)后,1987年该疗法即被应用于皮肤T细胞淋巴瘤(CTCL)的姑息性治疗。经多中心实验证实该疗法对CTCL的早期病例,主要是红皮病性Sézary综合征有效。2008年,通过在CTCL及一系列其他T淋巴细胞介导的疾病中疗效的体现,该治疗方法建立了其确切的治疗价值。因此,这种物理疗法在美国、欧洲、亚洲、拉丁美洲的200多个医疗中心得以应用。本章将回顾该疗法的步骤及应用,包括持续但仍然快速发展的应用,如在骨髓移植后顽固性的急性、慢性移植物抗宿主疾病(GvHD)中的使用[12-30]。

为了解决待治疗的血浆/白细胞层部分中存在持续性可重复操作的补骨脂素水平,治疗程序从第一例施行开始就不断地进行微调。当前的治疗的治疗程序共有两处改良,一处是治疗中将口服给药转变为将药物直接导入淋巴细胞,另一处即是新近在治疗过程中使用连续循环的淋巴细胞收集和照射的装置,使得所有包含8-甲基补骨脂素(8-MOP)的淋巴细胞都可以均衡分配相同照射剂量的UVA。ECP平均治疗时间为连续2天,每2~4周重复疗程。在治疗无效的患者之中可选定一些患者,在有限的周期内用更短的间隔周期进行重复治疗。1次治疗可以治疗T细胞池中10%到15%的循环T细胞,UVA总剂量为$2J/cm^2$细胞。

自从Edelson等人的多中心研究报道,紧随其后的报告也基本证实了最初的观察:ECP就被认为是治疗红皮病型CTCL的一线疗法[39]。就目前所有可获得的文献资料来看,ECP治疗对于CTLT及其他一些适应证似有较小的毒副作用,因此在过去几年中,很多治疗中心广泛开展关于ECP治疗其他适应证的相关评价工作。得到一些关于评价ECP对免疫系统影响的实验室研究的支持[40-54]。基于ECP可抑制对机体有害的相关T细胞克隆及相关多肽的产生这个假设,为了评估ECP在CTCL以外,以自身免疫性T淋巴细胞为主导的炎症反应性疾病中的治疗价值,相关人员做了一系列研究。最新的研究进展也提示ECP的重要功能与调节性T细胞的诱导密切相关。目前,医疗界已经获得了一系列疾病谱的治疗经验,如系统性硬化、寻常型天疱疮、类风湿性关节炎、关节病型银屑病、系统性红斑狼疮及特应性皮炎等,大量的研究提示ECP可能在器官移植中急性、慢性排斥反应及骨髓移植后GvHD、以及顽固性激素依赖性炎性肠病(如溃疡性结肠炎、Crohn病)的治疗中起重要作用[12,22-24,28]。

除了评估其他可能适应证的临床研究以外,治疗程序的改进可使治疗费用降低和疗程缩短,而给药方式的改进也使相关副作用减少。

皮肤 T 细胞淋巴瘤

皮肤 T 细胞淋巴瘤(CTCL)是第一种接受 ECP 治疗评估的疾病。充分的临床研究证据及 FDA 的批准都强烈支持 ECP 在保守治疗红皮病性 Sézary 综合征中作为一线疗法。第一份在 1987 年由 Edelson 等人[1]发表的相关研究中,37 例患者中有 27 例对治疗有部分或完全的缓解,在随访中,接受 ECP 治疗的患者缓解期延长,生存时间中位数由 30 个月延长到 66 个月[36]。即使考虑到存在的争议以及将获得的结果同历史对照相比较过程中的统计效度问题,延长的缓解效应依然具有统计学意义。

后期的研究肯定了对于疗效的早期猜测[17,34,39,55,56]。研究显示 ECP 治疗该病的疗效显著,且治疗应答率达 75%,完全缓解率达 25%,无效率为 25%。有利于观察患者较好预后的标准是 CD4/CD8 比值,外周血 CD8 细胞计数的绝对值,较短的疾病周期[38,39]但是,这些指标并不足以预测有效反应,有效反应者和无效反应者均可出现两极分化。

作为单一疗法,ECP 治疗 CTCL 最常见的反应是部分缓解。免疫抑制因素如化疗及系统性激素用药等可干扰 ECP 疗效,因此,放疗在最终摧毁疾病阶段便显得有意义,有 1 例文献显示当接受 ECP 同时联合全身照射的患者完全反应率有所增加[52],另一种方案是联合注射干扰素进一步免疫刺激疗法。而另 1 例报道显示两种免疫调节疗法的协同作用很强,因而足以让我们在治疗初期即考虑联用两种物理疗法[58]。1 例有明显的淋巴结及血液系统并发症的 CTLT 患者在经过联合物理疗法的治疗后病情得到缓解[69]。该实践方案将观察与每日的实际操作相结合,被认为是多学科性疗法的启蒙。对于先前有肿瘤或显著血液系统疾病的患者,单用 ECP 疗法将无法达到症状的完全缓解。这些患者应该在开始就接受辅助治疗。而对于那些有红皮病的患者,应在单一疗法进行 3~6 个月后再接受辅助治疗,从而最大限度地提高疗效。目前很明确的是,我们仍需要将来进行前瞻性随机研究去确定联合治疗在总生存时间以及治疗反应方面的价值。

T 细胞介导疾病的体外光化学免疫疗法

以前和目前的少量临床试验数据提示体外光化学免疫疗法可应用于其他 T 细胞介导疾病,如系统性硬化症、寻常型天疱疮、类风湿性关节炎、较轻程度的系统性红斑狼疮、皮肌炎、关节型银屑病、溃疡性结肠炎、特应性皮炎等。从已发表的文献来看,ECP 在器官移植中受体对供体的抗原敏感问题呈现出可被有效治疗的趋势,如果在更大设计性试验中得到证实,将对心脏、肺、肝移植以及较轻程度的肾移植产生潜在的巨大效益。近来的数据也提示,体外光化学免疫疗法对异基因骨髓移植后 GvHD 有显著的作用。给药装置系统的改进及不断出现的临床与实验的新数据,有助于阐明其疗效机制,促进了治疗方案的改进,以期确定该疗法在治疗领域中长期和短期的治疗角色。

寻常型天疱疮

寻常型天疱疮是继皮肤 T 细胞淋巴瘤后最早采用 ECP 治疗进行评估疗效的自身免疫性疾病。Rook 等[5]总结了早期阳性结果,他们报道的初期试验中,4 个人中有 3 个存在药物抵抗,最初,这 4 个患者,病情表现出极大的改善,其特异性抗体的滴度明显下降,临床症状亦得到缓解。这主要归功于 ECP 与其他治疗相比,治疗没有毒副作用。伴随着糖皮质激素与免疫抑制剂的大幅度减量,4 个患者中有 3 个,明显缓解的周期达 6 个月。2 篇随后发表的报道和本医疗中心也验证了该治疗效果。

Liang 等报道了 1 例 31 岁的患者,接受了体外光化学免疫疗法后随着免疫抑制剂的明显减少,接近完全缓解[21]。Gollnick 等[8]报道了 1 例 37 岁的女性,她有 5 年的严重治疗抵抗病史,对有严重的副作用的药物如强的松(40 ~ 300mg/天)、硫唑嘌呤(100 ~ 150mg/天)、间歇性使用甲氨蝶呤(25mg/周)没有反应,该患者使用了 ECP 治疗,经过 4 轮 ECP 治疗,血清抗 IgG 从 1∶800 降至 1∶100,经 6 轮治疗后,95% 的皮肤黏膜损害消退。

基于以上 6 例 ECP 治疗病例和在 ECP 治疗过程中观察到的疗效,看起来有充分的证据或理由去组织能够验证该疗法在顽固性患者中疗效的多中心Ⅲ期临床随机试验。但由于它没能够纳入足够数量的患者去满足统计分析的要求,相对少见的情况甚至少见的顽固类型使更大规模的研究难于开展,在临床实践中,认为顽固性的天疱疮患者应接受 3 ~ 4 个月的 ECP 治疗。有关 ECP 对天疱疮抗体滴度的影响及其减少免疫抑制剂用量的效能应继续报告。而这 2 个参数代表了 ECP 疗法对顽固性天疱疮患者的改善程度。

进行性系统性硬化症

进行性系统性硬化症(PSS)也叫硬皮病,是以胶原在皮肤、脏器(如心、肺、肾、胃肠道)中的过多沉积为特点的自身免疫性疾病。PSS 与硬化性 GvHD 的类似之处说明它可能是由 T 细胞介导的疾病。早期 T 淋巴细胞在受损器官中的浸润,同时有自身反应性抗体的出现,都提示疾病的中心环节是自身免疫。有 ECP 的个案研究报道了 2 个对治疗抵抗快速进展的 PSS 患者[60],接受 ECP 治疗后都显示有所改善。

受这些报道的鼓舞,开展了1个单盲、随机、8中心的试验,比较体外光化学免疫疗法与D-青霉胺疗效。79个近期有系统性硬化症状发作(症状持续时间的中位数为1.83年)或入组前有6个月前即有进行性皮肤损害的患者入组进行平行、单盲的临床试验。每间隔4周便连续2天进行ECP的治疗,与接受D-青霉胺最大剂量750mg/天的治疗进行比较,由单盲的临床测试者用统一的量表评估[61],如皮损的范围与严重程度、受累面积、口腔孔、手掌闭合等,以重复活检评估皮肤变化,为评估肺部病变的影响与病程,定期进行肺功能检查。在基线观察时与治疗后6月、12月时随访血清学指标。患者的排除标准:随机化之前或之后D-青霉胺治疗失败及广泛的全身脏器受累患者。

在10个月的研究中,显示ECP疗效优于增加剂量使用的D-青霉胺治疗。它显示能逆转皮肤病理变化及阻止病情发展。56个患者坚持了最少6个月的治疗,其中31例患者接受ECP治疗,25例接受D-青霉胺治疗。47例完成了10个月的治疗,其中有29个接受了ECP治疗。在6个月疗程的评价初期,31例接受ECP疗法患者中有21例(68%)显示皮肤明显软化,而接受D-青霉胺治疗的25例患者中只有8例有皮肤软化。在6个月里,31例接受ECP治疗的患者中有3例(10%)显示皮肤评分明显恶化,而25例接受D-青霉胺治疗的患者中有8例(32%)显示病情明显进展。所有接受ECP治疗的患者都完成了疗程的治疗,而有25%接受D-青霉胺治疗的患者由于副作用或病情进展而退出实验。

一方面,这些观察结果近期受到了对照研究的质疑,因为对照研究显示ECP治疗组疗效并没有优于安慰剂组。另一方面,在治疗累及皮肤和关节的疾病中取得的一些微小却意义重大的进展或可被文献收录。我们仍然需要更多的研究资料去进一步证实或推翻这个观察结论。

同样的,Zachariae等[4]关于8个患者的小样本观察显示在初期采取免疫抑制疗法后用单一ECP治疗严重的PSS患者取得令人鼓舞的结果。

类风湿性关节炎

为使治疗在达到最佳疗效的同时副作用最小,Malawista等人[19]对7个治疗抵抗的类风湿性关节炎患者进行试点试验。由于自身免疫性疾病的相似性,研究者受到了ECP可诱导出可能致病性的循环T细胞单克隆的免疫反应的启发,设计6个月的研究。研究中患者在2次连续治疗期间每月进行随访,而对治疗无反应者则每2周进行随访。排除安慰剂效应的影响后观察到,7个患者中有4个在经过4个月的治疗后呈现出症状的改善。从这个意义上讲,这些经过ECP治疗的患者在几个月后疾病复发的情况进一步支持ECP对疾病病程有影响这个论断。作者报道了7个人中的4个患者在接受了12到16周的治疗后受累关节数与关节症状评分明显改善,其中4个患者中的3个改善情况可确诊,上述测量分别提高了平均值为71%和80%的基线值。另一个间接的临床反应的测量结果是其他方面的改善,如7个人中有2个握力改善、1个50步行走时间缩短、2个人晨僵情况改善。这些小样本的初步研究提示ECP治疗短期内可为类风湿性关节炎带来益处,同时与传统的治疗药物相比有更低的毒副作用。ECP是否推荐应用于治疗类风湿性关节炎及相关疾病,如关节病性银屑病[10,11,25]、莱姆关节炎[18],在实施之前,需要ECP治疗这些相关疾病的支持性的证据,需要进行双盲、安慰剂对照试验,其中也许有不同治疗方案,以及有无其他药物辅助性治疗方案。

移植物抗宿主病

光免疫疗法在器官移植显示重要的应用价值,是其最鼓舞人心的发展领域。多组临床研究显示,与目前常用的免疫抑制疗法相比,ECP没有其经典的副作用,是控制与预防器官排斥反应很有用的辅助治疗方法。Loyola大学的Constanzo-Nordin等人[23]对7例接受了三联免疫抑制剂(环孢素、糖皮质激素、硫唑嘌呤)的心脏移植的患者进行体外光化学免疫疗法疗效评价,结果发现他们有9段适度的非血液动力学的排斥。9段中的8段经体外光化学免疫疗法治疗后成功逆转(治疗后1周行心内膜心肌活检(EMB))。另外,与ECP治疗前相比,治疗后免疫组化中与排斥反应有关的T细胞、B细胞及巨噬细胞计数明显减少。随访研究评估ECP逆转排斥的能力,观察国际心肺移植协会(ISHLT)所制定的没有血液动力学障碍的2、3A及3B级排斥反应。16例患者随机入组接受体外光化学免疫疗法治疗或糖皮质激素疗法研究显示,ECP逆转了9段排斥反应中的8段,而糖皮质激素只逆转了7段。ECP在初始治疗后逆转排斥反应的中位时间25天,糖皮质激素组是17天。作者通过对这些前瞻性随机患者的初步短期结果认为ECP对治疗ISHLT排斥反应2、3A及3B级可能与糖皮质激素同样有效,而且有较低的副作用[24]。

哥伦比亚大学的Rose等评价了ECP治疗4例患者的疗效[26]。其中,2例多次接受器官移植的患者有先存高水平的群体反应性抗体,2例经产的妇女被认为有高敏感风险。在常规的免疫抑制疗法中加入ECP治疗,有1例高水平的群体反应性抗体的抗体水平下降,1例排斥反应的段数下降,4例患者中没有出现感染并发症。特别的是,2例以前曾接受过移植的患者中,出现群体反应性淋巴细胞毒抗体的下降,而另外2个患者也观察到淋巴细胞毒抗体表达的受阻。作者认为ECP的研究应扩展到阻止急性排斥反应的领域。

随着研究的进行,另外有 2 个欧洲研究组证实了前面早期的研究。Dall Amico 等人的第一组,治疗 4 例心脏移植后由于多发性急性排斥反应需要增加糖皮质激素剂量的患者。体外光化学免疫疗法治疗联合免疫抑制疗法,帮助控制了反复发作的排斥反应,减少了激素用量[62]。第二组德国慕尼黑大学在心脏移植后的头 6 个月,在免疫抑制疗法中辅以体外光化学免疫疗法治疗,研究了 15 例原位心脏移植的患者[63],他们被分为 3 组:1 组接受标准的 3 联免疫抑制药物(环孢素、硫唑嘌呤、糖皮质激素)治疗,第 2 组接受 10 个单天的 ECP 辅助治疗,第 3 组接受 20 个疗程的 ECP 治疗。每个治疗都一致由 2 个背靠背治疗组成。在最后 2 组中有高频度的体外光化学免疫疗法治疗,在移植后 24 小时内早期术后阶段及随后 4 周的间歇共 6 月的时间内进行研究显示,就移植后头 4 周的急性排斥反应发作的总次数而言,第 3 组接受标准背靠背治疗比单独治疗更引人关注。所有的体外光化学免疫疗法治疗治疗组比对照组更有效,减少了超过50%的排斥反应[64]。

最后一项 Knobler 等人的研究是加入体外光敏药物 8-MOP 的实验[31]。尽管每组患者人数少,药物浓度低于目前研究所建议的 ECP 疗效的理想浓度(~100ng/ml),这些观察与其他已披露的研究一起,确切的显示了该治疗方法在器官移植领域中的应用价值。最近,相关研究人员已完成了一个囊括了 12 个中心 60 个初次接受心血管移植患者的多中心、前瞻性、平行设计性研究,评估关于持续 6 个月 ECP 治疗有效性与安全性。患者经过年龄与性别的分层与平衡后入组,接受单独的标准三联药物疗法或联合 ECP 治疗。尽管两组的生存率相似,ECP 组为 94%[3,31],标准疗法组为 96%[26,27]。研究中值得注意的是 ECP 组比标准组在时间上有 2.13 倍的免疫排斥缓解期。研究显示 ECP 组能显著降低心血管免疫排斥反应而不增加感染风险[64]。在肺、肾、小肠、骨髓移植等方面,标准的免疫抑制疗法没有那么成功或有显著的威胁生命的副作用,而这项研究肯定地支持了 ECP 免疫调节的效果,肯定了其在移植等应用的前景[12,13,27-30],关于这方面,进展中的一系列试验将为确定 ECP 疗法的治疗指南而做铺垫。

系统性红斑狼疮

系统性红斑狼疮(SLE)是 T 细胞介导的自身免疫性疾病。目前没有无副作用的特别疗法,控制该病需使用非特异性免疫抑制治疗,包括长期使用糖皮质激素和细胞毒类药物。前面提到,这些药物的长期使用会导致人体器官功能受限和使人衰弱的副作用及并发症。为评估 ECP 在治疗 SLE 中的安全性、可行性及效果,相关人员进行了一个开放性的为期 2 年的临床试验[6,7]。10 个符合美国风湿协会(ARM)诊断标准的红斑狼疮患者入组观察,基于试点研究的目的,如果系统损害还没到威胁到生命的程度;仅有轻到中度用包括非甾体类抗炎药、低剂量激素、氯喹、口服硫唑嘌呤、环孢素等传统治疗就足以控制的病情;在3个月内减少或停用这些药物但疾病活动持续存在的患者优先入组。10个患者中有8个完成实验,其中7个对治疗有明显反应。

临床活动性评分从中位数7(1~9)降至中位数1(0~5)($P<0.05$),与已知的SLE评分系统相比,利用率评分(SIS)可信。实验的遗传学指标没有明显变化,但是正如作者所说的,在初期是轻度的。与其他小型的研究一样,该研究报道了ECP在治疗SLE方面的安全性。该结果被认为是鼓舞人心的进步,尤其是在应用于治疗SLE患者关节与皮肤损害的相关临床症状。也许该观察中最令人感兴趣的是ECP可应用于有光敏的患者而没有导致病情加重。同样,建议进一步评估该疗法,不仅仅是在所选择病例的治疗上,而且还要在临床对照试验设计之前[20]。

口腔扁平苔藓

扁平苔藓与GvHD的相似性反映了其共同致病特性。Becherel报道了一系列有严重顽固性糜烂的口腔扁平苔藓患者,经6个月的ECP治疗有效[65],并观察了最小毒性,但此后没有追踪报道。尽管我们中心已经治疗过1例严重的口腔扁平苔藓,在2轮ECP治疗后得到迅速缓解,这个反应的机制尚不清楚,我们的患者同时患有丙肝。另外,研究显示ECP可以诱导对干扰素抵抗丙肝患者的有益反应[66],这可能与其加强抗病毒的免疫有关,也使得有疑似感染症状的口腔扁平苔藓患者得到改善。

多发性硬化症

由于干扰素在临床中应用的不良反应影响,ECP被寄望对T细胞介导的严重疾病——多发性硬化症产生作用。在一项有良好对照的双盲研究中,16名患者接受ECP治疗或非ECP治疗,随后的1年追踪性研究中,未见神经或MM评分的变化[67]。

总结

CTLT中成熟T细胞的控制机理应被临床工作者应用至其他T细胞介导的疾病治疗之中。以最小的急性与慢性毒性,这种治疗方法在许多情况下,包括进行性系统硬化的皮肤症状、对治疗抵抗的寻常型天疱疮、心脏移植急性排斥反应、急性与慢性GvHD、类风湿性关节炎、系统性红斑狼疮、关节型银屑病、扁平苔藓等疾病中可以最低程度的急性或慢性毒性而发挥积极的作用。不单局限于以上所介绍的病种,这种创新性的光免疫疗法治疗显然为治疗 T 细胞介导性疾病提供了新的思路。这种低副作用的治疗方法比目前使用的化疗与免疫抑制剂更引人注意,一旦明确其作用机制,其应用可造福更多患者,这将不单是科学研究者的责任。恰当的研究其与不同治疗方法联合应用的方案将极大地发挥 ECP 的作用,并取得更有意义的进步。

(黄茂芳 译,高方铭　陈荃 校,朱慧兰 审)

参考文献

1. Edelson RL, Berger C, Gasparro F, Jegasothy B, Heald P, Wintroub B, Vonderheid E, Knobler R, Wolff K, Plewig G, McKiernan G, Christensen I, Oster M, Hoenigsmann H, Wilford H, Kokoschka E, Rehle T, Perez M, Stingl G, Laroche L (1987) Treatment of cutaneous T-cell lymphoma by extracorporeal photochemotherapy. N Engl J Med 316:297–303
2. Rook AH, Freundlich B, Jegasothy BV, Perez ML, Barr WG, Jiminez SA, Rietschel RL, Wintroub B, Kahaleh B, Varga J, Heald PW, Steen V, Massa MC, Murphy GF, Perniciaro C, Istfan M, Ballas SK, Edelson RL (1992) Treatment of systemic sclerosis with extracorporeal photochemotherapy—results of a multicenter trial. Arch Dermatol 128:337–346
3. DiSpaltro F, Cotrill C, Cahill C, Degnan E, Mulford J, Scarborough D, Franks A, Klainer A, Bisaccia E (1993) Extracorporeal photochemotherapy in progressive systemic sclerosis. Int J Dermatol 32:1–5
4. Zachariae H, Bjerring P, Heickendorff L, Moller B, Wallevik K (1992) Photopheresis and systemic sclerosis. Arch Dermatol 128:1651–1653
5. Rook AH, Jegasothy BV, Heald P, Nahass GT, Ditre C, Witmer WK, Lazarus GS, Edelson RL (1990) Extracorporeal photochemotherapy for drug-resistant pemphigus vulgaris. Ann Intern Med 112:303–305
6. Knobler RM, Graninger W, Graninger W, Lindmaier A, Trautinger F, Smolen J (1992) Extracorporeal photochemotherapy for the treatment of systemic lupus erythematosus. A pilot study. Arthritis Rheum 35:319–324
7. Knobler RM, Graninger M, Lindmaier A, Trautinger F (1991) Photophereses for the treatment of lupus erythematosus. Ann NY Acad Sci 636:340
8. Gollnick H, Owsianowski M, Taube K, Orfanos C (1993) Unresponsive severe generalized pemphigus vulgaris successfully controlled by extracorporeal photopheresis. J Am Acad Dermatol 28:122–124
9. Prinz B, Nachbar F, Plewig G (1994) Treatment of severe atopic dermatitis with extracorporeal photopheresis. Arch Dermatol Res 287:48–52
10. Wilfert H, Hönigsmann H, Steiner G, Smolen J, Wolff K (1990) Treatment of psoriatic arthritis by extracorporeal photochemotherapy. Br J Dermatol 122:225–232
11. Vahlquist C, Larsson M, Ernerudh J, Berlin G, Skogh T, Vahlquist A (1996) Treatment of psoriatic arthritis with extracorporeal photochemotherapy and conventional psoralen-ultraviolet A irradiation. Arthritis Rheum 39(9):1519–1523
12. Owsianowski M, Gollnick H, Siegert W, Schwerdtfeger R, Orfanos EE (1994) Successful treatment of chronic graft-versus-host disease with extracorporeal photopheresis. Bone Marrow Transpl 14:845–848
13. Gerber M, Gmeinhart B, Volc-Platzer B, Kahls P, Greinix R, Knobler R (1997) Complete remission of lichen-planus-like graft-versus-host disease (GVHD) with extracorporeal photochemotherapy (CP). Bone Marrow Transplant 19:517–519

14. DeWilde A, DiSpaltro F, Geller A, Szer L, Klainer A, Bisaccia E (1992) Extracorporeal photochemotherapy as adjunctive treatment in juvenile dermatomyositis. A case report. Arch Dermatol 128:1656–1657
15. Rosetti F, Zulian F, Dall'Amico R, Messina C, Montini G, Zacchello F (1995) Extracorporeal photochemotherapy as single therapy for extensive cutaneous, chronic graft-versus-host disease. Transplantation 59:149–151
16. Vonderheid EC, Kang C, Kadin M, Bigler RD, Griffin TD, Rogers TJ (1990) Extra-corporeal photopheresis in psoriasis vulgaris: clinical and immunologic observations. J Am Acad Dermatol 23:703–712
17. Zachariae H, Bjerring P, Brodthagen U, Sogaard H (1995) Photopheresis in the red man or pre-Sezary syndrome. Dermatology 190:132–135
18. Randazzo J, DiSpaltro F, Cottrill C, Klainer A, Steere A, Bisaccia E (1994) Successful treatment of a patient with chronic lyme arthritis with extracorporeal photo-chemotherapy. J Am Acad Dermatol 30:908–910
19. Malawista S, Trock D, Edelson R (1991) Treatment of rheumatoid arthritis by extracorporeal photochemotherapy: a pilot study. Arthritis Rheum 34:646–654
20. Licht-Mbalyohere A, Heller A, Stadler R (1996) Extracorporeal photochemotherapy of therapy-refractory cases of systemic lupus erythematosus with urticarial vasculitis and pemphigus foliaceus. Eur J Dermatol 6:106–109
21. Liang G, Nahas G, Kerdel FA (1992) Pemphigus vulgaris treated with photopheresis. J Am Acad Dermatol 26:779–780
22. Berkson M, Lazarus GS, Uberti-Benz M, Rook AH (1991) Extracorporeal photochemotherapy: a potentially useful treatment for scleromyxedema. J Am Acad Dermatol 25:724
23. Costanzo-Nordin MR, Hubbell EA, O'Sullivan EJ, Johnson MR, Mullen GM, Heroux AL, Kao WG, McManus BM, Pifarre R, Robinson JA (1992) Successful treatment of heart transplant rejection with photopheresis. Transplantation 53:808–815
24. Costanzo-Nordin MR, Hubbell EA, O'Sullivan EJ, Johnson MR, Mullen GM, Heroux AL, Kao WG, McManus BM, Pifarre R, Robinson JA (1992) Photopheresis versus corticosteroids in the therapy of heart transplant rejection. Circulation 86:242–250
25. Hilliquin P, Andreu G, Heshmati F, Menkes CJ (1993) Treatment of refractory rheumatoid arthritis by extracorporeal photochemotherapy. Rheumatol Rev 60:125–130
26. Rose EA, Barr ML, Xu H, Peoino P, Murphy MP, McGovern MA, Ratner AJ, Watkins JF, Marboe CC, Berger CL (1992) Photochemotherapy in human heart transplant recipients at high risk for fatal rejection. J Heart Lung Transpl 11:746–750
27. Sunder-Plassman G, Druml W, Steininger R, Hönigsmann H, Knobler R (1995) Renal allograft rejection controlled by photopheresis. Lancet 346:506
28. Wolfe J, Tomaszewski J, Grosman R, Gottlieb S, Naji A, Brayman K, Kobrin S, Rook A (1996) Reversal of acute renal allograft rejection by extracorporeal photopheresis: a case presentation and review of the literature. J Clin Apheresis 11:36–41
29. Slovis BS, Loyd JE, King LE (1995) Photopheresis for chronic rejection of lung allografts. N Engl J Med 332:962
30. Andreu G, Achkar A, Couteil JP, Guillemain R, Heshmati F, Amrein C, Chevalier P, Guinvarch A, Dore MF, Capron F et al (1995) Extracorporeal photochemotherapy treatment for acute lung rejection episode. J Heart Lung Transplant 14(4):793–796
31. Knobler RM, Trautinger F, Graninger W, Macheiner W, Gruenwald C, Neumann R, Ramer W (1993) Parenteral administration of 8-methoxypsoralen in photopheresis. J Am Acad Dermatol 28:580–584
32. Knobler RM, Edelson RL (1986) Cutaneous T-cell lymphoma. Med Clin North Am 70:109–138
33. Knobler RM (1987) Photopheresis—extracorporeal irradiation of 8-MOP containing blood—a new therapeutic modality. Blut 54:247–250
34. Armus S, Keyes B, Cahill C, Berger C, Crater D, Scarborough D, Klainer A, Bisaccia E

(1990) Photopheresis for the treatment of cutaneous T-cell lymphoma. J Am Acad Dermatol 23:898–902
35. Heald PW, Perez MI, Christensen I, Dobbs N, McKiernan G, Edelson RL (1989) Photopheresis therapy of cutaneous T-cell lymphoma: the Yale-New Haven Hospital Experience. Yale J Biol Med 62:629–638
36. Heald P, Rook A, Perez M, Wintroub B, Knobler R, Jegasothy B, Gasparro F, Berger C, Edelson R (1992) Treatment of erythrodermic cutaneous T-cell lymphoma with extracorporeal photochemotherapy. J Am Acad Dermatol 27:427–433
37. Heald P, Knobler R, LaRoche L (1994) Photoinactivated lymphocyte therapy of cutaneous T-cell lymphoma. Dermatol Clin 12:443–449
38. Knobler R (1995) Photopheresis and the red man syndrome. Dermatology 190:97–98
39. Zic J, Arzubiaga C, Salhany KE, Parker RA, Wilson D, Stricklin GP, Greer J, King LE Jr (1992) Extracorporeal photopheresis for the treatment of cutaneous T-cell lymphoma. J Am Acad Dermatol 27:729–736
40. Berger CL, Perez MM, Laroche L, Edelson R (1990) Inhibition of autoimmune disease in a murine model of systemic lupus erythematosus induced by exposure to syngeneic photoinactivated lymphocytes. J Invest Dermatol 94:52–57
41. Berger CL Wang N, Christensen I, Longley J, Heald P, Edelson RL (1996) The immune response to class I-associated tumor-specific cutaneous T-cell lymphoma antigens. J Invest Dermatol 107:392–397
42. Edelson R (1988) Light activated drugs. Sci Am 259:68–75
43. Gasparro FP, Song J, Knobler RM, Edelson RL (1986) Quantitation of psoralen photoadducts in DNA isolated from lymphocytes treated with 8-methoxypsoralen and ultraviolet a radiation (extracorporeal photopheresis). Curr Probl Dermatol 15:67–84
44. Gasparro F, Dall'Amico R, O'Malley M, Heald PW, Edelson RL (1990) Cell membrane DNA: a new target for psoralen photoadduct formation. Phochem Photobiol 52:315–321
45. Perez M, Edelson R, Laroche L, Berger C (1989) Inhibition of antiskin allograft immunity by infusions with syngeneic photoinactivated effector lymphocytes. J Invest Dermatol 92:669–676
46. Vowels BR, Cassin M, Boufal MH, Walsh LJ, Rook AJ (1992) Extracorporeal photo-chemotherapy induces the production of tumor necrosis factor-α by monocytes: implications for the treatment of cutaneous T-cell lymphoma and systemic sclerosis. J Invest Dermatol 96:686–692
47. Gasparro FP, Berger CL, Edelson RL (1984) Effect of monochromatic UVA light and 8-methoxypsoralen on human lymphocyte response to mitogen. Photodermatol 1:10–17
48. Santella RM, Dharmaraja N, Gasparro FP, Edelson RL (1985) Monoclonal antibodies to DNA modified by 8-methoxypsoralen and ultraviolet a light. Nucleic Acids Res 13:2533–2544
49. Schmitt I, Moor A, Patrignelli R, Chimenti S, Beijersbergen van Henegouwen G, Edelson R, Gasparro F (1995) Increased surface expression of class I MHC molecules on immunogenic cells derived from the xenogenization of P815 mastocytoma cells with 8-methoxypsoralen and long-wavelength ultraviolet radiation. Tissue Antigens 46:45–49
50. Sumpio BE, Phan SM, Gasparro FP, Deckelbaum LI (1993) Control of smooth muscle cell proliferation by psoralen photochemotherapy. J Vasc Surg 17:1010–1016
51. Trautinger F, Knobler RM, Macheiner W, Grünwald C, Miksche M (1991) Release of oxygen-free radicals by neutrophils is reduced by photopheresis. Ann NY Acad Sci 636:383–385
52. Van Iperen HP, Beijersbergen van Henegouwen GMJ (1992) Animal model for extracorporeal photochemotherapy based on contact hypersensitivity. J Photochem Photobiol B Biol 15:361–366
53. Yamane Y, Lobo FM, John LA, Edelson RL, Perez MI (1992) Suppression of anti-skin-allograft response by photodamaged effector cells—the modulating effects of prednisone and cyclophosphamide. Transplantation 54:119–124
54. Rook A, Prystowsky M (1991) Combined therapy for Sezary syndrome with extracorporeal

photochemotherapy and low-dose interferon alfa therapy. Arch Dermatol 127:1535–1540
55. Duvic M, Hester P, Lemak A (1996) Photopheresis therapy for cutaneous T-cell lymphoma. J Am Acad Dermatol 35:573–579
56. Zic J, Stricklin G, Greer J, Kinney M, Shyr Y, Wilson D, Kind L Jr (1996) Long term follow-up with cutaneous T-cell lymphoma treated with extracorporeal photochemotherapy. J Am Acad Dermatol 356:935–945
57. Gottlieb S, Wolfe T, Fox F, DeNardo B, Macey W, Bromley P, Lessin S, Rook A (1996) Treatment of cutaneous T-cell lymphoma with extracorporeal photopheresis monotherapy and in combination with recombinant interferon alpha: a 10 year experience at a single institution. J Am Acad Dermatol 35:946–957
58. Haley H, Davis D, Sams W (1999) Durable loss of a malignant T-cell clone in a stage IV cutaneous T-cell lymphoma patient treated with high dose interferon and photopheresis. J Am Acad Dermatol 41:880–883
59. Wilson LD, Licata AL, Braverman IM, Edelson RL, Heald PW, Feldman AM, Kacinski BM (1995) Systemic chemotherapy and extracorporeal photochemotherapy for T3 and T4 cutaneous T-cell lymphoma patients who have achieved a complete response to total skin electron beam therapy. Int J Radiat Oncol Biol Phys 32:987–995
60. Rook AH, Freundlich B, Nahass G, Washko R, Macelis B, Skolnicki M, Bromley P, Winter W, Jegasothy B (1989) Treatment of autoimmune disease with extracorporeal photochemotherapy: progressive systemic sclerosis. Yale J Biol Med 16:639–645
61. Kahale MB, Suttany GL, Smith EA et al (1986) A modified scleroderma skin scoring method. Clin Exp Rheumatol 4:367–369
62. Dall'Amico R, Livi U, Montini G et al (1994) Successful treatment of heart transplant (HT) patients with multiple rejection. J Heart Lung Transplant 2:S81
63. Meiser BM, Kur F, Reichenspurner H et al (1994) Reduction of the incidence of rejection by adjunct immunosuppression with photochemotherapy after heart transplantation. Transplant 57:563–568
64. Barr ML (1996) Immunomodulation in transplantation with photopheresis. Artif Org 20/8:971–973
65. Becherel P, Bussel A, Chosidow O, Rabian C, Piette J, Frances C (1998) Extracorporeal photochemotherapy for chronic erosive lichen planus (letter). Lancet 351(9105):805
66. O'Brien C, Henzel B, Moonka D, Inverso J, Rook A. (1999) Extracorporeal photopheresis alone and with interferon alpha 2a in chronic hepatitis C patients who failed previous interferon therapy. Dig Dis Sci 44:1020–1026
67. Rostami A, Sater R, Bird S, GalettaS, Farber R, Kamon M, Silberberg D, Grossman R, Pfohl D (1999) A double blind, placebo controlled trial of extracorporeal photopheresis in chronic progressive multiple sclerosis. Multiple Sclerosis 5:198–203

第 13 章 UVA-1 光疗：适应证和作用机制

J. Krutmann, H. Stege, A. Morita

内容

引言 ··· 259
UVA-1 光疗法治疗 T 细胞介导的皮肤病 ······························ 260
UVA-1 光疗法治疗色素性荨麻疹 ··· 263
UVA-1 光疗法治疗结缔组织病 ·· 264
UVA-1 光疗法治疗 HIV 阳性患者 ·· 266
UVA-1 光疗法的各种适应证 ··· 268
UVA-1 光疗法的副作用 ··· 269
展望 ··· 269

要点

- UVA-1 光疗法的适应证主要分为四类：T 细胞介导的皮肤病、肥大细胞介导的皮肤病、结缔组织疾病以及针对 HIV 病人的光疗法。
- UVA-1 射线诱导的辅助 T 细胞凋亡是 UVA-1 光疗法治疗特应性皮炎的机制。
- UVA-1 光疗法可能代替 PUVA 成为色素性荨麻疹的首选疗法。
- UVA-1 光疗法是治疗 HIV 病人银屑病的有效方法。
- 对 UVA 敏感的光线性皮肤病患者或光敏性特应性皮炎患者病人不宜采用 UVA-1 光疗法。
- UVA-1 光疗法不宜用于儿童，但特殊病例如硬皮病患儿在其他治疗方法无效的情况下可采用。

引言

1981年，MutzHas等人报道了一种新的放射装置，基本只发射波长在长波紫外线(UV)的A段的光线，即UVA-1(340~400nm)[36]。首次发现的配有新型过滤系统的金属卤化物灯让人类皮肤接触高剂量的UVA-1照射而不引起晒伤成为可能。此后，UVA-1放射线装置被证实了在光激发实验中对UVA敏感的光线性皮肤病患者是有效的，尤其是多形性日光疹。但是，过了十年的时间这些新型放射装置的治疗潜力才被认可和系统应用。1992年，Krutmann与Schöpf报道了高剂量的UVA-1照射对于严重的急性过敏性皮炎患者是有益的[22]。这些观察促使人们对UVA-1放射的治疗使用产生了越来越多的兴趣。所以，现在有大量文献表明，在一些特定的适应证下，UVA-1光疗法比传统的光疗方式更加有效[27]。UVA-1和UVB或UVA/UVB放射的主要区别在于，UVA-1可以穿透真皮获得治疗效果，但不会像穿透力较差的UVB和与其作用类似的UVA-2波段那样产生常见的副作用[16]。另外，UVA-1放射有一些独特的免疫调节特征，适当的情况下，它甚至可能会比补骨脂素加UVA(PUVA)疗法更有效[24]。UVA-1光疗法一开始是用来治疗特应性皮炎患者，但之后发现它在治疗其他皮肤疾病也有效，比如局限性和系统性硬皮病，而这些病的其他治疗选择有限。UVA-1光疗法的光生物和分子基础研究分析促进了这一进展。目前，UVA-1光疗法的适应证主要分为四类：T细胞介导的皮肤病，肥大细胞介导的皮肤病，结缔组织疾病以及针对HIV病人的光疗法(表13.1)。

表13.1　UVA-1治疗的适应证

适应证	研究类型	结论
特应性皮炎	数个开放性实验，1个多中心实验	已建立标准
色素性荨麻疹	2个开放性实验	有效,"长期疗效",缺乏对照研究
局限性硬皮病	2个开放性实验	疗效显著,"有突破性",需要大量的对照实验
系统性硬化	1个开放性实验	疗效显著,"有突破性",需要大量的对照实验
皮肤T细胞淋巴瘤	2个开放性实验，1个对比实验	有效的多中心实验正在进行中
银屑病(HIV阳性)	1个开放性实验	疗效显著,"治疗的选择"需要大量的研究
银屑病(HIV阴性)	病例报告	效果不佳
斑秃	非公开实验	无效
日光性荨麻疹	数个病例	无效
扁平苔藓	数个病例	无效

UVA-1 光疗法治疗 T 细胞介导的皮肤病

体外研究证明了 UVA-1 照射可有效诱导人类 T 淋巴细胞的细胞凋亡[9]。在分子水平,UVA-1 照射诱导的细胞凋亡与 UVB-照射或 PUVA-治疗所诱导的细胞凋亡不同,因为它是通过通路介导而不需要蛋白质的合成。这就是所谓的程序性细胞死亡或早期细胞凋亡,似乎只是在 UVA-1 照射下发生,而且是通过单线态氧的产生而介导作用的。这些体外的结果在体内的相关性,是对特应性皮炎患者进行 UVA-1 光疗后导致的浸润皮肤的 T 辅助细胞的细胞凋亡的观察所发现的[33]。T 细胞出现凋亡,随之被耗尽,促炎 T 细胞分泌的细胞因子干扰素 γ 的原位表达减少,皮疹被清除[12,13]。所以,现在普遍认为 UVA-1 照射诱发的 T 辅助细胞凋亡是 UVA-1 光疗法治疗特应性皮炎的基础。作为一个临床结果,UVA-1 光疗法已经延伸到治疗其他 T 细胞介导的皮肤疾病,包括皮肤 T 细胞淋巴瘤[38]。

UVA-1 光疗法治疗特应性皮炎

UVA-1 照射治疗特应性皮炎患者的治疗效果首次通过对急性严重恶化患者的开放式研究进行评估[23]。这些患者每天接受辐照强度为 70mW/s 的辐射 130J/cm² (图 13.1),连续 15 天。治疗效果是通过一套临床评分系统以及对其嗜酸性粒细胞阳离子蛋白的血清水平的监测来评估的[4,7]。后者代表一个可以被客观测量的实验室参数,且已经证实是与疾病活动密切相关的。在这个研究中,UVA-1 光疗法被证实可以迅速而高效改善临床症状。这与升高的嗜酸性粒细胞阳离子蛋白血清水平降低有关。当时普遍认为 UVA/UVB 是对特应性皮炎最好的光疗方法,研究者比较了 UVA-1 光疗法治疗和 UVA/UVB 光疗法,发现两者之间存在显著的差异且 UVA-1 光疗法更胜一筹。研究结果表明 UVA-1 光疗法是严重的特应性皮炎患者的治疗首选。

在随后几年已经有许多报告证实了这些最初的观察[19,21,31]。值得注意的是,Krutmann 等人在他们的初步研究中使用 UVA-1 光疗作为单一治疗方法,以此证明它可代表一种治疗选择,相对于糖皮质激素治疗严重的特应性皮肤炎这一金标准[23]。实际上,通过直接比较 UVA-1 光疗法与已作为标准的外用糖皮质激素疗法,其结果提示:针对严重的 AD 患者,UVA-1 光疗的效果至少与局部糖皮质激素治疗效果相当[26]。到目前为止,这项研究也是唯一一个通过对照随机研究大量严重 AD 患者 ($n=53$),提供 UVA-1 光疗多中心评价治疗效果的研究。患者接受 UVA-1 ($10\times130J/cm^2$),UVA/UVB(最小红斑量)或局部氟考松外涂治疗。在接受 10 次治疗后,三个组的患者症状都有改善,但 UVA-1 照射疗法及氟考松局部疗法的效果比长波紫外线 UVA/UVB 光线疗法更明显。而在

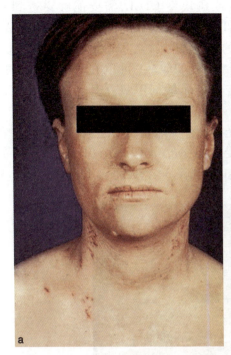 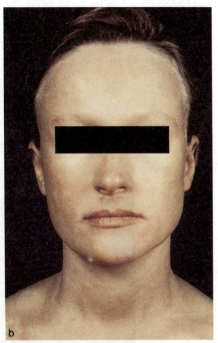

图 13.1 严重的急性特应性皮炎治疗前(a);接受 15 次的 130J/cm² UVA-1 光疗后(b)

UVA-1 疗法及糖皮质激素局部疗法中可观察到嗜酸细胞阳离子蛋白的血清水平显著降低。多中心试验证实,UVA-1 光疗可给严重的 AD 患者带来极大的益处。

目前对于 UVA-1 的治疗效果是否取决于剂量仍有争论。近期研究发现,与 130J/cm² 高剂量方案相似,中等剂量的 UVA-1 也比 UVA/UVB 的治疗效果好[19]。另外,在 UVA-1 波段里的治疗效果似乎是取决于剂量大小,因为 50J/cm² 照射量比 20J/cm² 的低剂量方案治疗效果更好[21]。最近,研究发现 130J/cm² 高剂量方案比 50J/cm² 中等剂量方案疗效更好,同时也比 20J/cm² 低剂量方案效果更好(J. C. simon 等人提交出版)。所以,使用低剂量的 UVA-1 并不比传统光疗法如 UVA/UVB 或 311nm UVB 更有优势,因此低剂量 UVA-1 疗法不被支持。相反地,中等或高等剂量 UVA-1 很明显地比传统光疗法效果更好。但是,为了达到一个最佳的治疗效果,130J/cm² 高剂量方案是必要的。

UVA-1 光疗法治疗皮肤 T 细胞淋巴瘤

皮肤 T 细胞肿瘤(CTCL)是辅助性 T 细胞肿瘤在皮肤上的最初体现。最常见的是蕈样肉芽肿。蕈样肉芽肿的辅助 T 细胞位于表皮内和表皮下,真皮带状浸润。因此,局部治疗斑片或斑块型 CTCL,需要能够穿透到真皮的治疗方法。对于 I A 和 I B 期 CTCL 患者,最佳的治疗方法是 PUVA,它和 UVA-1 一样,可以诱发 T 细胞的细胞凋亡[27]。理论上来说,UVA-1 光疗法可以代替 PUVA,因为和 PUVA 相比,UVA-1 可以在高强度下到达更深层的真皮,而且 UVA-1 光疗法避免了光敏剂甲氧补骨脂素产生的副作用。

　　Plettenberg 等人单独使用 UVA-1 光疗治疗 3 名组织学上被诊断为 I A 和 I B 期的 CTCL 患者[38]。患者每天接受 $130J/cm^2$($n=2$)或 $60J/cm^2$($n=1$)的 UVA-1 照射(图 13.2)。经过几次 UVA-1 照射后,3 名患者的皮损开始消退。无

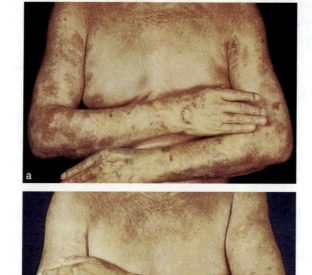

图 13.2　I A 阶段的 CTCL I A 期的患者接受 UVA-1 光疗($20×130J/cm^2$)治疗前(a)及治疗后(b)

论是高剂量还是中等剂量治疗,在经过 16~20 次光照之后,患者的皮损都完全清除。这些临床数据经过了组织学证实。3 名患者在治疗之前都具有有蕈样肉芽肿的组织学特征,而在 UVA-1 光疗之后,表皮几乎正常,只有少数淋巴细胞浸润真皮。在第二个研究里,患有早期 CTCL 的十名患者每天接受 $100J/cm^2$ 剂量

的 UVA-1 治疗．在经过 20~25 次光照之后，所有患者的症状都完全缓解[3]。在最近一次对比研究里，CTCL 患者随机接受 UVA-1($n=10$)或 PUVA($n=10$)的治疗[39]。UVA-1 光疗法再次被证实在 CTCL 早期阶段有效，而且与 PUVA 疗法没有显著的差异性。

目前ⅠA 到ⅠB 期 CTCL 的主要治疗方法是 PUVA 疗法。从实用的观点来看，UVA-1 光疗比 PUVA 疗法具有显著的优势，因为它可以完全避免因为系统性应用光敏剂造成的不必要的副作用。因此，一个国际的(杜塞尔多夫，越南，布雷西亚，明斯特，名古屋和爱丁堡)多中心试验已经开始启动，比较 UVA-1 和 PUVA 在治疗早期 CTCL 功效的对照研究。

这项试验还将证实了 UVA-1 光疗可以延长缓解期持续时间。在这项研究中使用的 UVA-1 是中等计量而非高剂量，而且是通过体外研究推断出的剂量[35]。这些实验证实肿瘤 T 细胞比正常 T 细胞对 UVA-1 辐照诱导细胞凋亡更敏感。这与之前的研究相符合，那就是对于 CTCL 患者来说，暴露于 $60J/cm^2$ 的 UVA-1 与 $130J/cm^2$ 的 UVA-1 方案同样有效。所以，治疗 CTCL 患者的最佳剂量可能会和治疗过敏性皮炎患者的剂量有所不同。

UVA-1 光疗法治疗色素性荨麻疹

UVA-1 光疗治疗色素性荨麻疹的主要机制是诱导皮肤浸润细胞凋亡及清除它们。最初，用 UVA-1 治疗前后患者皮肤的组织化学和免疫组织化学改变来评估 UVA1 对肥大细胞的影响[10]。研究发现，UVA-1 光疗能够使真皮肥大细胞密度下降，它与临床症状改善密切相关。这些研究表明，真皮肥大细胞数量和功能的改变是其产生临床疗效的原因。因此，UVA-1 光疗对皮肤肥大细胞增多症患者有效并奇怪。

一项初步研究中，仅用高剂量 UVA-1 治疗 4 例严重的泛发型色素性荨麻疹患者。UVA-1 照射每天 1 次，每周 5 次，连续 2 周[48]。初始剂量为 $60J/cm^2$，随后，每日剂量为 $130J/cm^2$/身体单侧。所有患者皮肤症状迅速改善，后者通过增加的尿组胺在 24 小时后减少到正常水平来反应。除了皮肤症状外，2 名患者出现全身表现，如腹泻和偏头痛。10 次治疗后，2 名患者的全身症状得到缓解，升高的血清 5-羟色胺减少到正常水平。停止 UVA-1 疗法两年后，所有患者均无复发。相比之下，PUVA 治疗色素性荨麻疹的特点是 5~8 个月后会复发。UVA-1 治疗色素性荨麻疹的持久有效性最近被另一个研究所证实[50]。总共有 15 个荨麻疹患者使用高剂量 UVA-1 治疗方案。其中 14 个患者对 UVA-1 光疗反应迅速，且在光疗结束后皮肤或/和全身症状消退。对这些病人的随访 2 年发现，

UVA-1 治疗 8 个月后 100% 的患者仍完全缓解。观察到有 70% 的患者缓解期为 1 年，这些患者中 40% 缓解期可延长到 18 个月。

UVA-1 和 PUVA 治疗的色素性荨麻疹患者复发率的差异，可能是因为 UVA-1 治疗可引起真皮肥大细胞数量减少，但 PUVA 治疗后并没有观察到此现象[5,11,20]。最近一项体内研究支持了这一假说，检验证明 UVA-1 治疗的患者真皮肥大细胞的数量明显减少，但 PUVA 治疗的患者并无减少。利用双重染色技术也可以证明色素性荨麻疹患者的病变皮肤肥大细胞凋亡处于低水平，而其比例因 UVA-1 光疗显著增加[50]。相比之下，PUVA 疗法并没有引起肥大细胞凋亡。综上所述，这些研究表明 UVA-1 光疗，通过诱导皮肤浸润的肥大细胞细胞凋亡而使色素性荨麻疹患者的肥大细胞消耗。因此，UVA-1 光疗的治疗反应更持久，因此 UVA-1 光疗有潜力取代 PUVA 成为治疗色素性荨麻疹患者的首选。

UVA-1 光疗法治疗结缔组织病

局限性硬皮病是一个或多个象牙白色萎缩性斑块，境界清楚，有时直径可达 20 厘米，被炎症边缘包围即淡紫色炎症环[41]。尽管本病具有自限性，但皮肤硬化可能会导致功能缺陷和不适。皮肤硬化可导致肌肉萎缩，从而导致躯干或脸的畸形。皮损也可能发展至关节并引起屈曲挛缩与功能障碍。局限性硬皮病的治疗包括青霉素、青霉胺、抗疟疾药物、环孢菌 A、γ 干扰素以及局部或全身用糖皮质激素，但总体来说，没有特效疗法。

硬化的皮肤损伤可能与 I 型和 III 型胶原蛋白合成的增加有关[8,28,40]。证据显示，这种过度胶原沉积的主要原因是真皮成纤维细胞异常，特别是胶原酶 I 表达的减少[52]。UVA-1 照射体外培养的人类皮肤成纤维细胞可以增加胶原酶 I 的合成[37,43]。在这些研究中，UVA-1 照射诱导胶原酶产生与胶原酶 I 的 mRNA 表达呈剂量依赖关系。UVA-1 体外照射剂量实现了最大感应，这相当于那些用大剂量 UVA-1 光疗治疗过敏性皮炎或色素性荨麻疹患者的感应。因此有人猜测 UVA-1 照射通过提高胶原酶 I 的表达能力而对局限性硬皮病患者产生有利作用[17,49]。这个假设已被一个开放性研究证实了，该研究对病理确诊为局限性硬皮病的 10 名患者进行 30 次，130J/cm^2 UVA-1 照射[49]（图 13.3）。UVA-1 疗法软化了所有患者的硬化斑块，其中 4 名患者皮疹完全消退。此外，20-MHz 超声显示 UVA-1 治疗显著降低斑块厚度且增加斑块的弹性（图 13.4）。这些变化并非患者自身缓解，因为它只在经 UVA-1 照射下患者身上的斑块上观察到，但在未经 UVA-1 照射的患者身上的对照斑块未观察到。

第 13 章　UVA-1 光疗:适应证和作用机制

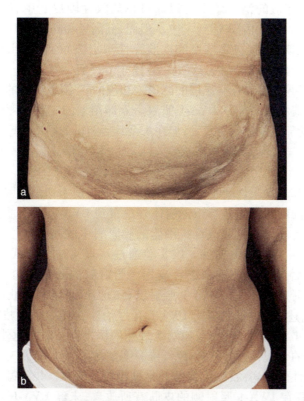

图 13.3　局限性硬皮病腹部硬化性斑块经 UVA-1 光疗(30 ×130J/cm^2)治疗前(a)和治疗后(b)

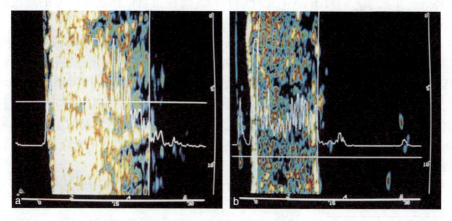

图 13.4　局限性硬皮病患者硬化斑块治疗前 20MHz 的超声图(a)和 UVA-1 光疗(30× 130J/cm^2)治疗后的超声图(b)

它也表明,相似的治疗效果可以通过将局限性硬皮病患者暴露在低剂量($20J/cm^2$)的 UVA-1 辐射来达到[14,18]。然而,低剂量和高剂量 UVA-1 光疗在所有参数评估(临床评估、斑块厚度和皮肤弹性测定法)的直接比较表明高剂量 UVA-1 疗法优于低剂量 UVA-1 疗法[49]。停止治疗后,随访三个月,所有患者停止 UVA-1 治疗不会导致有益作用的减退。相应的,7 例患者中的 6 例在随访结束时皮肤厚度值和其高剂量 UVA-1 照照后立即测量的皮肤厚度值相同。其中有 1 例患者,局部皮肤症状有复发,但在 3 个月后随访期间皮肤厚度仍明显低于光疗前的厚度。全部患者的皮肤症状在 UVA-1 治疗停止后并没有被观察到有进一步的改善。

UVA-1 光疗在局限性硬皮病精确的作用机制目前未知。使用高剂量 UVA-1 照射方案治疗的理论基础是基于先前体外观察到 UVA-1 照射通过剂量依赖的方式诱导了人工培养的皮肤成纤维细胞的胶原酶 I 的表达[37,43]。这一概念得到最近的研究结果的有力支持。该实验通过病理活检的方式研究了高剂量 UVA-1 治疗前后局限性硬皮病患者皮损。照射后的硬化性斑块中胶原酶 I mRNA 表达上调 20 倍,这与 UVA-1 照射诱导的临床改善和皮肤厚度的减少有关[49]。综上所述,这些研究表明 UVA-1 光疗治疗对局限性硬皮病是有效的。有效性依赖于 UVA-1 剂量,与胶原酶 I 表达的诱发有关联。此外,UVA-1 可能影响胶原蛋白的合成,从而使胶原原纤维厚度正常化[42]。

除了局限性硬皮病,胶原束松解和出现小胶原纤维。1 个病人自身对照显示,这些参数只在 UVA-1 照射侧的皮肤有所改善,未经 UVA-1 照射侧则无改善[34]。本研究进一步支持这一观点,UVA-1 光疗对于硬皮病患者来说是一种有价值的治疗选择。目前没有其他治疗能证明对于与皮肤硬化相关疾病有疗效。这将进一步激发人们对 UVA-1 光疗的兴趣。现在也有证据表明成年的硬皮病患者可受益于 UVA-1 光疗[53]。

应该指出的是除了 UVA-1 疗法之外,已有报道显示全身以及局部 PUVA 疗法对局限性硬皮病和系统性硬化症患者有效[32,44]。因此,未来的研究将比较 UVA-1 与 PUVA 治疗的效果和副作用。至少在体外,PUVA 治疗可诱导人工培养的成纤维细胞终端分化,而 UVA-1 照射无此作用,这表明 PUVA 疗法可能有极大的光老化风险。此外,系统性硬化症患者需要在 4~5 月的时间里接受平均 50 次 PUVA 治疗临床症状才能得到改善[32]。相比之下,UVA-1 光疗只需 30 次就能达到最大疗效[35]。和 PUVA 疗法相比,UVA-1 每日照射一次,故其总疗程可缩减至 1~1.5 个月,因此 UVA-1 光疗会比 PUVA 疗法起效用的时间快得多。

UVA-1 光疗法治疗 HIV 阳性患者

UVB 或 PUVA 治疗皮肤病患者的安全性目前仍存在争议。一方面,临床研究没有显示在免疫状态或血浆病毒载量有显著副作用。另一方面,实验室研究表明 UVB 或者 PUVA 可以激活培养的细胞内和转基因动物体内的艾滋病病毒。这场争论最近已经通过 PCR 半定量的方式分析被激活的 HIV 病毒在人类皮肤的表达而进一步证实。以往的体外实验已经证明亚红斑量的 UVB 照射可以激活血清 HIV 病毒阳性的银屑病或嗜酸性毛囊炎患者皮损及非皮损处皮肤病毒的表达。在之前的体外研究显示 UV 波长范围内唯有 UVA-1 波长范围内的紫外线不激活艾滋病毒启动子[54]。

由于银屑病目前被认为是 T 细胞介导的皮肤疾病,且 UVA-1 光疗已经被证明可以有效治疗 T 细胞介导的炎症反应性皮肤病,故对 UVA-1 光疗法是否可用于治疗 HIV 阳性的银屑病患者的评估结果显而易见。在一个公开的非对照试验中,对 HIV 阳性的病人($n=3$)每日进行高剂量 UVA-1 光疗并得到很好的治疗效果[6](图 13.5)。全身 UVA-1 光疗治疗开始前,评估 UVA-1 光疗对 HIV 阳性

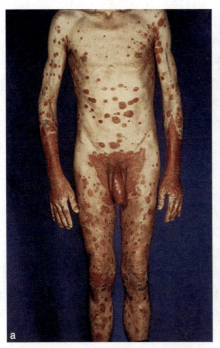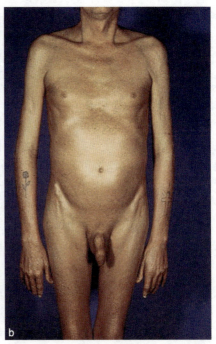

图 13.5 HIV 阳性的银屑病患者治疗前(a)和经过 UVA-1($20\times130J/cm^2$)光疗治疗后(b)

病人的安全性。为此,实验配对三组分别接受 UVB($150mJ/cm^2$)、UVA-1($130J/cm^2$)或安慰性光照病人的皮损和非皮损处的皮肤标本,采用 PCR 定量检测艾滋病毒数量,观察到 UVB 照射组皮肤艾滋病毒数比非辐照的皮肤增加 6~15 倍。相

比之下,UVA-1 治疗组则与安慰剂治疗组在艾滋病病毒数上无差异。此外还观察到,这些患者经 20~30 次 UVA-1 辐照治疗后银屑病皮损完全清除。更重要的是,在 UVA-1 辐照治疗(41 个患者接受 UVA-1 辐照)后 HIV 阳性的银屑病患者经 20~30 次 UVA-1 照射后皮肤上的 HIV 病毒数完全无增加。这些研究表明,UVA-1 可有效治疗 HIV 阳性的银屑病患者,且 UVA-1 不同于 UVB,前者不激活人类皮肤中的艾滋病病毒。至少从安全的角度来看,UVA-1 光疗几乎可成为 HIV 阳性患者光疗法的首选。

UVA-1 光疗法的各种适应证

在一个公开试点研究中,12 例慢性水疱型手部湿疹急性加重的患者接受 UVA-1 光疗[45]。手掌和手背接受每天剂量为 $40J/cm^2$ 的 UVA-1 照射三周。治疗 1 周后,除了一个患者无改善外其他患者均明显缓解瘙痒症状。经过 3 周治疗后其中 10 例患者临床症状显著改善。这份报告与观察到的 UVA-1 光疗对特应性皮炎和其他 T 细胞介导的皮肤病治疗的有效率是一致的[25,33]。对于慢性水疱型手部湿疹的患者,局部 UVA-1 光疗被证实是一种有效的治疗方法。

最近的一个报告表明,UVA-1 光疗对瘢痕疙瘩和肥厚性瘢痕的患者有效[1]。1 例 37 岁男患者(皮肤类型Ⅳ),胸部继发于严重痤疮的瘢痕疙瘩 17 年,接受了 22 次剂量为 $130J/cm^2$ 的 UVA-1 照射。其中三分之二面积的瘢痕疙瘩进行治疗,剩余三分之一面积的瘢痕则作为对照。UVA-1 治疗 3 周后以及 6 周后,观察发现 UVA-1 光疗部分瘢痕疙瘩软化变平,而对照组则无改变。组织学观察到接受光疗后瘢痕疙瘩重新出现正常外观的胶原蛋白和弹性纤维。这些初步的实验结果令人兴奋,它表明,UVA-1 光疗法可以用来治疗那些大的瘢痕,如手术重塑困难或病灶内注射皮质类固醇效果不佳的烧伤瘢痕。

已有报道 UVA-1 联合阿维 A 疗法治疗 1 例毛发红糠疹患者[15]。这个病例报告中 UVA-1 及阿维 A 疗法的治疗机制尚不明确。

已有观点提出,每日低剂量 UVA-1 照射对红斑狼疮患者有治疗效果。为了证实这个观点,一个公开的研究报告了 10 例接受单剂量为 $6J/cm^2$ 的 UVA-1 治疗(15 天~8 个月)的系统性红斑狼疮病例[29]。结果表明接受治疗后的 SLE 疾病活动的临床指标以及抗 SSA 或抗核抗体滴度较前降低。在这项研究为期 18 周,2 阶段的双向实验的双盲,安慰剂对照实验中[30],26 名女患者被分为两组:A 组患者接受 $6J/cm^2$ 的 UVA-1,B 组患者接受等量时间的可见光照射。各组治疗 3 周,而后 12 周行第 2 周期治疗方案,病人和医生知情,患者接受的 UVA-1 辐射剂量逐渐减小。在 A 组的患者,疾病的活动性在为期 3 周的 UVA-1 治疗后显著下降,而 3 周可见光治疗的患者则出现复发。与此相反,B 组患者初始 3 周可见光治及之后 3 周的 UVA-1 疗法均无显著效果。然而在第二阶段,两组为期 6 周的 UVA-1 光疗均显著改善了临床症状。可是这些单中心研究没有被其他研究组证实。此外，对紫外线治疗敏感的自身免疫性疾病，例如红斑狼疮与 UVA-1 光疗也不一定没有风险，尤其是当较高剂量 UVA-1 被运用于亚急性皮肤红斑狼疮（sCLE）的患者时，可能会因光疗引发一个全身反应[47]。

UVA-1 光疗可治疗外阴硬化性苔藓[2]。在一个非对照性研究中，7 例对外用强效糖皮质激素无效的严重外阴硬化性苔藓的女性患者，UVA-1 光疗治疗后 5 人症状改善。

UVA-1 光疗法的副作用

UVA-1 光疗法不可用于治疗对紫外线敏感的光线性皮肤病或患有光敏性皮炎的患者。在光疗前可用光敏试验筛除此类患者。目前已观察到经 UVA-1 治疗的患者除疱疹性湿疹外均无急性副作用。虽然 UVA-1 有潜在的致癌风险，但除此之外并无观察到其他副作用。已有报道称高剂量的 UVA-1 照射可诱导无毛白化病 sKH-HR1 小鼠发生鳞状细胞癌[51]。UVA-1 照射可促进人体恶性黑色素瘤生长的论点目前虽还存在争议，但不能排除[46]。与这些理论问题相关的主要是年轻的特应性皮炎患者。UVA-1 光疗只限用于特应性皮炎患者的急性发作，且一个治疗周期不应超过 10～15 次，每年 1～2 个治疗周期。一般来说，除其他治疗效果不佳的严重硬皮病患儿外，儿童患者不宜使用 UVA-1 光疗治疗[14]。对于其他适应证，如 CTCL，色素性荨麻疹和结缔组织疾病，UVA-1 光疗对疾病的治疗效果很可能超过其潜在的长期治疗风险。为了以更系统的方式解决这个问题，对于 UVA-1 光疗（EFUP-研究）的患者欧洲随访研究已经启动。这种纵向的，前瞻性的研究旨在监测每个经 UVA-1 治疗的患者，经此中心的登记，并收集资料作为 UVA-1 光疗对增加皮肤癌的风险的调查依据。

展望

UVA-1 光疗几乎总是被用作单一疗法以明确地证明其疗效。然而 UVA-1 光疗的联合治疗方案同样有明显的临床疗效和实践意义，因其可达到治疗效果及安全性同时最大化。

UVA-1 的联合治疗方法：适应证及应用包括 UVA-1 与外用糖皮质激素或免疫抑制剂的联合应用于治疗特应性皮炎，或 UVA-1 与维 A 酸或干扰素 α 联合系统治疗 CTCL。

研究 UVA-1 光疗的作用机制可迅速扩大其应用范围。预期在不久的将来有更多发展空间。在这方面，特别令人感兴趣地得知，由 UVA-1 照射产生的单态氧的光生物学机制是治疗有效的中心依据。策略针对于放大单态氧介导的效果及在人类皮肤单态氧产生的发展替代模式所提出的假设[33]，例如，通过辐射光谱的使用，甚至可以研究出比 UVA-1 更具选择性的治疗光线，且其将被证明优于目前所采用的 UVA-1 光疗法。所有这些研究结果最终将有助于 UVA-1 光疗的进一步发展，且其将成为未来光医学的驱动力之一。

（黄茂芳 译，潘乔林　周欣　校，朱慧兰 审）

参考文献

1. Asawonando P, Khoo LSW, Fitzpatrick TB, Taylor CR (1999) UVA-1 for keloid. Arch Dermatol 135:348–349
2. Beattie PE, Dawe RS, Ferguson J, Ibbotson SH (2006) UVA-1 phototherapy for genital lichen sclerosus. Clin Exp Dermatol 31:343–347
3. Calzavara Pinton P (2000) High-dose UVA1 therapy of large plaques and nodular lesions of cutaneous T-cell lymphoma. J Am Acad Dermatol (in press)
4. Costa C, Rillet A, Nicolet M, Saurat JH (1989) Scoring atopic dermatitis: the simpler the better. Acta Derm Venereol (Stockh) 69:41–47
5. Christophers E, Hönigsmann H, Wolff K, Langner A (1978) PUVA treatment of urticaria pigmentosa. Br J Dermatol 98:701–702
6. Cruz P Jr, Dougherty I, Dawson B, Krutmann J (2000) Unlike UVB, UVA-1 radiation does not activate HIV in human skin. J Invest Dermatol (in press)
7. Czech W, Krutmann J, Schöpf E, Kapp A (1992) Serum eosinophil cationic protein is a sensitive measure for disease activity in atopic dermatitis. Br J Dermatol 126:351–355
8. Fleischmajer R (1993) Localized and systemic scleroderma. In: Lapiere CM, Krieg T (eds) Connective tissue diseases of the skin. Dekker, New York, pp 295–313
9. Godar DE (1999) UVA 1 radiation mediates singlet-oxygen and superoxide-anion production which trigger two different final apoptotic pathways: the S and P site of mitochondria. J Invest Dermatol 112:3–12
10. Grabbe J, Welker P, Humke S, Grewe M, Schöpf E, Henz BM, Krutmann J (1996) High-dose UVA1 therapy, but not UVA/UVB therapy, decreases IgE binding cells in lesional skin of patients with atopic eczema. J Invest Dermatol 107:419–423
11. Granerus G, Roupa G, Swanbeck G (1981) Decreased urinary histamine levels after successful PUVA treatment of urticaria pigmentosa. J Invest Dermatol 76:1–3
12. Grewe M, Gyufko K, Schöpf E, Krutmann J (1994) Lesional expression of interferon-γ in atopic eczema. Lancet 343:25–26
13. Grewe M, Bruijnzeel-Koomen CAFM, Schöpf E, Thepen T, Langeveld-Wildschut AG, Ruzicka T, Krutmann J (1998) A role for Th1 and Th2 cells in the immunopathogenesis of atopic dermatitis. Immunol Today 19:359–361
14. Gruss C, Strucker M, Kobyletzki G, Kerscher M, Altmeyer P (1997) Low dose UVA1 phototherapy in disabling pansclerotic morphea. Br J Dermatol 136:293–294
15. Herbst RA, Vogelbruich M, Ehnis A, Kiehl P, Kapp A, Weiss J (2000) Combined ultraviolet A1 radiation and acitretin therapy as a treatment option for pityriasis rubra pilaris. Br J Dermatol 142:574–575
16. Jekler J, Larkö O (1990) Combined UV-A-UV-B versus UVB phototherapy for atopic dermatitis. J Am Acad Dermatol 22:49–53
17. Kerscher M, Dirschka T, Volkenandt M (1995) Treatment of localized scleroderma by UVA1 phototherapy. Lancet 346:1166

18. Kerscher M, Volkenandt M, Gruss C, Reuther T, Kobyletzki G, Freitag M, Dirschka T, Altmeyer P (1998) Low-dose UVA₁ phototherapy for treatment of localized scleroderma. J Am Acad Dermatol 38:21–26
19. Kobyletzki G, Pieck C, Hoffmann K, Freitag M, Altmeyer P (1999) Medium-dose UVA1 cold-light phototherapy in the treatment of severe atopic dermatitis. J Am Acad Dermatol 41:931–937
20. Kolde G, Frosch PJ, Czarnetzki BM (1984) Response of cutaneous mast cells to PUVA in patients with urticaria pigmentosa: histophotometric, ultrastructural, and biochemical investigations. J Invest Dermatol 83:175–178
21. Kowalzick L, Kleinhenz A, Weichenthal M, Ring J (1995) Low dose versus medium dose UVA-1 treatment in severe atopic dermatitis. Acta Derm Venereol (Stockh) 75:43–45
22. Krutmann J, Schöpf E (1992) High-dose UVA1 therapy: a novel and highly effective approach for the treatment of patients with acute exacerbation of atopic dermatitis. Acta Derm Venereol (Stockh) 176:120–122
23. Krutmann J, Czech W, Diepgen T, Niedner R, Kapp A, Schöpf E (1992) High-dose UVA1 therapy in the treatment of patients with atopic dermatitis. J Am Acad Dermatol 26:225–230
24. Krutmann J (1995) UVA1-induced immunomodulation. In: Krutmann J, Elmets CA (eds) Photoimmunology. Blackwell Science, Oxford, pp 246–256
25. Krutmann J (1996) Phototherapy for atopic dermatitis. Dermatol Ther 1:24–31
26. Krutmann J, Diepgen T, Luger TA, Grabbe S, Meffert H, Sönnichsen N, Czech W, Kapp A, Stege H, Grewe M, Schöpf E (1998) High-dose UVA1 therapy for atopic dermatitis: results of a multicenter trial. J Am Acad Dermatol 38:589–593
27. Krutmann J (1999) Therapeutic photomedicine: phototherapy. In: Freedberg IM, Eisen AZ, Wolff K, Austen KF, Goldsmith LA, Katz SI, Fitzpatrick TB (eds) Fitzpatrick's dermatology in general medicine, 5th edn. McGraw-Hill, New York, pp 2870–2879
28. LeRoy EC (1979) Increased collagen synthesis by scleroderma skin fibroblasts in vitro. J Clin Invest 54:880–889
29. McGrath H Jr (1994) Ultraviolet-A1 irradiation decreases clinical disease activity and autoantibodies in patients with systemic lupus erythematosus. Clin Exp Rheumatol 12:129–135
30. McGrath Jr H, Martinez-Osuna P, Lee FA (1996) Ultraviolet A-1 (340–400nm) irradiation in systemic lupus erythematosus. Lupus 5:269–274
31. Meffert H, Soennichsen N, Herzog M, Hutschenreuther A (1992) UVA-1 cold light therapy of severe atopic dermatitis. Dermatol Monatsschr 78:291–296
32. Morita A, Sakakibara S, Sakakibara N, Yamauchi R, Tsuji T (1995) Successful treatment of systemic sclerosis with topical PUVA. J Rheumatol 22:2361–2365
33. Morita A, Werfel T, Stege H, Ahrens C, Karmann K, Grewe M, Grether-Beck S, Ruzicka T, Kapp A, Klotz LO, Sies H, Krutmann J (1997) Evidence that singlet oxygen-induced human T helper cell apoptosis is the basic mechanism of ultraviolet-A radiation phototherapy. J Exp Med 186:1763–1768
34. Morita A, Kobayashi K, Isomura I, Tsuji T, Krutmann J (2000) Ultraviolet A-1 (340–400nm) phototherapy for systemic sclerosis. J Am Acad Dermatol 43:670–674
35. Morita A, Yamauchi Y, Yasuda Y, Tsuji T, Krutmann J (2000) Malignant T-cells are exquisitely sensitive to ultraviolet A-1 (UVA-1) radiation-induced apoptosis. J Invest Dermatol 114:751
36. Mutzhas MF, Hölzle E, Hofmann C, Plewig G (1981) A new apparatus with high radiation energy between 320–460nm: physical description and dermatological applications. J Invest Dermatol 76:42–47
37. Petersen MJ, Nasen C, Craig S (1992) Ultraviolet A irradiation stimulates collagenase production in cultured human fibroblasts. J Invest Dermatol 99:440–442
38. Plettenberg H, Stege H, Megahed M, Ruzicka T, Hosokawa Y, Tsuji T, Morita A, Krutmann J (1999) Ultraviolet A1 (340–400nm) phototherapy for cutaneous T-cell lymphoma. J Am Acad Dermatol 41:47–50

39. Plettenberg H, Stege H, Mang R, Ruzicka T, Krutmann J (2001) A comparison of Ultraviolet A-1 and PUVA therapy for early stages of cutaneous T-cell lymphoma. Photodermatol Photoimmunol Photomed 17:149–155
40. Rodnan GP, Lipinski I, Luksick J (1979) Skin collagen content in progressive systemic sclerosis (scleroderma) and localized scleroderma. Arthritis Rheum 22:130–140
41. Rosenwasser TA, Eisen AZ (1993) Scleroderma. In: Fitzpatrick TB, Eisen AZ, Wolff K, Freedberg IM, Austen KF (eds) Dermatology in general medicine, 4th edn. McGraw-Hill, New York, pp 2156–2167
42. Sakakibara N, Sugano S, Morita M (2008) Ultrastructural changes induced in cutaneous collagen by ultraviolet-A1 and psoralen plus ultraviolet A therapy in systemic sclerosis. J Dermatol 35:63–69
43. Scharffetter K, Wlaschek M, Hogg A, Bolsen K, Schothorst A, Goerz G, Krieg T, Plewig G (1991) UVA irradiation induces collagenase in human dermal fibroblasts in vitro and in vivo. Arch Dermatol Res 283:506–511
44. Scharfetter-Kochanek K, Goldermann R, Lehmann P, Hölzle E, Goerz G (1995) PUVA therapy in disabling pansclerotic morphea of children. Br J Dermatol 132:830–831
45. Schmidt T, Abeck D, Boeck K, Mempel M, Ring J (1998) UVA1 irradiation is effective in treatment of chronic vesicular dyshidrotic hand eczema. Acta Derm Venereol (Stockh) 78:318–319
46. Setlow RB, Grist E, Thompson K, Woodhead AD (1993) Wavelengths effective in induction of malignant melanoma. Proc Natl Acad Sci USA 90:6666–6670
47. Soennichsen N, Meffert H, Kunzelmann V (1993) UV-A-1 Therapie bei subakut-kutanem Lupus erythematodes. Hautarzt 44:723–725
48. Stege H, Schöpf E, Ruzicka T, Krutmann J (1996) High-dose-UVA1 for urticaria pigmentosa. Lancet 347:64
49. Stege H, Humke S, Berneburg M, Klammer M, Grewe M, Grether-Beck S, Dierks K, Goerz G, Ruzicka T, Krutmann J (1996) High-dose ultraviolet A1 radiation therapy of localized scleroderma. J Am Acad Dermatol 36:938–943
50. Stege H, Budde M, Kürten V, Ruzicka T, Krutmann J (1999) Induction of apoptosis in skin-infiltrating mast cells by high-dose ultraviolet A-1 radiation phototherapy in patients with urticaria pigmentosa. J Invest Dermatol 112:561
51. Sterenbroigh HCJM, van der Leun JC (1990) Tumorigenesis by a long wavelength UV-A source. Photochem Photobiol 51:325–330
52. Takeda K, Hahamochi A, Ueki H, Nakata M, Oishi Y (1994) Decreased collagenase expression in cultured systemic sclerosis fibroblasts. J Invest Dermatol 103:359–363
53. Tuchinda C, Kerr HA, Taylor CR, Jacobe H, Bergamo BM, Elmets C, Rivard J, Lim HW (2006) UVA1 phototherapy for cutaneous diseases: an experience of 92 cases in the United States. Photoderm Photoimmunol Photomed 22:247–253
54. Zmudzka BZ, Olvey KM, Lee W, Beer JZ (1994) Reassessment of the differential effects of ultraviolet and ionizing radiation on HIV promoter: the use of cell survival as the basis for comparisons. Photochem Photobiol 59:643–649

第4篇

日常生活中的光防护

第14章 光(化学)疗法和日晒所致的急性和慢性光损伤

B. H. Mahmoud, I. H. Hamzavi, H. W. Lim

内容

引言	276
光疗和PUVA引起的光损伤	276
日光辐射引起的光损伤	287
总结	289

要点

- 紫外线辐射(ultraviolet radiation, UVR)引起皮肤多种急性和慢性损伤。
- 急性UVR反应包括红斑、色素加深、免疫抑制和影响维生素D的合成。
- 慢性UVR影响包括光老化和致癌性。
- 光穿透的深度和UVR影响的强度取决于波长。
- UVB辐射产生红斑的效力是UVA辐射的1000倍。
- PUVA引起的不良反应与补骨脂素的给药方式和种类不同而不同。
- 光损伤程度、色素变化以及罹患皮肤癌的风险大小都与长期UVR有关。
- UV治疗的风险效益比因种族和皮肤类型而有所不同。
- UV治疗引起的不良反应应记录在案以留后续分析使用。
- 制定UV治疗指南十分重要;治疗中心应依照其指南使治疗更标准化。

引言

到达地球表面的紫外线辐射(UVR)中95%是长波紫外线(UVA)(320~400nm),只有5%是中波紫外线(UVB)(290~320nm)。短波紫外线(UVC)(200~290nm)被臭氧层吸收。UVR能够引起皮肤各种急慢性损伤。急性损伤包括红斑、色素加深、晒伤、免疫抑制、影响维生素D的合成[1]。慢性损伤包括光老化和致癌性,后者部分是由突变和免疫抑制所致[2]。

UVB,UVA1及补骨脂素和UVA结合的PUVA疗法可用于治疗如银屑病、多形性日光疹、特应性皮炎、白癜风和蕈样肉芽肿等多种皮肤病。急性不良反应可在UV暴露后立即出现或几天后出现。光疗的不良反应与众多因素有关,如医疗设备的类型和操作人员的技术。UV治疗和计量指南将会使治疗更加标准化。尽管各个治疗中心都有其治疗方案,但是目前对应光疗相关的不良反应的应对并没有一个共同的指导方案,使其被高度忽视[3]。

本章简要介绍UVR引起的光损伤,重点是UVB,UVA-1和PUVA所引起的光损伤。

光疗和PUVA引起的光损伤

UVB辐射引起的急性光损伤

当UVR到达皮肤时,部分被角质层散射和反射,部分被表皮吸收,部分则进入了真皮。UVR穿透的深度取决于波长;波长越长穿透的越深。大部分波长较短的UVB都被表皮吸收;然而,还有一些UVA则进入了较深的皮肤部位——真皮[4,5]。

以往发表的光疗不良反应发生率根据实验设置不同而不同。在众多研究中,根据所用的协议,UVB所致红斑比例从10%到94%[6,7]。其他炎症表现包括疼痛、发热和肿胀。此外,还有色素加深、表皮增厚、免疫和维生素D的合成改变等[1]。所报告的其他急性不良反应包括瘙痒、多形性日光疹发作、感染病毒激活和角膜炎等。

宽谱UVB引起的红斑出现在照射后3~5小时,6~24小时可达高峰,72小时消退;其峰值和强度均呈剂量依赖性。与Ⅲ型皮肤和Ⅳ型皮肤相比,Ⅰ型皮肤产生的红斑持续的时间更长。窄谱UVB(NB-UVB)引起的红斑呈陡峭的剂量-效应曲线,换言之,照射剂量的小幅增加即可引起红斑显著增加[7]。同宽谱UVB相比,窄谱UVB诱导皮肤延迟晒黑更快更强。采用最小红斑量(MED)的测定和逐渐增加治疗剂量的方法可以将UVB引起的红斑降至最低。在治疗过程中,患者应佩戴护目镜以防引起结膜炎和角膜炎。

UVA 辐射引起的急性光损伤

UVA 引起皮肤红斑的效力低于 UVB 的千分之一。仅由 UVA 引起的急性不良反应罕见。对美国四所治疗中心中接受 UVA-1 治疗的 92 位患者进行回顾发现其不良反应包括晒伤、瘙痒、红斑、刺痛感和烧灼感;然而,治疗的耐受性较好[8]。2003 年,Dawe[9]描述了 UVA-1 导致的主要急性不良反应,并提到,UVA-1 引起的红斑整体上远远少于宽波 UVA 或者 UVB;其他不良反应包括色素沉着、多形性日光疹、瘙痒和单纯疱疹复发。尤其是硬皮病,在经过几次治疗,临床症状改善尚不明显前皮损边缘较正常皮肤出现较明显的色素沉着。

补骨脂素和 UVA 导致的红斑在照射后 24~36 小时出现,36~48 小时达高峰;也可延迟至 72~96 小时,7 天消退。PUVB 治疗后的几个小时内,一些患者会出现瘙痒,有时甚至比较严重。光照性甲剥离和摩擦性水疱亦有报道。10%的患者由于光毒性而中断治疗[10]。如果治疗过程未保护眼睛,则很容易导致结膜炎和角膜炎;适当的眼保护措施可避免这些不良反应。

PUVA 治疗所引起的亚急性光毒反应并不常见,表现为刺痛感或烧灼感,随后在 PUVA 照射区出现银屑病样皮炎,常发生于长期接收 PUVA 治疗的Ⅰ、Ⅱ型皮肤类型的患者[11]。

PUVA 治疗所引起的不良反应根据补骨脂素的给药途径和种类不同而有所不同。PUVA 浴可引起过敏性或光接触性皮炎。欧洲使用的 5-甲氧补骨脂素(5-MOP)潜在的光毒性较 8-甲氧补骨脂素(8-MOP)小,前者未在美国使用。系统使用 8-MOP 较 5-MOP 更常引起全身症状,主要为肠胃不适[3]。

光疗和 PUVA 引起急性不良反应的机制和频率

UV 引起红斑的机制不清,认为 UVB 照射后能诱导 DNA 产生红斑的色基。这是因为人类皮肤细胞中的 DNA 产生嘧啶二聚体的频率光谱和红斑光谱非常相似。UVA 引起红斑的色基目前尚不清楚[1]。

回顾以往的 16 506 例口服 8-MOP PUVA 疗法病例,由于光毒性反应太过剧烈而中止治疗的仅占 0.3%[3]。2007 年,Martin 等对 NB-UVB 和 PUVA 治疗疗程超过 12 个月的患者进行随访发现急性不良反应发生比例很低,8784 例中只有 70 例,占 0.8%,其中 4 例较严重(占所有病例的 0.05%)。只有 2 例与治疗操作有关。研究中有关不良反应的数据可具体到计量表,后者是根据治疗前测定每位患者的最小红斑量(MED)和最小光毒量(MPD)来制定的。最小光毒量(MPD)是指应用药物后,用 UVA 照射,引起皮肤刚可见的红斑所需的光辐射量[12]。很明显,不同的光疗中心的数据有所不同。

2004年,对67家英国光疗中心的一项调查表明,只有28%的光疗中心在UVB治疗之前进行MED测试[3]。因此,光疗引起的严重不良反应事件就不足为奇了。在苏格兰,1989—2001年之间,27%的法律诉讼是关于光疗的,医疗人员都将其称为合法诉讼[13]。所以,遵从已公布的治疗条约对于光疗是非常重要的[3]。

2008年,Alkali等评估了一家光疗中心单一接受光疗的患者出现急性不良反应的比例,并将其与已发表的数据进行对比。这项研究对一年内光疗产生的不良反应事件进行了回顾性分析。治疗方法包括口服PUVA、PUVA浴、手/足局部的PUVA和NB-UVB治疗。这项研究总共包括了7383例光疗记录:518例口服PUVA(7%),136例PUVA浴(2%),811例手/足局部的PUVA(11%),5918例NB-UVB治疗(80%)。治疗之前由专门护士例行进行MPD和MED测试。所有的光疗不良反应事件总计105例(1.4%)。这个数据比起之前的0.84%略高(8688例治疗后不良反应有73例)。

在所有的治疗方式中,口服PUVA占2.5%,PUVA浴占0.74%,手/足局部的PUVA占0.36%,NB-UVB治疗占1.49%。只有4例不良反应属于严重类型(红斑疼痛或溃烂),占所有治疗案例的0.054%,其中NB-UVB疗法中有3例,手/足局部的PUVA中有1例,这些不良反应都是由于患者不配合造成的。所有不良反应中4例是由操作者错误造成(4%),15例由于患者不配合造成(14%)。研究者发现其所在的光疗中心光疗恶性事件比较少。据报道,大多数恶性事件都与口服PUVA有关,其次是NB-UVB疗法,手/足局部的PUVA所引起的不良反应最少。研究者认为通过记录和分析不良反应可以增加光疗的安全性和有效性[14]。

Herr等在2007年对PUVA光化学疗法引起的意外不良反应的研究显示,偶尔也会出现如大面积烧伤等反应。据观察,6例是由医务人员的失误所致,还有6例是由于患者在未受到监督的情况下所发生错误所致。需要进行PUVA治疗的患者中7例白癜风,3例银屑病,2例商业美容晒黑者。5名患者本应接受局部UV治疗,却照射了口服PUVA的计量。1名患者使用8-MOP药膏的同时服用了5-MOP片剂。另外3名患者在PUVA治疗后进行了1~3小时的日光浴。一对夫妇为了增加晒黑效果使用了5-MOP,并在用药后1小时进行了日光浴。另外1名患者PUVA治疗停止6个月后开始重新治疗,并未采用初始计量而是沿用了以前的计量。所有的患者在接受PUVA后的36~72小时内全身皮肤5%~25%出现了二度烧伤类似的红斑、水疱所有患者均在1~3周内痊愈,除了炎症后色素沉着外均未进行植皮或出现严重的后遗症。

慢性光损伤

光致癌

近年来,一些研究表明,长期口服 PUVA 治疗会增加罹患皮肤鳞状细胞癌(SCC)和基底细胞癌(BCC)的风险,这使人们开始关注 UV 治疗的长期副作用。stern 等也发现[16],在首次接受 PUVA 治疗的 15 年后罹患恶性黑素瘤的风险会增加,尤其是已经接受了 250 次或者更多次治疗的患者。动物实验已经证明无论是宽谱 UVB、NB-UVB 或 UVA-1 疗法均有潜在的致癌风险,但它们对人类的致癌性目前还不明确[17,18]。

在明尼苏达州的罗切斯特,玛雅诊所针对 280 位接受了 Goeckerman 疗法的银屑病患者进行了长达 25 年的追踪研究,分析原焦油结合 UV 辐射(Goeckerman 疗法)的致癌性。这项研究结果表明,患者使用原焦油药膏并不会增加罹患皮肤癌的风险。作者认为治疗银屑病使用 Goeckerman 疗法诱发皮肤癌的风险极小[19]。

由于这些接受治疗的患者分布于全世界各地,所以没有关于 UVA-1 潜在光致癌性的数据。同样,也没有关于外用 PUVA 光致癌性的数据。

光致癌性是由于 UV 辐射后 DNA 结构损伤续而突变等系列级联反应而诱发的。UV 诱导的某些细胞防御机制可减少这种级联反应的可能性。这些反应均由信号通路介导,多数与抑癌基因 p53 有关,UV 辐射诱导 p53 突变,随后中断细胞损伤应答是大多数日光诱导的皮肤 sCC 的原因。激活损伤应答信号通路导致受到紫外线辐射损伤的细胞凋亡,这样就阻止了 DNA 受损的细胞存活,也就阻止了紫外线辐射引起突变的细胞数量增加。最终,大部分受损的细胞就会被免疫介导的细胞毒作用清除。

2007 年,Ibuki 等在小鼠体内试验的一项研究表明,连续增加 UVA(67,110,和 168 kJ/m^2)辐射剂量和极高剂量 UVB(3780 J/m^2)会减少皮肤表皮细胞凋亡。通过日晒细胞,caspase-3 阳性细胞减少以及凋亡 DNA 碎片减少而被观察到;这些结果可以从两个方面来解释。首先,日晒细胞数量减少反映了 DNA 受损程度降低,这也是 Ibuki 等赞成的观点[21]。第二种解释是 UV 辐射诱导的凋亡可被看作一种保护性、抗突变及抗癌变的细胞反应。用后一种解释,当同时接受 UVA 和 UVB 辐射可抑制凋亡,会增加细胞突变的风险,最终增加皮肤癌变的几率。在 UVA 对 UVA/UVB 诱导小鼠皮肤癌的影响的其他研究中,有两项研究显示 UVA 照射增强了 UVA 联合 UVB 的致癌作用,其他两项研究则显示降低其致癌作用或无影响。后两项研究中的一项观察到低剂量 UVA 辐射降低 UVB 诱导的癌变几率,而高剂量 UVA 则无此作用[20]。

UV 剂量在皮肤癌发生中的重要作用

2004 年，Ramos 等[22]的一项研究表明，UV 剂量对非黑素皮肤癌（nonmelanomaskin cancer，NMSC）的三个重要特征有影响，BCC/SCC 比率，患病部位和肿瘤数量。一个重要的发现是在接受了极高 UV（包括 UVA 和 UVB）剂量（>145 000kJ/m）的患者中，BCC/SCC 比率下降。接受 15 年以上的高强度紫外线辐射的人被列为极高 UV 暴露组。研究这些参与者发现，降低 BCC/SCC 比的最小累积剂量为 145 000kJ/m^2。接受低剂量（<29 000kJ/m^2）和高剂量（29 000～145 000kJ/m^2）UV 照射的患者其 BCC/SCC 比为 4.2∶1，是接受极高 UV 剂量组的两倍（BCC/SCC 2.1∶1），这与临床相关且有显著统计学意义。在动物模型中，随 UV 辐射剂量的增加 SCC 和光化性角化的数量越来越多。这可能是由于 DNA 损伤的累积和 p53 基因突变[22]。

第二个观察是在参与者接受极高剂量 UVA 和 UVB 比照射组 NMSC 数量翻了一倍，极高剂量是指 UV 的累积剂量至少达 145 000kJ/m^2。这是在人口研究中使 MSC 肿瘤数量增加的有效 UV 剂量。暴露于极高剂量 UV 导致 BCC 和 SCC 数量增加，而 SCC 增加更明显，因此降低了 SCC/BCC 的比。暴露于极高剂量的 UV 导致发生第二种肿瘤的风险增加 13%，具有显著统计学差异，并与每名参与者肿瘤数量的增加相关。由动物模型的研究结果显示，损害的程度及随后进展为皮肤癌取决于 UV 辐射的剂量。在无毛小鼠中，DNA 损伤增加以及 p53 突变与 UV 剂量增加有关[22]。

第三个研究的 NMSC 特征是 UV 辐射和肿瘤位置关系。接受高 UV 辐射的患者中肿瘤发生于日光暴露部位的几率高，如头部、颈部和手臂外部。这说明了与受到保护的皮肤相比，受到较高 UV 辐射的皮肤，DNA 损伤和突变累及嘧啶二聚体累积的更多。澳大利亚的一项研究表明长时间暴露与高 UV 辐射水平下，面部较身体其他部位出现的损伤更多。促使 NMSC 更容易在日光照射部位发生所需的最小 UV 剂量是 29 000kJ/m^2，比加倍肿瘤数量或降低 BCC/SCC 率的剂量小[22]。

UVB 引起的慢性变化

自从 20 世纪 80 年代引进了 TL-01 灯光技术（飞利浦，艾恩德赫温，荷兰），NB-UVB 治疗银屑病和其他皮肤病的数量显著增加。以小鼠为实验对象的研究结果表明 TL-01 的致癌风险和宽谱 UVB 一样，可能比 PUVA 小。2004 年，Weischer 等[24]对使用 TL-01 治疗的 126 名银屑病患者进行了平均 68.4 个月的随访并未发现皮肤癌的风险增加。

2006 年，苏格兰的 Hearn 等观察了 1985 年至 2002 年间 4050 名接受 NB-

UVB疗法的患者,平均随访时间5.8年(最长16.7年)。这项研究调整了调查对象的年龄和性别,将其与一般苏格兰人口中的肿瘤数目进行比较。研究人员并没有发现预期中那么多的黑素瘤或者SCC。但是在接受了NB-UVB治疗和PUVA治疗以及只接受NB-UVB治疗的患者中,BCC较预期中的多。研究人员建议,如果对这些患者进行仔细监视,更多的BCC能被更早的发现。最后,他们认为NB-UVB对人类的致癌性不容忽视。

2006年北爱尔兰的Black和Gavin[26]的一项研究表明,接受TL-01 UVB光疗的患者未罹患皮肤癌。德国一项类似的研究将192名接受TL-01 UVB光疗的患者的资料与当地的癌症登记处的资料做了对比,结果并未发现皮肤癌增加。尽管Black和Gavin的研究规模远远大于德国的研究规模,但却小于Hearn的研究规模[25]。令人欣慰的是,Black的研究中并未发现罹患皮肤肿瘤的病例,因为他们人口中Ⅰ和Ⅱ型皮肤类型比例非常高(92%)。Hearn的苏格兰研究群体大都是Ⅰ~Ⅲ型皮肤,德国的研究对象并未记录皮肤类型。Black和Gavin[26]认为,TL-01 UVB光疗目前看来是相对安全的治疗方式,尽管还需要长期随访资料[16]。Flindt-Hansen等[17]对小鼠的研究很值得一提,这项研究表明,同传统的宽谱UVB光疗相比,窄谱UVB光疗法每最小红斑量致癌的可能性可能是前者的2~3倍,与国际照明委员会(CIE)的非黑素瘤标结论相同,同宽谱源(TL-12)相比,窄谱UVB光疗法每最小红斑量带来的致癌性也是前者的2~3倍。然而,要指出的另外一个因素是NB-UVB比BB-UVB在治疗银屑病方面更为有效;因此,同BB-UVB相比,NB-UVB有效治疗所需的最小红斑量小[27]。

2007年,Diffey和Farr通过对各个年龄段的患者进行大规模队列研究,随访时间为5~20年,分析了UVB光疗的整体危险度。研究表明,若患者在年轻时开始UVB光疗,并且在之后的几十年接受了多次治疗,尤其是在治疗过程中脸部没有做好防护措施的情况下,罹患NMSC的终身风险增加三分之一。研究者通过计算得出结论,NB-UVB发生NMSC的风险要远远高于日光辐射,而且在相同的红斑暴露下,其发生NMSC的风险也高于其他UVB。结论的证实需要大量诊疗中心以及每年数以千计的新患者和长达十多年的追踪调查;也许这就是NMSC风险增加至今没有定论的原因[27]。

评估风险一个行之有效的方法是将人们所受的日光辐射和治疗中的UVB辐射结合起来。剂量-反应关系和光谱反应数据对于量化评估窄谱UVB导致的非黑素瘤案例很有效,但并不针对恶性黑素瘤。基于人口的黑素瘤流行病学的多变量分析,结合来自小鼠实验的光肿瘤模型数据,确定决定患病风险的的两大因素:年龄和环境中的UV量。针对面部有防护和无防护措施的窄谱UVB暴露量,人们都做了风险计算评估。研究指出窄谱UVB光疗辐射和日光对于产生红斑有相同效果。所以结论便是,患者接受窄谱UVB光疗辐射的次数不仅与皮肤癌风险评估有关(与窄谱 UVB 光疗辐射的不确定性评估有关),也与其他因素比如在治疗过程中有没有采取面部防护措施,参加治疗的次数以及患者对待治疗风险的态度有关。

要减少 NB-UVB 治疗后罹患 NMSC 的方法是将治疗疗程控制在一年一次,如果可能,在治疗过程中尽量对面部采取防护措施。最后,应该认识到这些评估需与临床判断相结合,对于重症银屑病患者可系统使用如甲氨蝶呤、环孢菌素或者其他的生物药剂来代替光疗[28]。

需要更多的对照研究来评估 NB-UVB 联合维 A 酸治疗的有效性和安全性。鉴于并没有确定的结论表明 NB-UVB 光疗与皮肤癌的增加有关,对于重症银屑病的治疗 NB-UVB 利大于弊[29]。尽管光疗对于皮肤有潜在致癌风险,但不会引起内在副作用;因此,光疗法也许比生物药剂更为安全。

PUVA 导致的慢性皮肤改变

补骨脂联合 UVA(PUVA)已在世界各地用于治疗各类皮肤疾病,如银屑病、白癜风、皮肤 T 淋巴瘤和特应性皮炎。补骨脂素的衍生物,如甲氧补骨脂素或者三甲基补骨脂,已被用于口服、外用或沐浴,然后再接受 UVA 辐射。PUVA 通常耐受性好,常见的副作用有恶心、红斑和瘙痒。然而,人们对其潜在的长期毒性还是有很多忧虑,尤其是它可能增加皮肤癌的风险[30]。

长期的 UVA 治疗可以导致日光性弹力组织变性、雀斑、日光性角化病和皮肤癌,尤其是 SCC。长期重复 PUVA 治疗和 UVA 计量的累积和皮肤癌变密切相关。长期 PUVA 治疗引起非黑素瘤皮肤癌的主要原因是 DNA 损伤和 PUVA 诱导的免疫应答下调。危险因素包括高剂量的 PUVA(超过 160 次的治疗或者 UVA 总量大 1000J/cm^2),电离辐射暴露史和严重光损伤病史,砷摄入,其他皮肤癌,以及某些基因缺陷,如着色性干皮病和 Fitzpatrick 皮肤类型。

PUVA 分别于 1974 年和 1976 年被用于治疗银屑病和白癜风。银屑病患者中 PUVA 相关的 SCC 有报道,而直到 1996 年,都没有在白癜风患者中发现与 PUVA 相关的皮肤肿瘤。直到最近,报道了 2 例白癜风患者出现与 PUVA 相关的 SCC,分别报道于 1996 年和 1998 年。一篇报道显示,与健康对照组相比,具有肿瘤抑制功能的野生型 p53 蛋白在白癜风患者中的表达更多,前者在降低皮肤癌风险中发挥作用。另一个解释是白癜风患者倾向于避免日晒。相反,接受高计量 PUVA 治疗的银屑病患者更有可能是重度型,并且之前有用致癌物质如焦油化合物和甲氨蝶呤进行治疗。因为银屑病是一种 T 细胞疾病,故更有可能恶变。这就很容易解释为什么和银屑病患者相比,白癜风患者发生 SCC 的几率更小[32]。

然而,最近一项对 479 名白癜风患者的研究表明,老年白人白癜风患者发生

NMSC 的危险度与历史对照相比类似[33]。

法国的 Doubs 地区,阴囊和阴茎的生殖器癌很罕见,平均每 100 000 个居民的年发病人数为 0.48[34]。但是这种现象因区域不同而有所不同。只有 2 项研究认为男性生殖器癌的风险更大。Stern 等[16]一项前瞻性研究(12.3 年随访 892 名男性)发现了生殖器肿瘤的发生率比基于人口基数的预期发生率高 100 倍。在一项长达 13 年的 PUVA 调查中,Perkins 等[35]调查了 130 名接受治疗的男性,其中有 3 名发生生殖器 SCC。白皙的皮肤类型和高剂量的 UVA 辐射(> 2000J/cm^2)都与高风险密切相关。Lindelöf[36]等调查了 2343 名接受 PUVA 治疗的瑞典男性,平均随访时间 6.9 年,发现了 24 例患有 SCC 的患者有 6 例发生在生殖器部位,这可能与瑞典在治疗时忽略了生殖器保护措施有关。

调查结果之间的差异可能是由于调查对象的特点不同(皮肤类型、职业暴露)和银屑病患者使用其他促进肿瘤发展的治疗(焦油、免疫抑制剂)。

种族变异

欧洲和美国的调查研究表明 PUVA 疗法可导致 SCC 风险显著增加并呈计量依赖性,但可降低发生 BCC 的风险[37,38]。伴随风险,如先前使用电离辐射、焦油、甲氨蝶呤、砷剂、既往皮肤癌病史或者 I 和 II 类型皮肤,更容易罹患 NMSC。大量的研究调查发现 PUVA 增加 NMSC 发生多出现在高加索人种、北美或者欧洲人中。英国指南建议口服 PUVA 疗法的最大安全剂量是 1000~1500J/cm^2,然而一项爱尔兰人的调查表明口服 PUVA 计量大于 250J/cm^2 或者接受 100 次治疗增加 NMSC 发生的风险极小。

种族差异会影响皮肤癌的发生率,故人们认为不同种族背景人群 PUVA 相关的皮肤癌的发生风险显著不同[30]。Medhat El Mofty 和 Abdel Monem El Mofty[30] 对 1763 名接受 PUVA 的埃及患者 5 年随访的数据进行分析,发现上千名阿拉伯患者在 25 年的 PUVA 治疗中没有发生皮肤癌。Kobayashi 等[39]建议日本人接受局部 PUVA 的相对安全的最高次数是 100~150 次;这是基于两个独立的日本调查组的数据分析得出的,他们的调查结果表明 PUVA 相关的良性痣的的增加取决于 UVA 的积累计量。Park 等[32]在一项针对非高加索人群的研究中,发现 1303 名接受局部和口服 PUVA 疗法的韩国人未观察到有恶性皮肤肿瘤的发生。在这项研究中,67% 的患者 UVA 积累计量为 0~200J/cm^2,15% 的患者 UVA 积累剂量为 201~400J/cm^2,8% 的患者为 401~600J/cm^2,还有 10% 的患者超过了 600J/cm^2。Park 等[40]认为对于需要长期接受 PUVA 治疗的韩国患者来说,很难决定是否中止治疗,因为在韩国并没有建立安全的 UVA 最大积累计量。

这些数据表明 PUVA 对于亚洲和阿拉伯-非洲国家等棕色到黑色人种产生的致癌性更小一些。即使从亚洲群体(日本[39]和韩国[40])采集到数据来看,PUVA 光化学疗法并未增加发生恶性肿瘤的风险。这些结论强调了基于种族和皮肤类型利弊比是不同的。当收集不同种族的数据时对于深色皮肤的保护措施必须要慎重考虑[30]。

UVR 引起的恶性黑色素瘤的风险

虽然皮肤 SCC 是一种潜在的威胁生命的肿瘤,但它生长缓慢,早期发现容易治疗。然而,恶性黑素瘤是一种生长快速并且致命的肿瘤。很多文献都有侵袭性黑素瘤的案例报道,但是很难确定这些肿瘤是由 PUVA 引起的还是偶发的[36]。

1975 年,美国的 16 所大学皮肤中心联合研究了 PUVA 治疗的功效和短期安全性。这次最初的临床协作研究表明 PUVA 是十分有效的治疗严重银屑病方法。基于其作用机制,PUVA 长期治疗的潜在风险,如 NMSC(特别是 SCC)、黑素瘤、加速皮肤老化、白内障以及增加非皮肤恶性肿瘤的风险可能与其抑制免疫应答有关。1977 年,一项前瞻性研究调查了 1450 名最初纳入 PUVA 治疗有效性测试的患者中的 1380 名,后者同意研究者对 PUVA 治疗的潜在风险及其他健康事件进行监督[16]。

Stern[16]发现接受 PUVA 治疗的患者罹患黑素瘤的风险增加,尤其是照射剂量过高的患者。甚至在大剂量 PUVA 照射组,直到首次治疗的 15 年后发生黑素瘤的风险才增加。虽然照射计量和照射时间均有影响,但时间的影响比剂量更重要。自从 1991 年以来,甚至在接受低剂量 PUVA 照射的患者中,黑素瘤的风险显著增加,几乎是普通人群的 5 倍。在接受低剂量的 PUVA 的患者中,调整年龄、性别和发生黑色素瘤人口的短暂增加等因素之后,同 15 年前相比,1991 年之后患黑素瘤的风险增加 10 倍。患者接受 PUVA 辐射越少,风险就越低。然而,作者认为罹患黑素瘤的风险并不完全与 PUVA 有关,但需权衡利弊[16]。

Lindelöf 等人[36]的研究并不能证明 Stern[16]所发现的关于黑素瘤风险增加的结论。他们在 4799 例患者中发现了 15 例恶性黑素瘤患者,其中包括接受全身 PUVA 治疗的 2477 名银屑病患者中的 11 例,这个发生率与他们预期的一致。他们确认接受 PUVA 治疗的患者容易长痣。Lindelöf 等人[36]通过对瑞典 4799 例患者平均随访 16 年得出结论,长期 PUVA 照射治疗会增加罹患 SCC 的风险,但不会增加罹患黑素瘤的风险。他们假定美国和欧洲的 PUVA 治疗管理或许有所不同。他们推荐接受 PUVA 治疗的患者应严格筛选,认真随访,若接受高剂量(>200 次)不应再进一步 PUVA 治疗[36]。

有关 PUVA 治疗和体内恶性肿瘤之间的可能关系,斯堪的纳维亚人和美国人在之前的研究中得出了不同的结论。Gach 等人[41]发现在英国接受 PUVA 治疗的患者发生体内恶性黑素瘤的风险并未增加,虽然他们资料对于得出严格的结论还太过局限。

UVA-1 的不良反应

研究已经表明 UVA-1 能够有效治疗特应性皮炎和硬皮病(尤其是硬斑病)。已知的 UVA-1 的作用包括诱导 T 细胞的凋亡,减少真皮中郎格罕细胞和肥大细胞数量,皮损处下调干扰素 α 表达,诱导胶原酶和基质金属蛋白酶。Tuchinda 等人[8]回顾了美国四个治疗中心接受 UVA-1 治疗的 92 名患者的资料,所有患者都有不同程度的晒黑,只有 1 例患者因出现多形性日光疹而中断治疗。其他患者未出现需要中断治疗的不良反应。92 例患者中发生不良反应的占 15%,其中包括红斑(7.5%)、瘙痒(3.2%)、刺痛(3.2%)和烧灼感(2.1%)[8]。

UVA 诱发光老化

皮肤过早老化或光老化是由 UV 辐射不良反应所引起的重要美容问题之一。随着年龄增长、日光辐射以及其他环境或治疗因素,皮肤的外观、组织及功能会出现改变。皮肤出现皱纹、色素变化和结构变化。随着年龄增长,真、表皮组织结构和皮肤主要成分也会发生改变。PUVA 照射 6 年所诱发的皮肤临床和组织改变与日光辐射类似。一项队列研究中一小部分接受 PUVA 治疗超过 5 年的患者出现了皮肤组织和外观变化,包括皱纹、毛细血管扩张和皮肤痕迹(光化学变性)。随访 6 年发现接受 PUVA 光疗的皮肤区域发生色素沉的几率增加,在 PUVA 光疗时间较长的病人中更严重。PUVA 诱发的痣与日光诱发的痣组织学表现不同,前者黑色素细胞更大,非典型细胞更常见。虽然这项研究缺乏量化,但作者临床上观察到接受大剂量 PUVA 照射的患者的痣颜色更深,边缘更不规则[42]。

20 多年后,接受超过 300 次 PUVA 治疗的患者臀部出现可见的色素改变的中至重度光化学变性的超过 40%。PUVA 暴露的积累计量在曝光区和非曝光区均是色素改变的信号。虽然 Stern 等人[42]的队列研究发现罹患黑色素瘤的风险增高,但色素沉着的程度和罹患黑色素瘤风险之间的关系未在其研究中体现。光化学改变和色素改变程度以及罹患 SCC 的风险与 PUVA 的积累计量密切相关。需要 PUVA 治疗的患者应被告知长期治疗会改变皮肤外观,并且这种变化很可能会持续数年。除了致癌风险,这些变化应该在长期 PUVA 光疗前就考虑到[42]。

UVB 诱发光老化

目前,还没有关于 UVB 光疗诱发光老化的研究。随着时间的推移,人类活动的影响导致臭氧系统损耗,含卤素化合物排放,导致地球上紫外线剂量增加及皮肤接受 UVB 辐射增多[43]。哺乳类动物细胞对 UV 辐射会产生一系列生物化学变化,包括与信号转导、抗氧化防御和细胞周期控制相关的基因表达改变,这种变化称为 UV 反应。UVB 诱导的基因包括数个蛋白水解酶,如基质金属蛋白酶(MMPS)。在 UVB 剂量恰好低于导致皮肤发红的情况下可诱发和激活金属蛋白酶蛋白。低剂量 UV 辐射激活特殊转录因子,真皮结缔组织中 MMP-1,MMP-9,MMP-3 蛋白增多,降解皮肤胶原和弹力纤维。UVR 的不断暴露,导致结缔组织不断修复引起日光损伤和皱纹形成。

哺乳类动物 UV 反应的两种信号转导通路已被识别。第一种信号转导通路是起源于细胞核的间接(氧化)或直接 DNA 损伤。环丁烷嘧啶二聚体的 UVB 剂量依赖性增加与由 DNA 依赖蛋白激酶介导的人皮肤成纤维细胞 MMP-1 和 MMP-3 mRNA 表达水平提高呈剂量依赖性相关,由 DNA 依赖蛋白激酶介导的第二种信号转导通路包括在细胞膜上或者附近由 UV 辐射产生的活性氧(ROS)。ROS 包括自由基、超氧化物歧化酶(阴离子)(O_2^-),活性中间体的形成中发挥核心作用,包括羟基自由基(HO·)和过氧自由基(ROO·),或非自由基的化合物如单线态氧($^1O_2$)、有机过氧化物(ROOH)、和过氧化氢(H_2O_2),这些都是由酶复合物在氧化磷酸化过程中产生的。ROS 的量通常由抗氧化剂控制。在许多疾病(如癌症、老化和神经退行性病变疾病)的起始和发展过程中及一定条件下发现,ROS(助氧化剂)和抗氧化剂失衡,助氧化剂多时会导致 DNA、线粒体、蛋白质和脂类(氧化压力)损伤。在皮肤病理学上完全信号通道和分子机制潜已得到确定,使用抗氧化剂阻止光老化和光致癌的结缔组织失调,是一种好的干涉选择[43]。

维 A 酸通过刺激皮肤或单层培养基中成纤维细胞和角质形成细胞的生长,改变 UVR 产生的某些有害作用。表皮细胞培养基、成纤维细胞培养基以及人类皮肤中,维 A 酸也可增加 ECM 胶原蛋白和纤维连接蛋白的合成。维 A 酸也抑制紫外线辐射诱导 MMP 激活。因此,维 A 酸通过促进 ECM 胶原蛋白合成以及抑制其分解来修复 UVR 引起的光损伤[44]。此外,近来发现人类皮肤无论是光保护区还是光暴露区,对维 A 酸治疗反应类似。最近维 A 酸疗法被认为是治疗皮肤光老化皮肤的特效方法,治疗慢性皮肤老化也同样有效[44]。

透明质酸(HA)通过控制上皮细胞表型在健康皮肤中发挥作用。不仅如此,HA 含量影响皮肤的一般功能,例如水含量、弹性和营养物的扩散。UVA 和 UVB 辐射可以减少小鼠表皮 HA。与此相反,很少生物化学和组织学研究涉及紫外线辐射对鼠类和人类真皮 HA 含量的作用。部分研究显示鼠类经紫外线辐射后皮肤 HA 含量增加,然而其他研究显示 HA 含量减少。这种矛盾结果或许会是由于 UV 辐射的计量和周期不同。另外,或许由于 UV 辐射对皮肤 HA 急性作用与慢性 UV 辐射的长期慢性作用不同。近来研究表明在经过 UVB 辐射(3 小时与 24 小时相比),角化细胞和成纤维细胞呈现出不同的 HAS 亚型表达、透明质酸酶表达和 HA 复合体相关细胞类型和次数。在 24 小时时,表皮 HA 含量增加,真皮 HA 含量减少。HA 新陈代谢的调控也与对 UVB 辐射的急性炎症反应有关。

Dai 等[45]证实慢性反复 UVB 辐射诱发鼠类 HA 丧失,通过减少依赖 TGF-β1-通路中 HAS 的表达转录激活。不仅如此,减少的 HAS2 表达抑制胞移行和增殖,这或许可以解释老化细胞稀释和减少再生能力[45]。

紫外线辐射对角蛋白表达的影响

对暴露皮肤最重要的环境刺激物之一是太阳紫外线辐射,它对皮肤产生如晒黑、晒伤等短期影响,也可产生如 UV 诱发肿瘤和光老化等长期影响。虽然 UV 辐射对皮肤生理学改变的影响已被广泛研究,但它对角蛋白基因表达的影响还知之甚少。Horio 等人[46]研究表明 UV 辐射导致豚鼠皮肤中角蛋白 5 和 14 增加。另一个人体体内研究发现,UVA 诱导角蛋白 1 和 10 减少,UVC 诱导角蛋白 5 和 14 增加,UVB 诱导角蛋白 5、14、1 和 10 增加。Bernerd 等人[2]发现 UV 辐射能够改变表皮角蛋白基因转录,它和波长相关,UVB 和 UVA 作用于不同的细胞靶点。UVB 可引起一些肿瘤相关角蛋白(如角蛋白 6 和 19)明显增加。这些数据强调了一个事实,在角蛋白家族中,每个成员都被严密管控,使上皮细胞对精确刺激做出相适的反应[2]。

日光辐射引起的光损伤

UV 辐射和皮肤癌

皮肤是接受环境中 UV 最多的器官,也是产生副作用最多的器官。皮肤暴露 UV 辐射导致突变。抑癌基因 *p53* 在皮肤癌中经常发生突变,它是 UV 辐射诱导肿瘤的早期标志。白化无毛小鼠中导致 SCC 的作用光谱最高峰值为 293nm,第二峰值为 354nm 和 380nm。影响黑素瘤发生的光谱波长在 UVB(290～320nm)范围[47];然而,在某些动物模型中,诱导黑色素瘤的发生的光谱波长可能大于 320nm[48]。对于对这些波长的更敏感的浅肤色的人种,以及通过晒黑沙龙增加人工 UV 暴露的人群发生皮肤癌的风险更高[47]。

NMSC 发生率和纬度有直接关联。越接近赤道,人体就会接受越多的 UV 辐射。已经证实 BCC 和 SCC 发生率与纬度有直接关系。Scotto 等人[49]证实,不论性别,纬度与 BCC 和 SCC 发生率之间有很强的逆相关。罹患黑色素瘤的风险和平均年 UVB 暴露联系密切且男女一致。虽然全球研究显示这种关联很弱,但 1950 到 1967 年间在美国和加拿大显示,黑色素瘤死亡率与年用太阳 UV 红斑剂量相当,两者联系密切。

NMSC 发生的部位可能与这些部位的 UV 平均暴露量有关。NMSC 好发生于曝光部位即头颈部。在很少受 UV 照射的区域,如臀部或女性的头皮,NMSC 发生率低。黑色素瘤好发于女性腿部,后者受到的 UV 辐射较男性多。深色皮肤的人更易患恶性肢端黑色素瘤,或许是由于这些黑色素瘤的不同基因变异。皮肤癌基本防护措施对降低皮肤癌发生率有积极效果[47]。

日光辐射导致 DNA 光损伤

UV 辐射最主要的急性作用是 DNA 光损伤。UVA 和 UVB 根据对皮肤的生物学效应表现出不同的特性。UVB 辐射较 UVA 辐射的细胞毒性和致突变性更强,根据波长依赖性学说,导致小鼠 DNA 光损伤、红斑、晒黑和皮肤癌,UVB 辐射较 UVA 辐射每单位物理计量(J/cm^2)高 3 至 4 个数量级。然而和 UVB 相比,UVA 不能被玻璃窗过滤,能穿透皮肤深层到达真皮。估计 50% 的 UVA 暴露发生在阴凉处。而 UVB 会直接被 DNA 吸收并导致 DNA 结构损伤。UVA 主要通过产生 ROS 而间接导致 DNA 损伤,ROS 包括超氧化物阴离子、过氧化氢、单线态氧,它可导致 DNA 及 DNA 蛋白质交联单链断裂。DNA 光损伤会导致各种关键基因产生高特异性基因突变[2]。

美国近十年卫生优先事项中,BCC 和 SCC 在内的 NMSC 位列第八。BCC 比 SCC 更常见,但是,SCC 可发生转移,在皮肤癌导致的死亡中 SCC 超过 20%[50]。慢性 UV 暴露或(和)先前存在的光化性角化病导致的皮肤 SCC 中 16% 发生现转移。如果皮损伴随慢性炎症其风险可高达 30%。UV 辐射是发生 NMSC 的主要危险因素。UVA(320~400nm)和 UVB(290~320nm)都有致癌和免疫抑制作用。强烈断续的 UV 暴露是发生 BCC 的主要危险因素,因为它可以通过促进产生环丁烷型嘧啶二聚体和 6-4 光化产物,引起 DNA 直接损伤和突变。而 UV 暴露的慢性累积是产生 SCC 的主要危险因素[22]。UVA 促进活性氧族和光敏自由基产生。光敏性 DNA 基质诱发单链断裂、氧化应激反应、环丁烷型嘧啶二聚体和 DNA 突变[51]。

大多数与慢性 UV 辐射相关的组织病理学变化发生在真皮中上层。经 UV 辐射皮肤,病理的切片在组织学下出现肿胀且含有许多在普通或正常老化皮肤中不存在的额外成分。这种物质弹力特染着色明显。因此,这种物质的堆积即所谓的日光性弹力组织变性。的确,这种弹性组织变性物质积累在组织学中被认为是皮肤光老化的标志之一。

晒伤

波长小于 290nm 最易引发皮肤红斑,波长越长作用越弱。为了产生相同的红斑,所需的 UVA 的计量是 UVB 的 1000 倍[52]。

UV 和免疫抑制

UV 辐射有局部和系统性的免疫抑制特性,可以降低机体对肿瘤和病毒抗原的监视能力。经过 UV 照射后,抗原递呈朗格汉斯细胞经历了无数次功能和形态改变,导致其消耗。UV 诱导的免疫抑制反应会抑制对炎症产物的免疫应答,炎症产物来源于 UV 介导的损伤(如,UV-损伤 DNA)。近来研究显示 UVA 辐射较 UVB 辐射免疫抑制作用更强。

小鼠实验证明,UV 诱导免疫抑制可能是皮肤肿瘤发生的一个危险因素[53]。经 80% 波长长于 285nm 的水银蒸汽灯辐射 3～4 小时后,幼龄小鼠表皮朗格汉斯细胞数目减少,24～72 小时后数量几乎为零。在老龄小鼠中,朗格汉斯细胞数量开始下降较慢,但 24 小时也可降至最低水平[54]。在所有年龄群中,任何时间段,真皮浸润的单核细胞数量超过中性粒细胞数量。照射后 11～21 小时,单核细胞增长到达稳定水平,48 小时上升。中性粒细胞在辐射后立即出现,4 小时达到峰值,之后数量减少。巨噬细胞增长在 24 小时达最高峰[1]。

由黑色素-UV 反应诱导的损伤

黑色素被认为可保护机体避免 UV 诱导的光损伤。然而,体外研究发现黑色素同样具有毒性,特别暴露于 UVR 后,它与 DNA 反应,并且在 UVA 照射后能够像光敏物质一样产生 ROS,导致皮肤细胞中断裂的单链 DNA 产生。与真黑素相比,褐黑素易于发生光降解并且和 UVR 的损伤作用有关。经过 UV 辐射的褐黑色素能够产生过氧化氢和过氧化物阴离子,这可能导致黑色素细胞或其他细胞产生突变。此外,褐黑素和大量凋亡细胞产生有关。黑素细胞暴露于 UV 后可加速肥大细胞和嗜碱粒细胞释放组织胺,这和皮肤白皙人群中日光诱导的红斑和水肿形成有关[55]。小鼠体内实验显示,黑色素,尤其是褐黑素,会成为 UVA 和 UVB 光敏剂,从而导致细胞死亡。

总结

本章的重点是 UVR 的急性和慢性的不良反应,重点探讨 UV 光疗和 PUVA 光化学疗法不同形式的不良反应。尽管有各种不良反应,UV 光疗和 PUVA 光化学疗法仍可产生良好的临床疗效。为了将不良反应(特别是急性不良反应)降至最低,我们同意 Martin 等人的观点[3],需要出版光疗指南,这将优化治疗效果和安全性。经过特殊训练的光疗医护人员与皮肤科医生密切合作是保证光疗安全的关键。

本章的重点是 UVR 的急性和慢性的不良反应，重点探讨 UV 光疗和 PUVA 光化学疗法不同形式的不良反应。尽管有各种不良反应，UV 光疗和 PUVA 光化学疗法仍可产生良好的临床疗效。为了将不良反应（特别是急性不良反应）降至最低，我们同意 Martin 等人的观点[3]，需要出版光疗指南，这将优化治疗效果和安全性。经过特殊训练的光疗医护人员与皮肤科医生密切合作是保证光疗安全的关键。

（肖常青 译，江娜　周欣 校，朱慧兰 审）

参考文献

1. Soter NA (1993) Acute effects of ultraviolet radiation on the skin. In: Lim H, Soter NA (eds) Clinical photomedicine. Dekker, New York, p 75–93
2. Bernerd F, Del Bino S, Asselineau D (2001) Regulation of keratin expression by ultraviolet radiation: differential and specific effects of ultraviolet B and ultraviolet A exposure. J Invest Dermatol 117:1421–1429
3. Martin JA, Laube S, Edwards C, Gambles B, Anstey AV (2007) Rate of acute adverse events for narrowband UVB and psoralen-UVA phototherapy. Photodermatol Photoimmunol Photomed 23:68–72
4. Coopman SA, Garmyn M, Gonzalez-Serva A, Glogau R (1996) Photodamage and photoaging. In: Arndt KA, Leboit P, Robinson J K, Wintroub BU (eds) Cutaneous medicine and surgery: an integrated program in dermatology. Saunders, Philadelphia, p 732–750
5. Gilchrest BA (1990) Actinic injury. Annu Rev Med 41:199–210
6. Green C, Ferguson J, Lakshmipathi T, Johnson BE (1988) 311 nm UVB phototherapy—an effective treatment for psoriasis. Br J Dermatol 119:691–696
7. Coven TR, Burack LH, Gilleaudeau R, Keogh M, Ozawa M, Krueger JG (1997) Narrowband UV-B produces superior clinical and histopathological resolution of moderate-to-severe psoriasis in patients compared with broadband UV-B. Arch Dermatol 133:1514–1522
8. Tuchinda C, Kerr HA, Taylor CR, Jacobe H, Bergamo BM, Elmets C et al (2006) UVA1 phototherapy for cutaneous diseases: an experience of 92 cases in the United States. Photodermatol Photoimmunol Photomed 22:247–253
9. Dawe RS (2003) Ultraviolet A1 phototherapy. Br J Dermatol 148:626–637
10. Morison WL, Marwaha S, Beck L (1997) PUVA-induced phototoxicity: incidence and causes. J Am Acad Dermatol 36:183–185
11. Morison WL (1997) Subacute phototoxicity caused by treatment with oral psoralen plus UV-A. Arch Dermatol 133:1609
12. Rafal ES, Hamilton TA, Gonzalez E (1991) Comparison of minimal phototoxic dose and skin type for determining initial UVA dose in oral liquid methoxsalen photochemotherapy for the treatment of psoriasis. J Invest Dermatol 97:1048–1052
13. Drummond A, Kane D, Bilsland D (2003) Legal claims in Scottish National Health Service Dermatology Departments 1989–2001. Br J Dermatol 149:111–114
14. Alkali AS, Owens L, Azurdia RM (2008) Rates of acute adverse events for psoralen ultraviolet A and narrow-band UVB phototherapy. Br J Dermatol 159:128–133
15. Herr H, Cho HJ, Yu S (2007) Burns caused by accidental overdose of photochemotherapy (PUVA). Burns 33:372–375
16. Stern RS (2001) The risk of melanoma in association with long-term exposure to PUVA. J Am Acad Dermatol 44:755–761
17. Flindt-Hansen H, McFadden N, Eeg-Larsen T, Thune P (1991) Effect of a new narrow-band

UVB lamp on photocarcinogenesis in mice. Acta Derm Venereol 71:245–248
18. Sterenborg HJ, van der Leun JC (1990) Tumorigenesis by a long wavelength UV-A source. Photochem Photobiol 51:325–330
19. Pittelkow MR, Perry HO, Muller SA, Maughan WZ, O'Brien PC (1981) Skin cancer in patients with psoriasis treated with coal tar. A 25-year follow-up study. Arch Dermatol 117:465–468
20. Runger TM (2007) How different wavelengths of the ultraviolet spectrum contribute to skin carcinogenesis: the role of cellular damage responses. J Invest Dermatol 127:2103–2105
21. Ibuki Y, Allanson M, Dixon KM, Reeve VE (2007) Radiation sources providing increased UVA/UVB ratios attenuate the apoptotic effects of the UVB waveband UVA-dose-dependently in hairless mouse skin. J Invest Dermatol 127:2236–2244
22. Ramos J, Villa J, Ruiz A, Armstrong R, Matta J (2004) UV dose determines key characteristics of nonmelanoma skin cancer. Cancer Epidemiol Biomarkers Prev 13:2006–2011
23. Czarnecki D, O'Brien T, Meehan CJ (1994) Nonmelanoma skin cancer: number of cancers and their distribution in outpatients. Int J Dermatol 33:416–417
24. Weischer M, Blum A, Eberhard F, Rocken M, Berneburg M (2004) No evidence for increased skin cancer risk in psoriasis patients treated with broadband or narrowband UVB phototherapy: a first retrospective study. Acta Derm Venereol 84:370–374
25. Hearn RMR, Dawe RS, Kerr A, Rahim K, Ibbotson SH, Ferguson J (2006) Is there a skin cancer risk with narrowband ultraviolet B phototherapy? Preliminary data from the second phase of the Dundee follow-up study. Br J Dermatol 155:866–867
26. Black RJ, Gavin AT (2006) Photocarcinogenic risk of narrowband ultraviolet B (TL-01) phototherapy: early follow-up data. Br J Dermatol 154:566–567
27. Diffey BL, Farr PM (2007) The challenge of follow-up in narrowband ultraviolet B phototherapy. Br J Dermatol 157:344–349
28. Diffey BL (2003) Factors affecting the choice of a ceiling on the number of exposures with TL01 ultraviolet B phototherapy. Br J Dermatol 149:428–430
29. Lee E, Koo J, Berger T (2005) UVB phototherapy and skin cancer risk: a review of the literature. Int J Dermatol 44:355–360
30. Murase JE, Lee EE, Koo J (2005) Effect of ethnicity on the risk of developing nonmelanoma skin cancer following long-term PUVA therapy. Int J Dermatol 44:1016–1021
31. Chuang TY, Heinrich LA, Schultz MD, Reizner GT, Kumm RC, Cripps DJ (1992) PUVA and skin cancer. A historical cohort study on 492 patients. J Am Acad Dermatol 26:173–177
32. Park HS, Lee YS, Chun DK (2003) Squamous cell carcinoma in vitiligo lesion after long-term PUVA therapy. J Eur Acad Dermatol Venereol 17:578–580
33. Hexsel C, Eide M, Johnson C, Krajenta R, Jacobsen G, Hamzavi I et al (2008) Incidence of nonmelanoma skin cancer in a cohort of 479 vitiligo patients. J Am Acad Dermatol 58:AB9
34. Aubin F, Puzenat E, Arveux P, Louvat P, Quencez E, Humbert P (2001) Genital squamous cell carcinoma in men treated by photochemotherapy. A cancer registry-based study from 1978 to 1998. Br J Dermatol 144:1204–1206
35. Perkins W, Lamont D, MacKie RM (1990) Cutaneous malignancy in males treated with photochemotherapy. Lancet 336:1248
36. Lindelof B, Sigurgeirsson B, Tegner E, Larko O, Johannesson A, Berne B et al (1999) PUVA and cancer risk: the Swedish follow-up study. Br J Dermatol 141:108–112
37. Stern RS, Laird N (1994) The carcinogenic risk of treatments for severe psoriasis. Photochemotherapy follow-up study. Cancer 73:2759–2764
38. Lindelof B, Sigurgeirsson B, Tegner E, Larko O, Johannesson A, Berne B et al (1991) PUVA and cancer: a large-scale epidemiological study. Lancet 338:91–93
39. Kobayashi H, Ohkawara A (1994) Long-term side effects of PUVA therapy. Jpn J Clin Dermatol 48(Suppl 5):144–148
40. Park SH, Hann SK, Park YK (1996) Ten-year experience of phototherapy in Yonsei Medical Center. Yonsei Med J 37

41. Gach JE, Madrigal AM, Hutton JL, Charles-Holmes R (2004) Retrospective analysis of the occurrence of internal malignancy in patients treated with PUVA between 1986 and 1999 in South Warwickshire. Clin Exp Dermatol 29:154–155
42. Stern RS (2003) Actinic degeneration and pigmentary change in association with psoralen and UVA treatment: a 20-year prospective study. J Am Acad Dermatol 48:61–67
43. Brenneisen P, Sies H, Scharffetter-Kochanek K (2002) Ultraviolet-B irradiation and matrix metalloproteinases: from induction via signaling to initial events. Ann NY Acad Sci 973:31–43
44. Varani J, Fisher GJ, Kang S, Voorhees JJ (1998) Molecular mechanisms of intrinsic skin aging and retinoid-induced repair and reversal. J Investig Dermatol Symp Proc 3:57–60
45. Dai G, Freudenberger T, Zipper P, Melchior A, Grether-Beck S, Rabausch B et al (2007) Chronic ultraviolet B irradiation causes loss of hyaluronic acid from mouse dermis because of down-regulation of hyaluronic acid synthases. Am J Pathol 171:1451–1461
46. Horio T, Miyauchi H, Sindhvananda J, Soh H, Kurokawa I, Asada Y (1993) The effect of ultraviolet (UVB and PUVA) radiation on the expression of epidermal keratins. Br J Dermatol 128:10–15
47. Rigel DS (2008) Cutaneous ultraviolet exposure and its relationship to the development of skin cancer. J Am Acad Dermatol 58:S129–132
48. Setlow RB, Grist E, Thompson K, Woodhead AD (1993) Wavelengths effective in induction of malignant melanoma. Proc Natl Acad Sci USA 90:6666–6670
49. Scotto J, Fears TR, Fraumeni JF (1983) Incidence of nonmelanoma skin cancer in the United States. US Department of Health and Human Services, Washington, DC
50. Rowe DE, Carroll RJ, Day CL Jr (1992) Prognostic factors for local recurrence, metastasis, and survival rates in squamous cell carcinoma of the skin, ear, and lip. Implications for treatment modality selection. J Am Acad Dermatol 26:976–990
51. Griffiths HR, Mistry P, Herbert KE, Lunec J (1998) Molecular and cellular effects of ultraviolet light-induced genotoxicity. Crit Rev Clin Lab Sci 35:189–237
52. Parrish JA, Jaenicke KF, Anderson RR (1982) Erythema and melanogenesis action spectra of normal human skin. Photochem Photobiol 36:187–191
53. Brenner M, Hearing VJ (2008) The protective role of melanin against UV damage in human skin. Photochem Photobiol 84:539–549
54. Gilchrest BA, Murphy GF, Soter NA (1982) Effect of chronologic aging and ultraviolet irradiation on Langerhans cells in human epidermis. J Invest Dermatol 79:85–88
55. Hruza LL, Pentland AP (1993) Mechanisms of UV-induced inflammation. J Invest Dermatol 100:35S–41S
56. Takeuchi S, Zhang W, Wakamatsu K, Ito S, Hearing VJ, Kraemer KH et al (2004) Melanin acts as a potent UVB photosensitizer to cause an atypical mode of cell death in murine skin. Proc Natl Acad Sci USA 101:15076–15081

第15章 光防护

P. Wolf, A. Young

内容

引言	294
局部使用防晒剂的原则	294
防晒系数	296
UVA 防护系数	298
防晒剂的赋形剂	299
防水防晒剂	300
紫外线滤光剂(UV Filters)	301
物理防晒剂	306
非传统局部光防护物质	308
系统性光防护剂	310
纺织品和光防护	311
局部使用光防护剂的不良反应	311
光防护对抗光老化、皮肤肿瘤和免疫抑制	312
预防光线性皮肤病和光敏性皮肤病	314
指南及总结	315

> **要点**
> - 化学性 UV 吸收剂将吸收的电子能量转换为热能,传递给邻近分子及细胞。
> - 物理防晒剂主要通过反射和散射作用来发挥保护作用。
> - 宽谱防晒剂包括化学性 UV 吸收剂和物理性防晒剂。
> - 防晒系数(sun protection factor,SPF)是衡量防晒剂有效性的指标。
> - 光稳定性对 UVA 防护剂非常重要。
> - 防晒剂本身有微小色素。
> - 自我晒黑乳剂含改变皮肤颜色的化学成分。
> - DNA 修复酶脂质体混悬剂是一种新型的光防护剂。
> - 口服 β-胡萝卜素可改善红细胞生成性原卟啉病的光敏性。
> - 纺织物的光防护能力主要取决纺织物的本质、结构和种类。
> - 防晒剂极有可能通过抑制 P_{53} 基因的突变来预防皮肤非黑色素瘤的发生。
> - 光线性皮肤病和光敏性皮肤病需要有效的 UVA 防护。

引言

这章将阐述使用防晒剂光防护基本原则——传统防晒剂包括化学和(或)物理 UV 滤光剂、SPF 测定。防晒剂主要用于预防日晒伤,除预防红斑出现外,本章还将探讨防晒剂的其他抗 UV 辐射作用——例如预防光老化、皮肤肿瘤、免疫抑制和导致光线性皮肤病。同时阐述新型局部光防护剂,例如自晒黑乳剂、DNA 修复酶脂质体注射混悬剂、抗氧化剂(包括维生素 C、E,青龙骨提取物和绿茶化合物表没食子儿茶素没食子酸酯)和系统性光保护剂 β-胡萝卜素,政府规范防晒剂测试和商标,也给临床医生提供光防护总指引。

局部使用防晒剂的原则

传统局部外用防晒剂的有效性取决于其混合有效成分,例如化学性 UV 吸收剂和物理性防晒剂[1],其化学结构如下(图 15.1),例如氨基苯甲酸酯、桂皮酸盐类、水杨酸盐类、二苯甲酮类、樟脑衍生物和其他吸收因子(图 15.2a),UV 辐射量子(例如电子)取决于其分子结构,从而由基态到激发态。以热能或荧光/磷光发射的形式将能量传递给周围的分子、细胞及组织。防晒剂的光防护水平

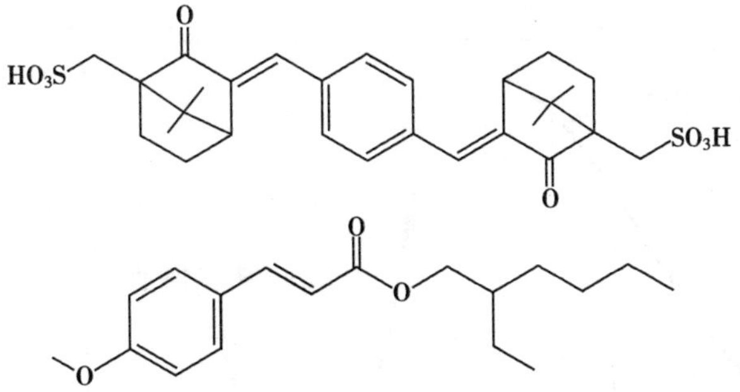

第15章 光防护

图15.1 甲氧肉桂酸辛酯(上)和对苯二甲基二樟脑磺酸(下)的化学结构

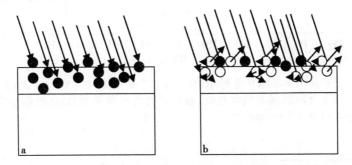

图15.2 化学性UV吸收剂(a)和物理性防晒剂(b)的作用机制

主要与每一种化学UV吸收剂的吸收峰值,吸收光谱或混合化学物质的吸收光谱相关。图15.3显示包含有UVB和UVA滤光剂的防晒剂联合吸收光谱。物理防晒剂例如二氧化钛、氧化锌及其他有机和无机颗粒剂主要通过反射、散射和吸收UV辐射而发挥光防护作用(图15.2b)。目前,宽谱防晒剂产品一般含有化学性UV吸收剂和物理性防晒剂。

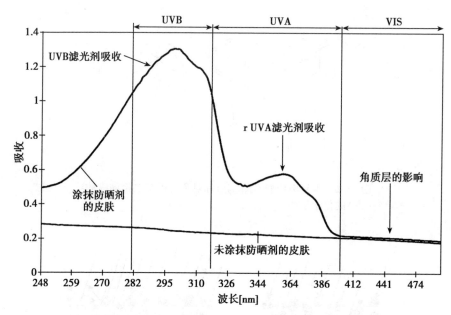

图 15.3 所示同时含有 UVB 滤光剂(4% 甲基亚苄基樟脑)和 UVA 滤光剂(1.5% 帕索 1789UV)混合防晒剂的吸收光谱,通过剥离的角质层测量。(吸收光谱图经 J. Lademann 和 H. J. Weigmann 允许)

防晒系数

防晒系数(sun protection factor, SPF)是衡量防晒剂有效性的指标。SPF 定义为使用防晒剂时 UV 照射皮肤产生的最小红斑量(minimal erythema dose, MED)与未使用防晒剂时产生 MED,两者间的比值。

即　　SPF = MED(使用防晒剂)/MED(未使用防晒剂)

多种方法和规范影响防晒剂的 SPF 值,测试方法中最重要的参数见表 15.1,其参数来自美国食品药品管理局(Food and Drug Administration, FDA)[2]、欧洲科利帕(墨西哥)[3] 和澳洲新西兰(AS/NZS2604:1998)。体外研究防晒剂吸收或传递可用于评估体内 SPF,事实上,体内 SPF 反过来与防晒剂在体外传递有关(见表 15.2)。

第15章 光防护

表15.1 比较发表在美国 FDA、欧洲科利帕（墨西哥）和澳洲新西兰3个不同地方 SPF 测试的重要参数

	FDA(1992)[2]	澳洲新西兰标准(As/NZs 2604:1998)	欧洲科利帕(1994)[3]
受试者数量	20~25	10	10~20
皮肤类型	Ⅰ,Ⅱ,Ⅲ	Ⅰ,Ⅱ,Ⅲ	Ⅰ,Ⅱ,Ⅲ 和比色值 ITA° 值 >28°
测试面积和部位	50cm²(后背)	30cm²(后背)	30cm²(后背)
产品使用量	2.0mg/cm²	2.0±0.1mg/cm²	2.0±0.4mg/cm²
产品干燥时间	15 分钟	15 分钟	15 分钟
防晒剂 sPF 标准(紫外线滤色器)	4.7(水杨酸三甲环己酯)	4.0(水杨酸三甲环己酯)	P1,低 SPF 标准,4.0~4.4;P2,高 SPF 标准,11.5~13.9;P3,高 SPF 标准,14.0~17.0
紫外线光源和光谱	人工灯源,持续发出 290~400nm 光谱,与海平面日光相似、10°天顶角;UVC(<290nm)<1%,可见光<5%	人工灯源,光谱 290~320nm,无峰值。持续光谱高达 400nm;UVC<1%	人工灯源,排出量受有效红斑决定,光谱在 290~400 337nm 之间,取决日光在北纬40°;相对有效红斑低于 290nm <1%
光源滤色器	WG320/1mm + UG5/1mm 或 UG11/1mm	WG320/1mm + 二色性或加热吸收滤光器	WG320/1mm+UG11/1mm
光源的剂量	5 个直径为 1.0cm 的区域;剂量按照 1.25 倍递增	5 个直径为 1.0cm 区域;每个区域剂量增加不超过 1.26 倍	5 个直径为 1.0cm 区域;剂量按照 1.25 倍递增
UV 光照射后判定 MED 值的时间	22~24 小时	16~24 小时	20±4 小时
SPF 计算	个体 SPF 的平均值-校正系数	个体 SPF 的平均值	个体 SPF 的平均值

表 15.2　防晒剂的防晒系数与其传递和吸收的关系

SPF[a]	传递	吸收(%)[b]
4	0.250	75
6	0.167	83.3
8	0.125	87.5
10	0.100	90
12	0.083	91.7
15	0.067	93.3
20	0.050	95
25	0.040	96
30	0.033	96.7
40	0.025	97.5
60	0.017	98.3

[a] SPF=1/传递

[b] 吸收%=(1-反射)×100

UVA 保护系数

经过 FDA 证实 UVB 和 UVA 照射均不利于身体健康：

UVA 持续照射可引起急性和慢性皮肤损伤，例如红斑、黑素形成、致癌作用、药物介导的光敏、光老化、及朗格罕氏细胞形态学改变……另外，消费者误认为使用高 SPF 的防晒剂后暴晒较长时间而无晒伤，反而增加 UVA 辐射时间，人们应认识到避免 UVA 辐射的重要性。它与避免 UVB 辐射同等重要。

由于 UVA 测试和贴商标事宜，FDA 已经延迟发表防晒剂相关论言，最后一篇专题论文有关防晒剂为非处方发表于 1999 年 5 月[2]。

通过 SPF 测试，将红斑作为评价 UVA 防护的指标是不合适的，因为引起皮肤红斑反应必须大剂量 UVA。当使用高 SPF 值的防晒剂，如采用标准的 UVA 照射光源，则 UVA 照射的时间长且不适合健康志愿者。UVA 照射出现即刻色素黑化 (Immediate Pigment Darkening, IPD) 和持续性色素黑化 (Persistent Pigment Darkening, PPD)，这两种方法也是目前体内试验测定 UVA 保护系数最广泛的方法（表格 15.3）。IPD 反应是 UVA 照射受试者皮肤 60 秒内产生一过性褐色改变，快速得出结果，照射 UVA 的剂量也相对较小，然而其结果多变，实验重复性不强。PPD 反应则在 UV 照射 2-24 小时后出现，产生长时间持续存在的黑斑，反应稳定，实验结果可重复性强，根据 SPF 实验方法，

UVA 保护系数的计算如下：

UVA 防护系数 PPD(IPD) = PPD(IPD)最小剂量(使用防晒剂)/

PPD(IPD)最小剂量(未使用防晒剂)

采用体外研究方法(表 15.3)，利用分光光度计测量 UVA 防护系数，从而得出 UVA 防护系数的理论值。根据 Diffey[4] 和 Cole[5]，计算 UVA 防护系数的公式如下：

$$UVA\ SsPF = \Sigma(CIE\lambda \times E\lambda)/\Sigma(T\lambda \times CIE\lambda \times E\lambda)$$

$T\lambda$ = 防晒剂反射波长 λ；$CIE\lambda$ = 按照国际发光照明委员会(CIE)规定波长为 λ 时作用光谱[6]；$E\lambda$ = 日光模拟器模拟的波长，UVA 范围 320～400nm。根据澳洲新西兰防晒剂的标准，防晒剂如被贴上或证实为广谱防晒剂，采用溶液或薄膜的方法，防晒剂的厚度为 8μm，它需至少滤过 90% 波长范围为 320～360nm UVA 光，或采用固体培养法，防晒剂的厚度为 20μm，需至少滤过 90% 波长范围为 320～360nm UVA 光。可是，直到 2009 年欧盟才建立新标准，UVA 防护系数至少需要是 SPF 的 1/3。

表 15.3　决定和(或)设计 UVA 保护系数的方法

体外实验
— UVA 照射出现即刻色素黑化(IPD)
— UVA 照射 2～4 小时出现持续性色素黑化(PPD)

体内实验
— 单色波保护系数[a]
— 临界波长[b]
— 英国星级评定系统(UVB/UVA 比率为 1～4 星)
— 澳洲新西兰标准(As/NZs2604:1998)

[a] 根据 Cole 和 Diffey[4-5]

[b] 根据 Cole 和 Diffey[4-5]；临界波长值定义为达到 290～400nm 光谱吸收曲线下积分面积的 90% 的波长数值。

防晒剂的赋形剂

防晒剂的剂型有多种形式，包括油包水、水包油、油剂、水凝胶、脂质体、酊剂和喷雾剂。防晒剂的基础成份对其直接属性很重要，例如其黏附性反映当薄薄涂抹一层时，粘附在皮肤的有效成分，弥散或渗透至皮肤角质层的能力。大多数防晒剂化学成分为亲脂性，因此它们与油脂有较好的亲和性，容易吸收。水溶性化合物例如对氨基苯甲酸目前不常用于防晒剂配方，因为(a)当皮肤大量出汗时水溶性防晒剂容易脱失。(b)低湿度、高温时,防晒剂容易剥落[1]。当防晒剂的配方掺入耐水活性成份丙烯酸盐聚合物时,其粘附性增强。脂质体也被用于防晒剂,其球形颗粒形成 1~2 层或多层磷脂双层膜,后者含有卵磷脂、胆固醇、神经酰胺类和脂肪酸类。脂质体亲角质层,能渗透至皮肤表层[7]。它们通过亲水物质被运载到内部或通过脂类物质被运载至脂膜。脂质体防晒剂配方具有高度防水性,可掺入或应用于化学 UV 吸收剂或新型光护防物质例如皮肤 DNA 修复酶。

防水防晒剂

防水防晒剂的特点:当游泳、持久运动和出汗时,使用防晒剂不易被擦除。FDA 将防水防晒剂分两大类:(a)"防水"和(b)"非常防水"。其标准测试需在室内带有涡旋或喷流式气泡浴的淡水游泳池,水温保持在 23~32℃(见表 15.4)。需强调即使防晒剂贴有"防水"或"非常防水"标签,由于皮肤机械摩擦,例如在海滩接触到沙或毛巾擦干时经常将防晒剂大部分擦掉。

表 15.4　FDA 协议的防晒剂防水测试[2]

a. 为给防晒剂贴上"防水"和"SPF"值标记。需在水中测试 40 分钟(防水测试具体步骤如下),再算出 SPF 值。

1. 涂防晒剂(按照防晒剂产品标签上标识的等待时间)
2. 在水中中度活动 20 分钟
3. 休息 20 分钟(不要用毛巾擦拭受试部位)
4. 在水中中度活动 20 分钟
5. 得出测试结果(风干测试部位,不能用毛巾擦拭)
6. 采用日光模拟器照射测试部位,开始测试 SPF 值

b. 为了防晒剂贴上"非常防水"、SPF 值标签。需在水中测试 80 分钟(防水测试具体步骤如下),再算出 SPF 值。

1. 涂防晒剂(按照防晒剂产品标签上标记的等待时间)
2. 在水中中度活动 20 分钟
3. 休息 20 分钟(不要用毛巾擦拭受试部位)
4. 在水中中度活动 20 分钟
5. 休息 20 分钟(不要用毛巾擦拭受试部位)
6. 在水中中度活动 20 分钟

7. 休息 20 分钟(不要用毛巾擦拭受试部位)

8. 在水中中度活动 20 分钟

9. 得出测试结果(风干测试部位,不能用毛巾擦拭)

10. 采用日光模拟器照射测试部位,开始 SPF 测试

紫外线滤光剂(UV Filters)

在美国,FDA 认为防晒剂是非处方药品,其在 1999 年 5 月发表专题论文[2]认为非处方药品防晒剂是安全有效的。防晒剂的组成成分(见表 15.5)可用于吸收、反射和散射波长范围为 290~400nm 紫外线。在美国,一款防晒剂产品可包含表 15.5 列出的 16 种任何一种成分及浓度,然而每种防晒剂最小 SPF 值不低于 2,一种防晒剂可包含 2 种或以上成分,并注明其含有的活性成份,每种防晒剂产品其 SPF 值不低于活性成份数量的 2 倍。表格 15.6 示在美国,FDA 拟定 UV 保护剂,例如氨基苯甲酸酯、桂皮酸盐类、水杨酸盐类、二苯甲酮类和混合类,以及它们有效的吸收范围。欧盟(European Community,EC)公布 28 种 UV 滤光剂。表 15.7 列出欧盟认可的 UV 滤光剂,包括其吸收范围、最大授权浓度。与美国相反,欧盟允许一些樟脑诱导药作为 UV 滤光剂(见表 15.7 中第 2,7,9,18 和 19 条)。在美国、欧洲和澳洲生产的大多数防晒剂包含 1 种或以上的化学性 UVB 吸收剂,宽光谱的防晒剂不仅包含 UVB 滤光剂,还包含至少 1 种有效的 UVA 吸收滤光剂(例如二苯酰甲烷、氰双苯丙烯酸辛酯、邻氨基苯甲酸甲酯、甲酚曲唑三硅氧烷、对苯二亚甲基二茨酮磺酸)或物理防晒剂(例如氧化锌或二氧化钛)。二苯甲酮诱导剂能有效吸收 UVB 和 UVA 辐射,常作为宽谱防晒剂的化学成分。

表 15.5 FDA 发表防晒剂的论著规定 FDA 认可防晒剂的成分及最大浓度

成分	最大浓度(%)
氨苯甲酸(PABA)	15
阿伏苯宗	3
西诺沙酯	3
二羟苯宗	3
胡莫柳酯	15
邻氨基苯甲酸甲酯	5
氰双苯丙烯酸辛酯	10
甲氧肉桂酸辛酯	7.5

续表

成分	最大浓度(%)
水杨酸辛酯	5
羟苯甲酮	6
二甲氨苯酸辛酯	8
苯基苯并咪唑磺酸	4
舒利苯酮	10
二氧化钛	25
水杨酸三乙醇胺	12
氧化锌	25

表 15.6　FDA 拟定化学性 UV 吸收剂

组别	化合物	UV 吸收波长范围(nm)
氨基苯甲酸酯	对氨基苯甲酸	260~313
	2-乙基己基苯甲酸	264~320
桂皮酸盐类	甲氧肉桂酸辛酯	280~320
	西诺沙酯	280~320
水杨酸盐类	胡莫柳酯	290~320
	水杨酸辛酯	280~320
	水杨酸三乙醇胺	260~355
二苯甲酮类	二羟苯宗	260~355
	舒利苯酮	260~360
	羟苯甲酮	270~360
混合类	阿伏苯宗	320~380
	邻氨基苯甲酸甲酯	300~370
	氰双苯丙烯酸辛酯	290~360
	苯基苯并咪唑磺酸	290~320
	二氧化钛	300~400
	氧化锌	300~400

化学成分吸收范围摘自 Pathak 等[1]

第15章 光防护

表 15.7 欧盟认可的化学性 UV 吸收剂

EC No.[a]	物质	INCI[b]	类似物,缩略语,或商品名	吸收[c]	最大浓度(g/100g)
1	4-氨基苯甲酸	PABA		UVB	5
2	N,N,N-三甲基-4-甲硫酸阿美铵	樟脑苯扎溴铵硫酸甲酯	Heliopan	UVB	6
3	胡莫柳酯	胡莫柳酯		UVB	10
4	羟苯甲酮	二苯甲酮-3	Eusolex 4360, Escalol 567, 羟甲氧苯酮,Neo Heliopan BB	UVB+UVA	10
6	2-苯基苯并咪唑-5-磺酸及其钾盐、钠盐,磺胺甲磺酸三乙醇胺盐	苯基苯并咪唑磺酸	Eusolex 232, Novantisol, Neo Heliopan Hydro	UVB	8
7	3,3'-(1-4-二亚甲基苯撑)双-(7,7-二亚基-2-氧代双环(2,2,1)庚烷 1-甲磺酸及其钠盐	对苯二亚甲基二樟脑磺酸	紫外线吸收剂	UVA	10
8	1-(4-叔丁基苯基)-3-(4-甲氧基苯基)-1-3 丙二酮	丁基甲氧基二苯甲酰甲烷	阿伏苯宗, Parsol 1789, Eusolex 920	UVA	5
9	α-(2-Oxoborn-3-亚基)-甲苯-4-磺酸及其盐	亚苄基樟脑磺酸	MexorylsL	UVB	6
10	2-氰基-3,3-二苯基丙烯酸,2-乙基己酯	氰双苯丙烯酸辛酯	Uvinul N539	UVB+UVA	10
11	氮聚合物-{(2-4)[(2-oxoborn-3-2-亚基-甲基]苯基}丙烯酰胺		MexorylsW	UVB	6

续表

EC No.[a]	物质	INCI[b]	类似物，缩略语，或商品名	吸收[c]	最大浓度（g/100g）
12	甲氧基肉桂酸辛酯	甲氧肉桂酸辛酯	Parsol MCX, Neo Heliopan AV	UVB	10
13	乙氧基化乙基 4-氨基苯甲酸（PEG-25 对氨基苯甲酸）			UVB	10
14	异戊基 4-甲氧基肉桂（异戊基对甲氧基）	Neo Heliopan E1000		UVB	10
15	2,4,6-三苯胺基-(对-羰基-2'-乙基己基-1'-氧基)-1,3,5-三嗪	辛烷基三嗪酮	Uvinul T150	UVB	5
16	酚,2-(2H-苯并三唑-2-基)-4-甲基-6-[2-甲基-3-[1,3,3,3,3-四甲基-1-[(三甲基甲硅烷基)氧基]-二硅氧烷]丙基]	甲酚曲唑三硅氧烷	Mexoryl XL, silatrizole	UVB+UVA	15
17	苯甲酸,4,4'-[[6-[4-((1,1-二甲基乙基)氨基羰基)苯基氨基]-1,3,5-三嗪-2,4-二基)二氨基]双(2-乙基己基)酯			UVB	10
18	3-(4'-甲基亚苄基)-樟脑	4-甲基亚苄基-樟脑	Eusolex 6300	UVB	4
19	3-亚苄基樟脑	3-亚甲基樟脑	Ultren 9 K, MexorylsD	UVB	2

第15章 光防护

续表

EC No.[a]	物质	INCI[b]	类似物，缩略语，或商品名	吸收[c]	最大浓度（g/100g）
20	水杨酸-2-乙基己酯	水杨酸辛酯		UVB	5
21	4-(二甲氨基)-苯甲酸-(2-乙基)己酯	辛基二甲基苯甲酸	Escalol 507, Eusolex 6007, Padimate O	UVB	8
22	2-羟基-4甲氧基二苯甲酮-5-磺酸及其钠盐	二苯甲酮-4，二苯甲酮-5	sulizobenzone and sulizobenzonesodium	UVB	5
23	2,2'-亚甲基双[6-(2H)-苯并三氮唑-2-基]-4-(2,4,4-三甲基戊-2-基)苯酚]	比索曲唑	Tinosorb M	UVB+UVA	10
24	2-2'-(1,4-亚苯基)双(1H苯并咪唑-4,6-二磺酸和单钠盐)	四磺酸钠苯基苯并咪唑	Bisimidazylate Neo Heliopan AP	UVA	10
25	2,4-双((((4-(2-乙基己氧基)2-羟基)-苯基)6-(4-甲氧苯基)-1,3,5-三嗪	贝曲嗪诺	Tinosorbs	UVB+UVA	10
26	聚硅氧烷-15（CAs-Nr. 207574-74-1)			UVA	10
27	二氧化钛	二氧化钛		UVB+UVA	25

[a] 第1～27，摘自 EEC 导则 76//768 EC 认可化学 UV 吸收剂
[b] 国际化妆品原料命名（international nomenclature cosmetic ingredient, INCI）
[c] 有效波长吸收范围

光稳定性

UV 辐射吸收引起光化学反应改变 UV 滤光剂的分子结构,从而导致 UV 吸收的物质减少,这个过程称为光不稳定性,这个过程会影响 UV 滤光器的有效性。例如,二甲氨苯酸戊酯 A 由于其光不稳定性及其光敏特性,已被 FDA 淘汰。同样,UVA 滤光器阿伏苯宗在光稳定性测试被证实丢失 36% 的活性[1]。而新型的 UV 滤光器例如甲酚曲唑三硅氧烷、贝曲嗪诺和比索曲唑即使经过长时间的 UV 辐射,其活性几乎不受影响,具有很好的光稳定性。

物理防晒剂

过去将有机或无机颗粒状防晒剂用于化妆品制备,这种方法沿用至今。物理性防晒剂包括二氧化钛和氧化锌,以及其他物质,如氧化钛、硫酸钡、金、滑石、瓷土、皂黏土、二氧化硅和云母。不同于化学性防晒剂,物理防晒剂可反射、散射和吸收紫外线(图 15.2b),当波长>400nm,物理防晒剂反射或散射 UV 辐射,当波长<400nm,物理防晒剂吸收 UV 辐射。

巨大色素颗粒

化妆品制备高浓度大色素颗粒(>200nm)(例如巨大色素颗粒)能完全拦阻宽光谱 UV 和可见光的辐射。例如,一些化妆品制备含有 20% 氧化锌或 20% 二氧化钛伴 1%~2% 氧化铁,这些防晒剂对一些光敏性皮肤病例如皮肤型红斑狼疮提供宽光谱的保护(见表 15.8)。它们还可用于制作防 UV 辐射的唇膏,可是,巨大色素颗粒的防晒剂并不受消费者的认可,由于使用它们时需要涂上厚厚的、似奶油状一层,容易引起毛孔阻塞和生成粉刺,使人产生不适感。

微色素颗粒

采用一种特殊技术将二氧化钛和氧化锌制成<100nm 的颗粒,例如微颗粒[8,9]。由于颗粒体积变小,色素颗粒反射及散射可见光和吸收 UV 波长范围的能力减弱。含有氧化锌和二氧化钛的乳化剂,并加入二甲基硅氧烷聚合物,后者能改变这些物理性防晒剂的展布系数,从而明显减少皮肤变白。含有微色素颗粒的防晒剂用于皮肤呈透明状;它们仅能避免 UVB 的辐射,很少防 UVA 辐射,对可见光无作用。微色素颗粒可用于制作防晒剂的成分,尤其是联合化学性 UV 滤光器。一些防晒剂包含微色素颗粒作为成分也可用于商用,例如,一款含有 5% 二氧化钛的防晒剂其 SPF≥15。经过长期的实践,二氧化钛安全无毒,FDA 建议将其作为儿童防晒剂成分。

表15.8 常见光敏性疾病、光线性疾病作用光谱和潜在有效的光防护剂

光线性皮肤病/光敏性皮肤病	作用光谱	化学性UVB滤光剂	化学性UVA滤光剂	巨大色素颗粒	微色素颗粒	羟基丙酮	β胡萝卜素
多形日光疹	UVA>UVB	是/不是	是/不是	是	是	是/不是	—
光化性痒疹	UVA, UVB	是/不是	是/不是	是	是	是/不是	—
牛痘样水疱病	UVA>UVB	是/不是	是/不是	是	是	是/不是	—
日光性荨麻疹	UVA, UVB, VIs	是/不是	是/不是	是	是/不是	—	—
慢性光线性皮炎	UVB>UVA>VIs	是/不是	是/不是	是	是	—	—
红斑狼疮	UVB>UVA	是/不是	是/不是	是	是	—	—
光敏性/光毒性药疹	UVA	不是	是	是	是	—	—
红细胞生成性卟啉病	UVA+VIS(>380nm)	不是	(是)	是	(是)	是	是
着色性干皮病	UVB>UVA	是	是	是	是	—	—

可见光(visible light, VIS);是:保护取决于作用光谱;不是:没有保护;是/不是患者个体保护或不保护取决于作用光谱;(是):低保护;—:对其作用无科学证据

非传统局部光防护物质

生物合成的黑素

某些防晒剂掺入生物合成的黑素,与天然黑素相似,合成黑素具有吸收、散射和反射 UV 辐射的作用[10,11]。另外,与天然黑素一样,生物合成黑素能清除活性氧。含有生物合成黑素产品,不同化学性或物理性防晒剂,其 SPF 最大仅为 6。如果将生物合成黑素掺入化学性防晒剂,可轻微提高 SPF 值,由于其自身棕黑色的颜色被限制用于防晒剂。

自我晒黑物质

自我晒黑或快速晒黑洗剂含有二羟丙酮(Dihydroxyacetone,DHA)成分[12],通过与皮肤的蛋白(例如角蛋白)发生化学反应,从而改变皮肤颜色,不与 UV 辐射发生交叉作用。DHA 是应用最广泛的自我晒黑剂活性成分[1]。将 DHA 涂皮肤后,通过与皮肤表面蛋白(可能是组氨酸和色氨酸)发生美拉德褐色反应,使皮肤由橙棕色改变为金褐色,多于搽完 DHA 3～10 小时后出现皮肤颜色改变,从而避免长波 UVA 和可见光范围的辐射[13]。二羟丙酮介导 UVA 防护指数为 3～5。由于表皮角蛋白脱屑,故搽完二羟丙酮后 5～7 天其保护作用也逐渐消失。临床上采用二羟丙酮治疗红细胞生成性卟啉病可能有效(见表 15.8)[1]。

晒黑物质

佛手柑的活性成分:5-甲氧基补骨酯素,过去常被用于商业晒黑物质中。5-甲氧基补骨酯素联合 UVA 介导光化学反应(例如 PUVA),可晒黑皮肤。年轻人和工人曾用 5-甲氧基补骨酯素晒黑发挥其光防护作用[14]。可是,由于已经证实 5-甲氧基补骨酯素和 UVA 治疗有潜在致突变和致癌作用,故很多国家(包括美国和欧盟)禁止向化妆品中加入 5-甲氧基补骨酯素。法国、比利时及德国的流行病学回顾性研究表明包括 5-甲氧基补骨酯素在内的晒黑物质可能增加黑素瘤的发生的风险,约为 2 倍。

另一种通过人工晒黑起光防护作用的物质是二酰基甘油,它不需要 UV 辐射的参与,即可激活蛋白激酶 D,增强酪氨酸酶的活性及增加黑素的形成[16]。但需要考虑通过晒黑达到光防护作用的安全性,某些肿瘤促成剂,例如佛波醇酯类可激活蛋白激酶 C。局部使用 DNA 修复酶 T4-内切核酸酶-V-脂质体可增加培养基中人类黑素细胞合成黑素[17]。Eller[18]等人进一步研究发现局部外用

DNA 碎片修复产品例如胸苷二核苷酸(pTpT)能增加培养基黑素细胞合成黑素，同时引起豚鼠皮肤晒黑反应，至少持续 60 天。市场上光防护化妆品含有 DNA 修复酶，例如光解酶或超微体，但这些产品介导人类皮肤晒黑起光防护的临床效果仍需进一步探讨。

DNA 修复酶脂质体

UV 辐射后局部使用 DNA 修复酶促进 DNA 修复，是一种新型的光防护方法。局部将包含 T4 脱氧核糖核酸酶的脂质体(T4N5 脂质体)涂在小鼠皮肤后，能对抗 UV 辐射介导 DNA 损伤(例如嘧啶二聚体的形成)和免疫学的改变，例如接触性皮炎、对某些抗原的迟发型超敏反应[20-22]及减少皮肤癌的形成[23,24]。Wolf 等人[7]研究表明曾患皮肤癌的人群在 UV 暴晒后局部使用 T4N5 脂质体后渗入皮肤，将 T4 切核酶渗入角质形成细胞和朗格罕氏细胞，它们能阻断 UV 介导的免疫抑制因子白介素-10 和肿瘤坏死因子-α 上调，避免 UV 介导的红斑反应。另一项相关研究中，Stege 等人[25]先在局部涂上包含有 DNA 修复酶蛋白的脂质体后暴露于可见光下，能避免 UVB 介导的 DNA 损伤、红斑、日晒伤细胞形成和免疫改变，例如抑制胞间黏附分子(Intercellular Adhesion Molecule，ICAM-1)和镍介导的超敏反应。

市面上可见包含 DNA 修复酶的脂质体，它们被一些厂家作为配方掺入光防护产品中。这些脂质体形成新型光防护产品，甚至在已经出现日晒伤反应的情况下仍有效。Yarosh 等学者[64]通过一项前瞻性、多中心、双盲和有安慰剂的研究发现，着色性干皮病的患者规律使用含有 T4N5 脂质体的日晒后防护产品超过 12 个月后，日光性角化和基底细胞癌的发生率减少 30% 和 68%。在初始治疗的 3 个月内即可见日光性角化的数量减少，提示 DNA 修复酶介导的免疫保护作用可在日晒后发挥作用。近期正在开展有关 T4N5 脂质体对肾移植患者和患皮肤癌高危人群的临床疗效的 II 期临床研究。

抗氧化剂和其他物质

防晒剂的产品，除了包含吸收或阻挡 UV 成分外，还包含其他物质，例如抗氧化物质，后者可防护 UV 滤光剂及赋形剂脂质氧化损伤并避免细菌定植。抗氧化剂，例如 VitC 和 VitE 本身不具有吸收 UV 的能力，但它们能中和活性氧而起到潜在光防护作用。近期有文献报道 VitC(15%) 和 VitE(1%) 联合使用能避免人类皮肤日晒伤、日晒伤细胞和胸腺嘧啶二聚体的产生[65]。在 4 天使用期间产生渐进式保护作用，产生 4 倍抗氧化剂保护因子。

芦荟提取物应用日晒后修复霜已有很长时间。芦荟提取物制成凝胶形式有冷却作用,常用于缓解日晒伤出现的疼痛反应。近期啮齿类的研究显示芦荟提取物包含寡糖类和多糖类,具有免疫保护能力,可抑制 UV 介导的接触性超敏反应、迟发型超敏反应和白介素-10 的产生[26-27]。

在西班牙和中美洲较流行用青石莲提取物治疗某些皮肤病,例如特应性皮炎、白癜风和银屑病[1],已经证实局部使用可避免急性光损伤、补骨脂素介导的光毒性反应和消除朗格罕氏细胞[28]。多足蕨属提取物可能起到抗氧化和清除自由基的作用[29]。在欧盟,防晒剂除了包含 UV 滤光剂,还有青石莲提取物。

Katiyar[66]等证实从绿茶提取出来的多酚类或其主要化学成分表没食子儿茶素-3-没食子酸酯(epigallocatechin-3-gallate,EGCG)能预防 UVB 介导的水肿反应和免疫抑制反应。Elmet 等[67]证实采用绿茶提取物抑制 UV 辐射导致的红斑反应,且呈剂量正相关。EGCG 和表儿茶素没食子酸酯(epicatechin-3-gallate,ECG)抑制红斑反应最有效,而表没食子儿茶素(EGC)和没食子酸酯(EC)其抑制红斑反应较弱。组织学显示,绿茶提取物能减少日晒伤细胞,减少 DNA 损伤和保护表皮朗格罕氏细胞细胞免受 UV 辐射的损害。

系统性光防护剂

口服 β-胡萝卜素可预防红细胞生成性原卟啉病的光毒性反应和光敏反应[30]。β-胡萝卜素是多种蔬菜(例如胡萝卜、西红柿、辣椒和橙子)的一种天然成分,可吸收 UVA 和可见光(360~500nm),其吸收峰值为 450~475nm[1]。β-胡萝卜素能有效灭活由光激发卟啉病产生的单态氧,这可能是治疗红细胞生成性原卟啉病的作用机制。临床采用 β-胡萝卜素治疗红细胞生成性原卟啉病的方案如下[1]:

β-胡萝卜素剂量:
- 儿童(低于 12 岁):30~120mg/d,口服
- 成人:120~180mg/d

口服 β-胡萝卜素治疗红细胞生成性原卟啉病,其最佳临床疗效在治疗后 6~8 周,其血药浓度为 600~800μg/100ml。虽然 β-胡萝卜素广泛用于作为口服光防护剂,但对于其保护作用的相关研究较少。近期 stahl 等[31]证实单独口服 β-胡萝卜素或联合 VitE 超过 12 周能避免 UV 辐射介导的红斑反应。口服 β-胡萝卜素治疗光敏性皮肤病(如多形性日光疹、种痘样水疱病和慢性光化性皮炎)的疗效是受质疑的,直到近期临床研究才被证实[1]。β-胡萝卜素对于预防皮肤肿瘤是无效的。

Mathews 等[32]采用双盲研究:将含硫氨基酸-半胱氨酸用为红细胞生成性原卟啉病患者的光防护剂,口服 500mg 半胱氨酸可有效预防儿童红细胞生成性原卟啉病。和 β-胡萝卜素光防护相似,半胱氨酸可灭活活性氧而起作用。

临床研究证实口服青石莲提取物(7.5mg/kg)具有光防护能力,可对抗 UV 辐射引起的红斑反应,微观水平可抑制日晒伤细胞形成,嘧啶二聚物产生,表皮细胞增殖及肥大细胞浸润[68]。

绿茶,含有未被氧化的多酚类复合物,如表没食子儿茶素-3-没食子酸酯(EGCG)(也被认为是抗氧化和混杂因子),也是系统性光保护剂的另一选择,研究发现:用绿茶水喂养小鼠能延迟由 UVB 和局部化学肿瘤促成剂诱导的皮肤肿瘤的发生[33]。口服这些化合物是否产生相同的效果,尚待进一步研究。

吲哚美辛,作为一种环加氧酶(cyclooxygenase,COX)抑制剂,可降低 UVB 介导的皮肤红斑反应[1]。各种物质,包括前列腺素抑制剂如乙酰水杨酸(阿司匹林)和抗组胺药,不能用于预防日晒伤反应[1]。目前尚无证据证实新型环加氧酶-2(COX-2)抑制剂能预防日晒伤。在小鼠实验中 COX-2 抑制剂被证实具有降低 UV 介导的肿瘤形成的作用。

纺织品和光防护

纺织品的光防护作用受一系列因素影响,包括纺织物的本质、编织物的结构和编织的类型[34]。纺织品的光防护范围较广,其 SPF 从 2 到超过 1000[34]。需要强调防 UV 辐射的能力衣服强于防晒剂。为了保证光防护效果,需要避免使用羊毛、一些人造纤维及疏松编织物例如绉纱,而应选择如棉布和绸缎,或高光泽的聚酯材料等排列紧凑的编织物[34]。美国服装行业联合美国材料试验学会和欧洲标准化委员会(CEN)[70]已经形成一种测试和光防护标签的新标准。在欧洲,符合这些标准的 UV 保护衣服需要经过严格测试、分类和标记,包括 UV 保护因子(UV Protection Factor,UPF)>40 和平均 UVA 传导<5%。外衣制造商和零售商需要按照这些官方指导方针标上 UV 保护衣服商标,以便光防护意识较强的消费者容易识别这些光防护衣服。

局部使用光防护剂的不良反应

局部使用防晒剂偶尔能出现一些不良反应,包括接触性皮炎、光毒性、接触性反应和光敏反应[1]。最常见不良反应为刺激反应,防晒剂中含有大量高浓度的光激发物质成分(防晒剂中的媒介、香料或光激发物质)。曾报道防晒剂出现光敏反应是由于防晒剂包含化学性 UV 滤光器某些特殊物质(例如对氨基苯甲酸及其酯类)。自从二十世纪 50 年代以来,在美国和欧洲,对氨基苯甲酸被广泛应用于防晒剂,但由于其刺激性、过敏反应和光敏反应,使用明显下降[1]。例如在美国,FDA 限制使用二甲氨苯酸戊酯作为 UVB 滤光器,主要是由于对氨基苯甲酸与其他包含氨基对位的位置的物质,例如对苯二胺、普鲁卡因、磺胺和对氨基苯甲酸乙酯发生相关的交叉过敏反应。樟脑的衍生物异丙基二苯甲酰甲烷已经不作为某些欧洲的防晒剂成分,主要由于其常见的光敏反应。羟苯甲酮也能引起光敏反应。欧盟规定,防晒剂如含有上述 UV 滤光器则需要在产品说明中特别注明。可是,其他 UV 滤光器,包括帕索 1789、二甲氨基苯甲酸异辛酯、苯基苯并咪唑磺酸等偶尔也会光敏反应[1,12]。化学 UV 滤光器的过敏反应和光敏反应可通过斑贴和光斑贴试验来测试,后者是通过局部皮肤贴上潜在光敏感的物质,然后通过 UVA 的标准剂量来照射,从而判断其结果。

光防护对抗光老化、皮肤肿瘤和免疫抑制

在动物实验研究中,化学性防晒剂能对抗光老化[35]和抑制肿瘤的发生发展[36-37]。在近期的分子生物学研究中[38],防晒剂保护啮齿类 *p53* 基因突变,后者是 UV 照射诱发发生皮肤癌的重要过程。人们采用防晒剂预防日晒伤目的是降低光老化和皮肤癌(包括黑素瘤)的发生率。例如,Sten 等[39]评估在儿童时期规律使用防晒剂后一生中发生非黑素瘤可能减少 80%。这些只是纯理论的结论,并未考虑到人类行为的影响,使用防晒剂可能增加日晒。

光老化

防晒剂能降低光老化的发生。Boyd 等[71]研究发现日光性角化患者每天规律使用防晒剂超过 2 年,日光性弹性组织变性的几率明显减少。一项短期的研究[72]显示防晒剂能预防紫外线介导人类皮肤老化的生物学改变(例如增加溶菌酶、α1-胰蛋白酶抑制剂和 I 型和 III 型胶原 mRNA)。目前尚缺少有关防晒剂在光老化保护作用长期疗效的相关研究。

光线性角化病

澳大利亚一项随机双盲研究,Thompson[40]等发现规律使用 SPF 为 17、其成分含有帕索 MCX 和阿伏苯宗的防晒剂能减少和预防新光线性角化病的发生,有

潜在形成鳞癌的风险。德克萨斯州一项随机双盲研究也得到同样结果,使用SPF为29的防晒剂能减少光线性角化病的发生。

非黑素瘤皮肤肿瘤

Green等[73]开展一项前瞻性、以社区为基础的研究,受试者每天使用SPF 15的防晒剂长达4.5年,同时口服β胡萝卜素预防基底细胞癌和鳞状细胞癌,结果每天规律使用和无使用防晒剂,有口服和无口服β胡萝卜素新发生皮肤肿瘤(基底细胞癌和鳞状细胞)的几率的差别均无统计学差异。使用防晒剂或口服β胡萝卜素对基底细胞癌的数目无影响,但使用防晒剂出现鳞状细胞癌的数目明显低于无使用防晒剂的数目[(1115/100 000vs1832/100 000;比率为0.61(0.46~0.81)]。相反,Hunter等[41]的前瞻性队列研究显示妇女规律使用防晒剂出现基底细胞癌的几率反而增加。

痣细胞痣

目前尚无有关防晒剂预防黑素瘤疗效的前瞻性研究,由于研究设计要考虑伦理方面的问题。但是已有前瞻性研究表明防晒剂能有效预防黑素细胞痣的形成。黑素细胞痣可潜在形成黑素瘤。过度暴晒与痣细胞形成有关。Gallagher等[74]报道一项随机研究:年龄为6~9岁的儿童在夏季使用防晒剂,超过3年能有效抑制痣细胞痣的形成。有项详细的分析表明使用宽光谱的防晒剂能明显减少痣细胞痣的数量,尤其是躯干部位[75]。另一方面,Autier等[44]做了回顾性研究表明规律使用防晒剂反而使儿童的痣细胞痣增多,有趣的是,同一研究采用衣服防护反而能减少痣细胞痣的数量[44]。

黑素瘤

目前为止,多项回顾性流行病学研究黑素瘤的危险因素与局部使用防晒剂的关系[42,43],除了两项相关研究,其他研究均显示防晒剂不能避免黑素瘤的产生。在多数研究中,使用防晒剂反而增加黑素瘤发生的风险,其危险系数约为2或3[42,43]。Roberts和Stanfield[45]指出在一些流行病学研究中有存在潜在选择性偏倚和一些混杂因素,可能影响黑素瘤与防晒剂的关系,他们认为那些曾有日晒伤的患者倾向更频繁使用防晒剂,使用防晒剂反而可能为危险因素,而真正的原因是在很长一段时间里出现过度暴晒。事实上,在先前一些研究,使用防晒剂与各种类型的黑素瘤呈正相关主要由于未考虑肤色和皮肤对日光的敏感性[46],而任何一种回顾性流行病学研究均不能完全排除一些混杂因素。近期一些有关使用防晒剂与黑素瘤危险因素研究中,越是详细排除一些复杂因素,包括对日晒风险的认识、日晒的行为、对日光的敏感度、对晒黑的反应与宿主的一些因素,结果越不容易受混淆[42,43]。

问题是为什么防晒剂能预防日晒伤,而对黑素瘤反而可能无效,甚至反而增加黑素瘤发生的风险呢?至今仍无明确答案,但可能考虑以下几种因素:例如目前介导、促进、导致黑素瘤发展的具体波长及机制尚不清楚,剑尾鱼属动物模型实验证实除了 UVB 波段其他波段也可能引起黑素瘤的形成[47-48],事实上曾有报道除了 UVB 可介导黑素瘤,UVA、短波和可见光不直接 DNA 吸收也可能介导黑素瘤的形成。如果导致人类黑素瘤的产生作用光谱与鱼类相似,则防护 UVB 优于 UVA 的防晒剂对预防黑素瘤的作用不大[48]。已有相关研究证实 UVA 是导致黑素瘤的重要因素,流行病学调查 UVA 日光浴是黑素瘤的危险因素[49-50]。

一些回顾性研究发现黑素瘤的发生与使用防晒剂有一定的关系,可能与不正确使用防晒剂相关:防晒剂能保护人们避免日晒伤,可能鼓励人们延长在日光中暴晒的时间,从而增加痣细胞痣和黑素瘤发生的风险,由于防晒剂不能有效防护非红斑现象,如突变,促进肿瘤的发生,和(或)免疫抑制[51]。

免疫抑制

UV 辐射介导的免疫抑制是促进包括黑素瘤在内的肿瘤形成的重要因素[42]。动物和人类有关防晒剂的免疫保护作用的研究结果不一致。这种差异因实验方案及所用防晒剂的不同而不同,能防御红斑的化学性防晒剂,对紫外线辐射的免疫抑制出现无作用、部分保护或完全保护[21,22,51-59]。有研究[52]评估了 3 种常见化学性 UV 滤光器的防晒剂对小鼠移植黑素瘤模型的作用,通过免疫系统评估对黑素瘤生长的影响。所有的防晒剂能完全避免小鼠日晒伤和降低组织学改变,但它们无法防御紫外辐射所导致的小鼠黑素瘤的生长。这项研究明确显示防晒剂能预防日晒伤,但无法阻止 UV 辐射所带来的影响,例如免疫抑制。

近期,一些科研团队进一步研究了化学防晒剂对人类的免疫保护作用[76-78]。这些研究明确提示化学性防晒剂对人类有免疫保护作用,至少阻止 UV 介导的局部免疫抑制[76-78]。尽管这些研究的设计和方法相似,其结果则不同[78]。Kelly 等[76]发现>50% 防晒剂对抗 UV 辐射介导的免疫抑制能力低于其预防红斑产生的能力。Wolf[78]等报道防 UVB 防晒剂的免疫保护系数与其防晒指数相近,而宽光谱 UVA+UVB 防晒剂其免疫保护能力高于其防晒指数。此外,Baron 等[77]发现宽光谱 UVA+UVB 防晒剂抗免疫抑制能力是抗日晒伤能力的 3 倍。

预防光线性皮肤病和光敏性皮肤病

临床上有潜在预防光线性皮肤病和光敏性皮肤病的物质见表 15.8。宽光谱的防晒剂包括一种或两种 UVB 滤光剂和其他有效的 UVA 滤光剂,例如阿伏苯宗(帕索 1789)、甲酚曲唑三硅氧烷、贝曲嗪诺或比索曲唑,还包括物理性防晒剂,例如二氧化硅或氧化锌,需要注意的是 UVA 和宽光谱滤光剂容易出现光敏感。防晒剂在光线性皮肤病或光敏性皮肤病中的保护能力取决于触发患者个体疾病的作用光谱,例如,大多数多形日光疹患者对 UVA 波段光敏感,但也对UVB、或 UVA 和 UVB 之间的波段敏感。日光性荨麻疹经常受 UVB、UVA 和可见光激发形成[60]。有些疾病例如红细胞生成性原卟啉病,光防护波段为长波 UVA(>380nm)或可见光范围,巨色素颗粒防晒剂或 DHA 介导肤色改变可能对其有用。

指南及总结

采用日光防护可避免急性和慢性皮肤损伤,全面光防护的方法如下:
- 在早上 11 点至下午 3 点,减少在太阳光下暴晒。
- 使用衣物防护:戴宽缘帽子、太阳伞和伞,穿具有光防护作用的编织物。
- 局部使用防晒剂。

局部使用防晒剂能有效降低日晒的影响。在美国,FDA 已建立一套新的有关防晒剂产品分类目录[2],从而有利于个体根据其肤色和期望更好地挑选防晒剂的种类,从而对抗紫外线辐射。FDA 设定防晒产品的最大 SPF 值为 30[2]。SPF>30 的防晒剂,即使增加 SPF 值,其保护作用的增加并不明显,SPF30 防晒剂能阻挡 96.7% 的紫外线,而 SPF60 防晒剂能阻挡 98.3% 的紫外线(表 15.2)。事实上,使用超高 SPF(SPF>60)的防晒产品可能产生一种错误的安全感。

FDA 规定的防晒剂标签:
- 低防晒产品:2<SPF<12
- 中度防晒产品:12≤SPF<30
- 高防晒产品:SPF≥30

在欧洲,科利帕已经规定 SPF50+防晒剂为高防护产品。截至 2009 年,欧盟防晒剂商品分类如下:
- 低保护:SPF6,10
- 中保护:SPF15,20 和 25
- 高保护:SPF30 和 50
- 超高保护:SPF50 以上

高防护(SPF>30)的防晒剂被推荐用于对光高度敏感、皮肤类型为 Ⅰ、Ⅱ、无晒黑的Ⅲ、Ⅳ的个体,尤其在高强度UV辐射的地区室外活动,例如热带、亚热带区域和高海拔山脉。SPF<12防晒剂仅能部分避免日晒伤和UV辐射的其他损害作用,不建议推荐给皮肤类型为Ⅰ～Ⅲ且试图暴晒的人群[1]。厂家制造和销售低SPF值的防晒剂主要针对化妆和那些试图去晒黑的人群。对于儿童,推荐使用物理性防晒剂,因为后者是最安全和无毒的。

使用一定量的防晒剂有利于预防急性光损伤[61,62]和避免紫外线的其他作用[63],例如免疫抑制。SPF测试实验中,防晒剂的使用浓度为$2mg/cm^2$(见表15.1)。如果使用防晒剂的浓度不足,则防晒剂的光防护作用明显下降,甚至可能出现日晒伤[61]。

尽管防晒剂的起效时间快,但也需要在日晒前10～15分钟使用。这个时间有利于:①防晒剂渗入皮肤角质层、增加其黏附性和防水性;②涂防晒剂时,避免无光防护情况下出现日晒伤(尤其是携带小孩的家庭在沙滩上使用防晒剂时)。需要提醒在户外时需要每2小时使用一次防晒剂。另外,当人们游泳时,即使防晒剂的商标标明"非常防水",由于擦干皮肤时经常将防晒剂擦掉,因此需要重新搽上防晒剂。

最后,需要再次强调:防晒剂是光防护的有效方法,但是,需要谨慎使用防晒剂,尤其是暴晒很长时间,因为目前除了证实防晒剂能预防日晒伤,尚没有明确的证据证实防晒剂能预防UV辐射带来的其他影响,例如免疫抑制和致癌[42]。

(马少吟 译,刘清　周欣 校,朱慧兰 审)

参考文献

1. Pathak MA, Fitzpatrick TB, Nghiem P, Aghassi DS (1999) Sun-protective agents: formulations, effects, and side effects. In: Freedberg IM, Eisen AZ, Wolff K (eds) Dermatology in general medicine, 5th edn. McGraw-Hill, New York, pp 2742–2763
2. Food and Drug Administration (1999) Sunscreen products for over-the-counter human use. Final monograph FR, federal register, vol 64, no 98, May 21, pp 27666–27693
3. COLIPA Sun Protection Factor Test Method (1994) Published by the European Cosmetic, Toiletry and Perfumery Association (COLIPA), Brussels, Belgium, October 1994
4. Cole C (1994) Multicenter evaluation of sunscreen UVA protectiveness with the protection factor test method. J Am Acad Dermatol 30:729–736
5. Diffey BL, Tanner PR, Matts PJ, Nash JF (2000) In vitro assessment of the broad-spectrum ultraviolet protection of sunscreen products. J Am Acad Dermatol 43:1024–1035
6. McKinlay A, Diffey B (1987) A reference spectrum for ultraviolet-induced erythema in human skin. CIE J 6:17–22
7. Wolf P, Maier H, Müllegger RR et al (2000) Topical treatment with liposomes containing T4 endonuclease V protects human skin in vivo from ultraviolet-induced upregulation of interleukin-10 and tumor necrosis factor-α. J Invest Dermatol 114:149–156

8. Robb JL, Simpson LA, Tunstall DF (1994) Scattering & absorption of UV radiation by sunscreens containing fine particle and pigmentary titanium dioxide. Drug Cosmet Ind 154:32–39
9. Woodruff J (1994) Formulating sun care products with micronised oxides. Cosmet Toiletries Manufacture Worldwide 1:179–185
10. Ahene AB, Saxena S, Nacht S (1994) Photoprotection of solubilized and microdispersed melanin particles. In: Zeise L, Chedekel MR, Fitzpatrick TB (eds) Melanin: its role in human photoprotection. Valdenmar, Overland Park, Kansas, pp 255–269
11. Césarini JP, Msika P (1994) Photoprotection from UV-induced pigmentations and melanin introduced in sunscreens. In: Zeise L, Chedekel MR, Fitzpatrick TB (eds) Melanin: its role in human photoprotection. Valdenmar, Overland Park, Kansas, pp 239–244
12. Schauder S, Schrader A, Ippen H (1996) Göttinger Liste 1996. Sonnenschutzkosmetik in Deutschland. Blackwell, Berlin
13. Johnson JA, Fusaro RM (1993) Therapeutic potential of dihydroxyacetone. J Am Acad Dermatol 29:284–285
14. Potten CS, Chadwick CA, Cohen AJ et al (1993) DNA damage in UV-irradiated human skin in vivo: automated direct measurement by image analysis (thymine dimers) compared with indirect measurement (unscheduled DNA synthesis) and protection by 5-methoxypsoralen. Int J Radiat Biol 63:313–324
15. Autier P, Dore JF, Schifflers E et al (1995) Melanoma and use of sunscreens: an EORTC case-control study in Germany, Belgium and France. Int J Cancer 61:749–755
16. Gilchrest BA, Park HY, Eller MS, Yaar M (1996) Mechanisms of ultraviolet light-induced pigmentation. Photochem Photobiol 63:1–10
17. Gilchrest BA, Zhai S, Eller MS, Yarosh DB, Yaar M (1993) Treatment of human melanocytes and S91 melanoma cells with the DNA repair enzyme T4 endonuclease V enhances melanogenesis after ultraviolet radiation. J Invest Dermatol 101:666–672
18. Eller MS, Yaar M, Gilchrest B (1994) DNA damage and melanogenesis. Nature 372:413–414
19. Darr D, Dunston S, Faust H, Pinnel S (1996) Effectiveness of antioxidants (vitamin C and E) with and without sunscreens as topical photoprotectants. Acta Derm Venereol 76:264–268
20. Kripke ML, Cox PA, Alas LG, Yarosh DB (1992) Pyrimidine dimers in DNA initiate systemic immunosuppression in UV-irradiated mice. Proc Natl Acad Sci USA 89:7516–7520
21. Wolf P, Yarosh DB, Kripke ML (1993) Effects of sunscreens and a DNA excision repair enzyme on ultraviolet radiation-induced inflammation, immune suppression, and cyclobutane pyrimidine dimer formation in mice. J Invest Dermatol 101:523–527
22. Wolf P, Cox P, Yarosh DB, Kripke ML (1995) Sunscreens and T4N5 liposomes differ in their ability to protect against UV-induced sunburn cell formation, alterations of dendritic epidermal cells, and local suppression of contact hypersensitivity. J Invest Dermatol 104:287–292
23. Yarosh D, Alas LG, Yee V et al (1992) Pyrimidine dimer removal enhanced by DNA repair liposomes reduces the incidence of UV skin cancer in mice. Cancer Res 52:4227–4231
24. Bito T, Ueda M, Nagano T, Fujii S, Ichihashi M (1995) Reduction of ultraviolet-induced skin cancer in mice by topical application of DNA excision repair enzymes. Photodermatol Photoimmunol Photomed 11:9–13
25. Stege H, Roza L, Vink AA et al (2000) Enzyme plus light therapy to repair DNA damage in ultraviolet-B-irradiated human skin. Proc Natl Acad Sci USA 97:1790–1795
26. Strickland FM, Pelley RP, Kripke ML (1994) Prevention of ultraviolet-induced suppression of contact and delayed type hypersensitivity by *Aloa barbadensis* gel extract. J Invest Dermatol 102:197–204
27. Strickland FM, Darvill A, Albersheim P, Eberhard S, Pauly M, Pelley RP (1999) Inhibition of UV-induced immune suppression and interleukin-10 production by plant oligosaccharides and polysaccharides. Photochem Photobiol 69:141–147
28. Gonzales S, Pathak MA, Cuevas J, Villarrubia VG, Fitzpatrick TB (1997) Topical or oral

administration with an extract of *Polypodium leucotomos* prevents acute sunburn and psoralen-induced phototoxic reaction as well as depletion of Langerhans cells in human skin. Photodermatol Photoimmunol Photomed 13:50–60
29. Gonzales S, Pathak MA (1996) Inhibition of ultraviolet-induced formation of reactive oxygen species, lipid peroxidation, erythema, and skin photosensitization by *Polypodium leucotomos*. Photodermatol Photoimmunol Photomed 12:45–56
30. Mathews-Roth MM, Pathak MA, Fitzpatrick TB, Harber LC, Kass EH (1970) Beta-carotene as a photoprotective agent in erythropoietic protoporphyria. N Engl J Med 282:1231–1234
31. Stahl W, Heinrich U, Jungmann H, Sies H, Tronnier H (2000) Carotenoids and carotenoids plus vitamin E protect against ultraviolet light-induced erythema in humans. Am J Clin Nutr 71:795–798
32. Mathews-Roth MM, Rosner B, Benfell K, Roberts JE (1994) A double-blind study of cysteine photoprotection in erythropoietic protoporphyria. Photodermatol Photoimmunol Photomed 10:244–248
33. Agarwal R, Mukhtar H (1996) Chemoprevention of photocarcinogenesis. Photchem Photobiol 63:440–444
34. Robson J, Diffey B (1990) Textiles and sun protection. Photodermatol Photoimmunol Photomed 7:32–34
35. Kligman LH, Akin FJ, Kligman AM (1982) Prevention of ultraviolet damage to the dermis of hairless mice by sunscreens. J Invest Dermatol 78:181–189
36. Kligman LH, Akin FJ, Kligman AM (1980) Sunscreens prevent ultraviolet photocarcinogenesis. J Am Acad Dermatol 3:30–35
37. Synder DS, May M (1975) Ability of PABA to protect mammalian skin from ultraviolet light-induced skin tumors and actinic damage. J Invest Dermatol 65:543–546
38. Ananthaswamy HN, Loughlin SM, Cox P, Evans RL, Ullrich SE, Kripke ML (1997) Sunlight and skin cancer: inhibition of p53 mutations in UV-irradiated mouse skin by sunscreens. Nat Med 3:510–514
39. Stern RS, Weinstein MC, Baker SG (1986) Risk reduction for nonmelanoma skin cancer with childhood sunscreen use. Arch Dermatol 122:537–545
40. Thompson SC, Jolley D, Marks R (1993) Reduction of solar keratoses by regular sunscreen use. N Engl J Med 329:1147–1151
41. Hunter DJ, Colditz GA, Stampfer MJ, Rosner B, Willet WC, Speizer FE (1990) Risk factors for basal cell carcinoma in a prospective cohort of women. Ann Epidemiol Publ Hlth 1:13–23
42. Donawho C, Wolf P (1996) Sunburn, sunscreen, and melanoma. Curr Opin Oncol 8:159–166
43. Wolf P (1999) What can sunscreens do against melanoma? Curr Pract Med 2:27–30
44. Autier P, Dore JF, Cattaruzza MS et al (1998) Sunscreen use, wearing clothes, and number of nevi in 6- to 7-year-old European children. European Organization for Research and Treatment of Cancer Melanoma Cooperative Group. J Natl Cancer Inst 90:1873–1880
45. Roberts LK, Stanfield JW (1995) Suggestion that sunscreen use is a melanoma risk factor is based on inconclusive evidence. Melanoma Res 5:377–378 (letter)
46. Holman CDJ, Armstrong BK, Heenan PJ (1986) Relationship of cutaneous malignant melanoma to individual sunlight-exposure habits. J Natl Cancer Inst 76:403–414
47. Setlow RB, Grist E, Thompson K, Woodhead AD (1993) Wavelengths effective in induction of malignant melanoma. Proc Natl Acad Sci USA 90:6666–6670
48. Setlow RB, Woodhead AD (1994) Temporal changes in the incidence of malignant melanoma: explanation from action spectra. Mutat Res 307:365–374
49. Autier P, Dore JF, Lejeune F et al (1995) Cutaneous malignant melanoma and exposure to sunlamps or sunbeds: an EORTC multicenter case-control study in Belgium, France and Germany. Int J Cancer 58:809–813
50. Westerdahl J, Olsson H, Masback A et al (1995) Use of sunbeds or sunlamps and malignant

melanoma in Southern Sweden. Am J Epidemiol 140:691–699
51. Wolf P, Donawho CK, Kripke ML (1993) Analysis of the protective effect of different sunscreens on ultraviolet radiation-induced local and systemic suppression of contact hypersensitivity and inflammatory responses in mice. J Invest Dermatol 100:254–259
52. Wolf P, Donawho CK, Kripke ML (1994) Effect of sunscreens on UV radiation-induced enhancement of melanoma growth in mice. J Natl Cancer Inst 86:99–105
53. Wolf P, Kripke ML (1996) Sunscreens and immunosuppression. J Invest Dermatol 106:1152–1153 (letter)
54. Granstein RD (1995) Evidence that sunscreens prevent UV radiation-induced immunosuppression in humans. Arch Dermatol 131:1201–1204
55. Wolf P, Kripke ML (1997) Immune aspects of sunscreens. In: Gasparro F (ed) Sunscreen photobiology: molecular, cellular and physiological aspects. Springer, Berlin, pp 99–126
56. Roberts LK, Beasley DG (1995) Commercial sunscreen lotions prevent ultraviolet-radiation-induced immune suppression of contact hypersensitivity. J Invest Dermatol 105:339–344
57. Bestak R, Barnetson RSC, Nearn MR, Halliday GM (1995) Sunscreen protection of contact hypersensitivity responses from chronic solar-simulated ultraviolet irradiation correlates with the absorption spectrum of the sunscreen. J Invest Dermatol 105:345–351
58. Walker SL, Young AR (1997) Sunscreens offer the same UVB protection factors for inflammation and immunosuppression in the mouse. J Invest Dermatol 108:133–138
59. Whitemore SE, Morison WL (1995) Prevention of UVB-induced immunosuppression in humans by a high sun protection factor sunscreen. Arch Dermatol 131:1128–1133
60. Mastalier U, Kerl H, Wolf P (1998) Clinical, laboratory, phototest and phototherapy findings in polymorphic light eruption: a retrospective study of 133 patients. Eur J Dermatol 8:554–559
61. Stenberg C, Larkö O (1985) Sunscreen application and its importance for the sun protection factor. Arch Dermatol 121:1400–1402
62. Bech-Thomsen N, Wulf HG (1992/1993) Sunbathers' application of sunscreen is probably inadequate to obtain the sun protection factor assigned to the preparation. Photodermatol Photoimmunol Photomed 9:242–244
63. Walker SL, Morris J, Chu AC, Young AR (1994) Relationship between the ability of sunscreens containing 2-ethylhexyl-4′-methoxycinnamate to protect against inflammation, depletion of epidermal Langerhans (Ia$^+$) cells and suppression of alloactivating capacity of murine skin in vivo. J Photochem Photobiol B Biol 22:29–36
64. Yarosh D, Klein J, O'Connor A, Hawk J, Rafal E, Wolf P (2001) Effect of topically applied T4 endonuclease V in liposomes on skin cancer in xeroderma pigmentosum: a randomised study. Xeroderma Pigmentosum Study Group. Lancet 357:926–929
65. Lin JY, Selim MA, Shea CR et al (2003) UV photoprotection by combination topical antioxidants vitamin C and vitamin E. J Am Acad Dermatol 48:866–874
66. Katiyar SK, Elmets CA, Agarwal R, Mukhtar H (1995) Protection against ultraviolet-B radiation-induced local and systemic suppression of contact hypersensitivity and edema responses in C3H/HeN mice by green tea polyphenols. Photochem Photobiol 62:855–861
67. Elmets CA, Singh D, Tubesing K, Matsui M, Katiyar S, Mukhtar H (2001) Cutaneous photoprotection from ultraviolet injury by green tea polyphenols. J Am Acad Dermatol 44:425–432
68. Middelkamp-Hup MA, Pathak MA, Parrado C et al (2004) Oral *Polypodium leucotomos* extract decreases ultraviolet-induced damage of human skin. J Am Acad Dermatol 51:910–918
69. Pentland AP, Schoggins JW, Scott GA, Khan KN, Han R (1999) Reduction of UV-induced skin tumors in hairless mice by selective COX-2 inhibition. Carcinogenesis 20:1939–1944
70. Gambichler T, Laperre J, Hoffmann K (2006) The European standard for sun-protective clothing: EN 13758. J Eur Acad Dermatol Venereol 20:125–130
71. Boyd AS, Naylor M, Cameron GS, Pearse AD, Gaskell SA, Neldner KH (1995) The effects of chronic sunscreen use on the histologic changes of dermatoheliosis. J Am Acad Dermatol

33:941–946
72. Seite S, Colige A, Piquemal-Vivenot P et al (2000) A full-UV spectrum absorbing daily use cream protects human skin against biological changes occurring in photoaging. Photodermatol Photoimmunol Photomed 16:147–155
73. Green A, Williams G, Neale R et al (1999) Daily sunscreen application and betacarotene supplementation in prevention of basal-cell and squamous-cell carcinomas of the skin: a randomised controlled trial. Lancet 354:723–729
74. Gallagher RP, Rivers JK, Lee TK, Bajdik CD, McLean DI, Coldman AJ (2000) Broad-spectrum sunscreen use and the development of new nevi in white children: a randomized controlled trial. JAMA 283:2955–2960
75. Lee TK, Rivers JK, Gallagher RP (2005) Site-specific protective effect of broad-spectrum sunscreen on nevus development among white schoolchildren in a randomized trial. J Am Acad Dermatol 52:786–792
76. Kelly DA, Seed PT, Young AR, Walker SL (2003) A commercial sunscreen's protection against ultraviolet radiation-induced immunosuppression is more than 50% lower than protection against sunburn in humans. J Invest Dermatol 120:65–71
77. Baron ED, Fourtanier A, Compan D, Medaisko C, Cooper KD, Stevens SR (2003) High ultraviolet A protection affords greater immune protection confirming that ultraviolet A contributes to photoimmunosuppression in humans. J Invest Dermatol 121:869–875
78. Wolf P, Hoffmann C, Quehenberger F, Grinschgl S, Kerl H (2003) Immune protection factors of chemical sunscreens measured in the local contact hypersensitivity model in humans. J Invest Dermatol 121:1080–1087
79. Fourtanier A, Moyal D, Maccario J et al (2005) Measurement of sunscreen immune protection factors in humans: a consensus paper. J Invest Dermatol 125:403–409

第 5 篇

临床实践中的光诊断学

第 16 章　光诊断学方法

N. J. Neumann, P. Lehmann

内容

引言 ·········· 323
材料和方法 ·········· 324
总结 ·········· 330

要点

- 至今尚无统一的光试验指南。
- 光线性皮肤病的诊断主要基于患者的病史、皮损的形态学、组织病理学、实验室检查和光试验结果。
- 最小红斑量(minimal erythema dose, MED)、即刻晒黑(immediate pigment darkening, IPD)和最小晒黑量(minimal tanning dose, MTD)的结果是判断是否存在光敏感性的筛查手段。
- 建立标准化的光照射流程是通过光激发试验重现光线性皮肤病的特异性皮损。
- 光斑贴试验和全身性的光激发试验是为了确定光致敏原。

引言

　　光线性皮肤病的诊断基于患者的病史、皮损的形态学、组织病理学和光试验的结果。但是目前尚无广泛一致接受的光试验指南。实验室检查可以帮助排除一些鉴别诊断,例如卟啉病。但是对于大多数光线性皮肤病,这些检查并不能帮助诊断。因为皮损可以在日光暴露后很快消失,所以需要通过合适的测试流程在指定测试部位诱导出皮肤病的表现。这对于诊断一个可疑日光敏感病史但缺乏相关皮损的患者是很重要的。医学进展已经使得在适当的部位诱发多种光线性皮肤病或者光加重性皮肤病都成为可能,例如多形性日光疹、种痘样水疱病、慢性光化性皮炎(包括持续性日光疹)、日光性荨麻疹和红斑狼疮[10-14,31]。

材料和方法

在我们工作的皮肤科,所有具有光敏感病史的患者都需要进行多步骤的光试验诊断方案,包括下列程序:

1. 判断红斑[30](中波紫外线照射的最小红斑量,MED-UVB)和色素沉着(即刻晒黑,IPD;最小晒黑量,MTD)产生的阈值剂量。
2. 通过标准化照射流程的激发性光试验重现特异性皮损。
3. 通过光斑贴试验和全身性光激发试验确定光致敏原。

在下面的章节,我们将具体描述这一诊断方案的操作经验。

UV 光源和测定

诊断日光性荨麻疹的作用光谱需要使用高强度的单色光源(Dermolum HI, Müller, Moosinning, Germany)。通过高压金属卤化物光源可以产生大剂量的多色 UVA(UVAsUN 3000, Mutzhas, Munich, Germany),具有 UVA 波段的高辐射剂量,同时检测不到产生 UVB 辐射[20]。这项设备很适合用于照射较大的检测部位。在 30cm 的距离,可以在 25 分钟产生 $100J/cm^2$ UVA。UVAsUN 对于重现 UVA 敏感性皮肤病是非常有用的工具。对于多色的 UVB 光源(UV 800, Waldmann, Villingen-schwenningen, Germany),一般使用一排十个荧光灯管(Philips TL 20W/12, Hamburg, Germany)。发射光谱可以从 285nm 到 350nm,最大强度在 310nm 到 315nm 处。在 30cm 距离处,40 秒之内的能量即可达到平均的 MED-UVB。如果装备了荧光 UVA 灯管(Philips TLK 40W/09N),UV800 还可以用于光斑贴试验的照射光源。它的能量光谱可以从 315nm 到 395nm,高峰在 355 到 365nm 处。在 30cm 的距离处,一般照射小于 25 分钟可达到 $10J/cm^2$ 的 UVA。

除了单色光源,装备卤素灯和滤光片的投影发光器(schott, Mainz, Germany)可以用于检测可见光敏感性皮肤病,例如日光性荨麻疹。

单色光源的剂量测定使用一种连接了电热堆和功率表的仪器(Müller, Moosinning, Germany)。UVAsUN 和 UV800 的 UV 辐射剂量测定使用一种 UV 测量表,具有分别测定 UVA 和 UVB 的探测器(Centra, Osram, Munich, Germany)。

多形性日光疹

所有怀疑多形性日光疹病史的患者都应该依照标准程序进行检查[5,14,22-24]。

最佳检查时间是出现强烈日晒前的早春季节(表16.1)。和皮肤类型匹配的正常对照相比较,患者的 MED-UVB、IPD 和 MTD 可以在正常范围之内。激发性光试验在85%的受试患者中是阳性的。其中80%是通过 UVA 诱发,8%是单独通过 UVB 诱发,12%是 UVA 和 UVB 均可以诱发典型皮损。激发性光试验还可以帮助评价不同的皮损类型。最常见的是丘疹型(70%),其次为斑块型(16%)。其他亚型少见,包括虫咬样型(6%)、多形红斑型(3%)、水疱大疱型(3%)和出血型(2%)。

红细胞生成性卟啉病

波长在400到600nm的UVA和可见光均可诱发红细胞生成性卟啉病(erythropoietic porphyria,EPP)的典型皮损[13,19]。但常用的辐射光源在这一波长范围内的辐射强度不足。根据我们的经验,采用 30～60J/cm² UVA(UVASUN3000)可以诱发EPP中典型的刺痛性晒伤反应(表16.2)[17]。但人工诱导的皮损常常是非特异的。

表16.1 重现多形性日光疹(polymorphous light eruption,PLE)的试验方案

参数	试验方案
测试部位	暴露部位
测试范围大小	5cm×8cm
光源	UVA:UVASUN 3000;UVB:UV 800,Philips TL 20W/12
剂量	3×(60～100)J/cm² UVA,3×1.5MED UVB
读取结果	照射后24～72小时

表16.2 重现红细胞生成性卟啉病(experimental reproduction of erythropoietic porphyria,EPP)的试验方案

参数	试验方案
测试部位	非日光暴露部位
测试范围大小	5cm×8cm
光源	UVA:UVASUN 3000,单色型
剂量	大于100J/cm² UVA,可提高至足以产生客观症状;波长在380～800nm的光线剂量为15J/cm²
读取结果	照射后即刻以及24小时后

种痘样水疱病

罹患这一疾病的患者罕见。文献报道 UVB 和 UVA 均可以诱发皮损出现。但似乎日光中的 UVA 部分包含了活性波长的光,可以诱发大多数患者种痘样水疱病。我们的团队报道了在背部和手臂重复照射 30、50 和 75J/cm² UVA,甚至在口腔黏膜照射 10J/cm² UVA 可以诱发皮损出现[3]。除了试验部位,种痘样水疱病的测试应该在背部和前臂伸侧进行以外,诊断试验采用的试验方案和表 16.1 中一致。

日光性荨麻疹

诊断日光性荨麻疹(solar urticaria,SU)相对简单,因为对于每个 SU 患者采用合适的测试后皮损可以很快诱发出现(表 16.3)。但是患者有不同的亚群。一部分只对 UVA 有反应,一部分只对可见光,其他可以对较广的光谱都有反应。在特定的条件下,可以研究抑制性和促进性的光谱。注射未经辐射的血浆或者血清也可以诱发皮损。最小风团剂量通常很低;一些患者可以对低至 0.5J/cm² UVA 或 1.5mJ/cm² UVB 照射出现反应。判断不同波长光线的最小风团剂量是有意义的,可以证实不同治疗手段的效果。对于任一患者,都建议进行作用光谱的检测[7,29]。

表 16.3 重现日光性荨麻疹(solar urticaria,SU)的试验方案

参数	试 验 方 案
测试部位	非日光暴露部位(骶尾部/臀部)
测试范围大小	小(2cm×2cm)
光源	UVA、UVB、UVC、可见光:单色型 Dermolum HI UVA:UVASUN 3000(330~460nm) UVB:UV 800 Philips TL 20W/12(285~345nm) 可见光:装备不同吸收滤光片的片状发光器(>400nm)(schott,Mainz,Germany)
剂量	因人而异
读取结果	照射后即刻以及 1 小时后

慢性光化性皮炎

慢性光化性皮炎(Chronic actinic dermatitis,CAD)临床上定义为皮肤日光暴露部位的慢性皮炎,组织病理学上表现为海绵状皮炎,光生物学试验可以通过

UVB或者更长波长的光线在缺乏光变应原的情况下激发出海绵状皮炎。传统的命名：持续性日光疹、光敏性湿疹、光敏性皮炎和光化性类网状细胞增多症，近来都被认为是CAD的不同亚型[18,25]。患者的典型临床表现是皮肤的极度光敏性，每位患者都可以通过光试验诱发湿疹样皮损（表16.4）。此外还应该进行斑贴试验和光斑贴试验的检测，这些患者通常可以发现阳性结果。和大多数其他光线性皮肤病相反，较低的MED-UVB也是一项常见的诊断标志。

表16.4 重现慢性光化性皮炎（chronic actinic dermatitis, CAD）的试验方案

参数	试验方案
测试部位	非日光暴露部位无皮损累及的皮肤
测试范围大小	5cm×8cm
光源	UVA：UVASUN 3000 UVB：UV 800 Philips TL 20W/12 可见光：装备合适吸收滤光片的片状发光器（Schott, Mainz, Germany）
剂量	$0.5, 1, 5, 10, 20, 30 J/cm^2$ UVA $0.5, 1, 1.5$ MED UVB $5, 10, 30 J/cm^2$ 可见光
读取结果	照射后24、48、72小时，可以长达一周
附加	斑贴试验和光斑贴试验

光变态反应

光变态反应的知名案例是类似流行病暴发的针对四氯水杨酰苯胺（tetra-chlorsalicylanilide, TCSA）的光变态反应，在1960到1963年间，它作为消毒剂被广泛应用在肥皂和其他清洁剂中。奥地利、瑞士和德国的光斑贴试验研究合作组（The Austrian, swiss, and German Photopatch Test study Group, DAPT）报道非甾体类抗炎药物、消毒剂、防晒剂、吩噻嗪类和香料是目前最常见的光敏物质[6,12,21,22]。

光斑贴试验

Stephan Epstein最早强调光斑贴试验（photopatch testing, PPT）确定光致敏原的重要作用[2]。但是，在1980年代早期，光斑贴试验的流程并不是标准化的，在不同国家和不同的皮肤病治疗中心中，测试用板、测试物质浓度、赋形剂以及测试反应结果的读取和分类都有很大的差异[4,6,26,27]。

最早的标准化光斑贴试验流程是斯堪的纳维亚光线性皮炎研究组（the scandinavian Photodermatitis Research Group, SPDRG）定义的[8]。由SPDRG领导，

来自奥地利、德国和瑞士的 45 个皮肤病学中心在 1984 年组建了 DAPT[12]。他们的标准化试验流程在表 16.5 ~ 表 16.7 中有总结。

表 16.5 光斑贴试验的操作方案

步骤	操作方案
测试材料	在上背部使用 Finn 小室用斑贴贴附受试材料达 24 小时
光照	移除斑贴后,用 10J/cm^2 UVA（UV 800, Philips TLK 40W/09, 320 ~ 395nm）照射
读取	即刻、24、48、72 小时时读取结果;如有必要,最晚的结果读取可以在三周后
对照	无光照的斑贴试验;无斑贴仅光照

表 16.6 光斑贴试验结果分级

分级	反应
0	无反应
1+	红斑
2+	红斑和浸润
3+	红斑和丘疹水疱
4+	红斑、大疱和糜烂

表 16.7 测试反应分类

类型	反应
接触性反应	对照区均有阳性反应,移除测试板后立即出现 1+ 的反应
光毒性反应	1+ 或者 2+ 反应,即刻或者延迟出现,反应程度渐弱
光变态反应	3+ 或者 4+ 反应,延迟出现,反应程度渐强

如果测试物质不能在试验期间穿透表皮角层,光斑贴试验可以表现为假阴性结果。在这些情况下,光搔刮（photopatch）或者光挑刺（photoprick）试验是检测这些光变应原的有效替代试验。

光搔刮和光挑刺试验

光搔刮和光挑刺试验是 PPT 的改良。和 PPT 不同,这两个测试的过程都需要在使用测试物质之前在表皮角层穿孔（例如使用柳叶刀）。可疑光致敏原可以不需要在角层渗透即可和表皮接触[1,28]。

系统性光激发试验

进行光斑贴试验时,系统使用的药物主要表现为假阴性的反应结果,因为其代谢后产物可能才是相应的光致敏原,而不是测试用的外用物质。因此系统性光激发试验可以应用于这种情况,其过程在表 16.8 中详述[10,11]。

表 16.8 系统性光激发试验方案

步骤	操 作 方 案
剂量	如果可行的话,用常用的给药方式(口服、皮下注射、肌肉注射)给予两倍治疗剂量
光照	在用药前以及根据药物动力学选取给药后不同时间点,通常为1、2、4、8小时,采用 10J/cm² UVA 照射不同的测试区域(5cm×5cm)
结果读取	连续3天读取结果,最长可以延迟至3周

红斑狼疮

已经明确日光可以加重和诱发所有亚型的红斑狼疮(lupus erythematosus, LE)[9,14-16]。光敏感性虽然很难定义,但是美国风湿协会(American Rheumatism Association)诊断系统性 LE 的十一条标准之一。1993 年,Kind 等人发表了一个专门针对 LE 的光试验标准化方案(表 16.9)[9]。在我们的系列报道中,64% 的亚急性 LE 患者可以诱发出临床和组织病理学符合 LE 的皮损,同时 42% 的盘状 LE 可以诱发,25% 的系统性 LE 可以诱发。最高的诱发阳性率见于肿胀型 LE,可达 78%,这种亚型的这一特征到目前为止常被低估。33% 的患者诱发皮损的作用光谱在 UVB 范围,14% 为 UVA,53% 则为 UVA 和 UVB 都可以诱发。行激发试验后,LE 的皮损诱发比其他的光线性皮肤病慢。一些患者中,典型的盘状皮损可以持续数周到数月的时间。红斑和色素沉着的阈值剂量一般在正常范围之类。

表 16.9 重现红斑狼疮(lupus erythematosus,LE)的试验方案

参数	试 验 方 案
测试部位	背部或者前臂上部
测试范围大小	5cm×8cm
光源	UVA:UVASUN 3000 UVB:UV 800, Philips TL 20W/12
剂量	3×60–100J/cm² UVA 3×1.5MED UVB
结果读取	照射后 24~72 小时,最迟可在 3 周后

总结

对于特定的光线性皮肤病诊断需要诱发特异性的皮损,特别是没有其他实验室诊断试验以及患者检查时没有相应的皮损时。在笔者实验室中,近年来主要的工作成就就是建立了一系列特异性标准化的光敏性疾病诊断试验方案。光激发试验是其中最重要的诊断手段,它不仅仅能作为确诊试验,还可以判断作用光谱以及作为监测治疗效果的客观指标。光斑贴试验和系统性光激发试验也属于光激发试验,可以在适当的部位重现皮损,甚至进一步明确光致敏原。判定红斑和色素沉着出现的阈值剂量主要作为高光敏感性的筛查,在进一步的其他光相关试验前应该进行。阈值剂量试验中,病理性反应主要发生在慢性光化性皮炎(包括持续性光反应)的患者。在其他的光线性皮肤病中,相较于正常皮肤匹配的对照,紫外线引起的红斑和色素沉着反应在正常的范围之内。

(陈荃 译,杨艳 周欣 校,朱慧兰 审)

参考文献

1. Bourrain JL, Paillet C, Woodward C, Beani JC, Amblard P (1997) Diagnosis of photosensitivity to flupenthixol by photoprick testing. Photodermatol Photoimmunol Photomed 14:159–161
2. Epstein S (1964) The photopatch test. Its technique, manifestations, and significance. Ann Allergy 22:1–11
3. Galosi A, Plewig G, Ring J, Meurer M, Schmöckel C, Schurig V, Dorn M (1985) Experimentelle Auslösung von Hauterscheinungen bei Hydroa vacciniformia. Hautarzt 36:449–452
4. Hölzle E, Plewig G, Hofmann C, Braun-Falco O (1985) Photopatch testing. Results of a survey on test procedures and experimental findings. Zentralbl Hautkr 151:361–366
5. Hölzle E, Plewig G, von Kries R, Lehmann P (1987) Polymorphous light eruption. J Invest Dermatol 88:32S–38S
6. Hölzle E, Neumann N, Hausen B, Przybilla B, Schauder S, Hönigsmann H, Bircher A, Plewig G (1991) Photopatch testing: the 5-year experience of the German, Austrian and Swiss photopatch test group. J Am Acad Dermatol 25:59–68
7. Horio T (1987) Solar urticaria—sun, skin and serum. Photodermatology 15:117
8. Jansen CT, Wennersten G, Rystedi I, Thune P, Brodthagen H (1982) The Scandinavian standard photopatch test procedure. Contact Dermatitis 8:155–158
9. Kind P, Lehmann P, Plewig G (1993) Phototesting in lupus erythematosus. J Invest Dermatol 100:53–57
10. Lehmann P, Hölzle E, Plewig G (1988) Photoallergie auf Neotri mit Kreuzreaktion auf Teneretic Nachweis durch systemische Photoprovokation. Hautarzt 39:38–41
11. Lehmann P, Hölzle E, von Kries R, Plewig G (1986) Übersicht—Neue Konzepte. Lichtdiagnostische Verfahren bei Patienten mit Verdacht auf Photodermatosen. Zentralbl Hautkr 152:667–682
12. Lehmann P (1991) Die deutschsprachige Arbeitsgemeinschaft Photopatch-Test (DAPT). Hautarzt 41:295–297
13. Lehmann P (1994) Photodiagnostische Testverfahren. Aktuel Dermatol 20:41–46
14. Lehmann P, Fritsch C, Neumann NJ (2000) Photodiagnostic tests. 2: Photoprovocation tests.

第 16 章　光诊断学方法

　　　Hautarzt 51:449–459
15. Lehmann P (1996) Photosensitivität des Lupus erythematodes. Aktuel Dermatol 22:47–51
16. Lehmann P, Hölzle E, Kind P, Goerz G, Plewig G (1990) Experimental reproduction of skin lesions in lupus erythematosus by UVB and UVA radiation. J Am Acad Dermatol 22:181–187
17. Lehmann P, Scharffetter K, Kind P, Goerz G (1991) Erythropoetische Protoporphyrie: Synopsis von 20 Patienten. Hautarzt 42:570–574
18. Milde P, Hölzle E, Neumann N, Lehmann P, Trautvetter U, Plewig G (1991) Chronische aktinische Dermatitis. Hautarzt 42:617–622
19. Murphy GM (2003) Diagnosis and management of the erythropoietic porphyrias. Dermatol Ther 16:57–64
20. Mutzhas MF, Hölzle E, Hofmann C, Plewig G (1981) A new apparatus with high radiation energy between 320–460 nm: physical description and dermatological applications. J Invest Dermatol 76:42–47
21. Neumann NJ, Hölzle E, Plewig G, Schwarz T, Panizzon RG, Breit R, Ruzicka T, Lehmann P (2000) Photopatch testing: the 12-year experience of the German, Austrian, and Swiss Photopatch Test Group. J Am Acad Dermatol 42:183–192
22. Neumann NJ, Fritsch C, Lehmann P (2000) Photodiagnostic test methods. 1: Stepwise light exposure and the photopatch test. Hautarzt 51:113–125
23. Neumann NJ, Lehmann P (2003) Photodermatoses during childhood. Hautarzt 54:25–32
24. Neumann NJ, Holzle E, Lehmann P (2004) Polymorphous light dermatoses. J Dtsch Dermatol Ges 2:220–224, 226
25. Norris PG, Hawk JLM (1990) Chronic actinic dermatitis. A unifying concept. Arch Dermatol 126:376–378
26. The European Taskforce for Photopatch Testing: Bruynzeel DP, Ferguson J, Andersen K, Gonçalo M, English J, Goossens A, Holzle E, Ibbotson SH, Lecha M, Lehmann P, Leonard F, Moseley H, Pigatto P, Tanew A (2004) Photopatch testing: a consensus methodology for Europe. J Eur Acad Dermatol Venereol 18:679–682
27. Rünger TM, Lehmann P, Neumann NJ, Matthies C, Schauder S, Ortel B, Münzberger C, Hölzle E (1995) Empfehlung einer Photopatch-Test Standardreihe durch die deutschsprachige Arbeitsgruppe, Photopatch-Test. Hautarzt 46:240–243
28. Schauder S (1990) Der modifizierte intradermale Test im Vergleich zu anderen Verfahren zum Nachweis von phototoxischen und photoallergischen Arzneireaktionen. Z Hautkr 65:247–255
29. Schauder S (2003) Solar urticaria. Hautarzt 54:952–958
30. Wucherpfennig V (1942) Zur Messung und Bemessung des Ultraviolett. Klin Wochenschr 21:926–930
31. Yashar SS, Lim HW (2003) Classification and evaluation of photodermatoses. Dermatol Ther 16:1–7

17

第 17 章 光斑贴试验

E. Hölzle

内容

引言 …………………………………………………… 333
光斑贴试验的历史 …………………………………… 333
光斑贴试验的指征 …………………………………… 333
方法 …………………………………………………… 334
测试品 ………………………………………………… 335
光照和剂量测量 ……………………………………… 337
结果读取 ……………………………………………… 337
结果相关性 …………………………………………… 339
针对临床医生的总结 ………………………………… 339

要点

> 进行光斑贴试验是为了确定外用的光变应原。
> 患者在光暴露部位有不明原因的"湿疹"或者有"晒伤加重"的情况,应该进行光试验。
> 国际上光斑贴试验的操作程序尚未标准化。
> 一般斑贴需要在后背部保留 48 小时,之后用 $5J/cm^2$ 宽谱 UVA 照射。光照前、光照后即刻和光照后 48 小时必须读取测试结果。
> 测试过程应该使用双份测试品,作为对照以排除单纯的接触性过敏。
> 最常见的光变应原包括防晒剂中的紫外线吸收剂。
> 如果患者自带产品有光致敏可能性,也应该进行测试。
> 鉴别光变态反应和光毒性反应十分困难。
> 评价试验阳性结果和患者临床症状的相关性至关重要。

引言

光斑贴试验对于光毒性反应或者光变态反应的患者是一种判定光致敏原的工具。光变态反应发生之前，患者须有致敏史。而光毒性反应是在刚开始接触致敏原时就发生反应。光毒性反应可以定义为一种光化学变化过程；但不同患者的易感性差异很大。

无论是光毒性反应还是光变态反应，试验的阳性结果都应该结合患者的临床相关性进行解读。因此，临床医生采集的临床症状和患者病史都需要结合考虑。

光斑贴试验的历史

发明了磺胺类药物之后，人们第一次观察到光变态反应现象[2,3,5]。随后，吩噻嗪类药物也作为光致敏原引起人们注意。为了诊断这些患者，1956年 Schutz 等人[19]以及 Epstein 和 Rowe[6]首次建立了光斑贴试验的检测方法。在1962年到1970年间的一场暴发流行的光变态反应中，水杨酰苯胺被认定是始作俑者[3,15,23]。这次的光敏流行与水杨酰苯胺广泛应用于除臭香皂和化妆品有关，前者主要用于抗菌剂。制造香皂的工人是最主要的发病人群。在这一情况下，人们首次描述了持续性光反应[24]。

现在，光斑贴试验已经是一个比较成熟的判定光变态反应和光毒性反应物质的试验。在1980年代早期之前，这个试验并没有标准化。最早开始进行标准化尝试的是斯堪纳维亚光敏性皮炎研究工作组（Scandinavian Photodermatitis Research Group，SPRG）[11,20]。在1984年，来自德国、奥地利和瑞士的著名光线性皮肤病专家建立了德国光斑贴试验工作组（Deutschsprachige Arbeitsgemeinschaft Photopatch-Test，DAPT）。他们建立一套标准化的试验方案，同时在一项大型研究中使用，这项研究在45个光生物学中心进行，囊括了1129名患者[10]。根据这项研究结果，试验方法得到进一步调整以优化，并应用于另外的1261名患者中[14]。英国光皮肤病学工作组（the British Photodermatology Group）在1997年发表了一个推荐意见，作为专题讨论的总结[1]。因为光皮肤病学的欧洲专家认为试验国际标准化的需求日渐增长，所以在2002年于阿姆斯特丹召开的国际特别工作组会议上提出光斑贴试验的方法学共识，并在2004年发表[7]。本书中对试验方案的描述主要基于标准化的德国方案，也包括欧洲方案共识的修正。

光斑贴试验的指征

当怀疑光毒性反应或者光变态反应存在时，即是进行光斑贴试验的指征。

慢性光化性皮炎病谱中的疾病也是指征。其他的光线性皮肤病，例如多形性日光疹、种痘样水疱病、日光性荨麻疹和卟啉病的诊断是根据各自的特异性标准，这些不是光斑贴试验的指征。

可能表现为不明的光反应，但又不能确诊真正的光线性皮肤病的患者也应该进行光斑贴试验。这种特别是对于光暴露部位分布的湿疹或者晒伤样反应患者也是适用的。这两种皮疹分别对应怀疑有光变态反应或者光毒性反应，应该仔细询问患者使用药物和外用制剂的病史。光斑贴试验可以判定其中存在的光致敏原。遵循这些严格的推荐意见，可以避免临床中不必要的检查，同时得到阳性的试验结果可以很好地与患者个人关联。

一项国际性的调查发现（P. Lehmann 2001），光斑贴试验平均在每个光生物学中心每年的检测量仅有16，相对较少。个人执业皮肤科医生更少应用光斑贴试验的检测。欧洲专家工作组讨论这一结果后认为，光斑贴试验显然在欧洲没有得到充分利用，应该鼓励促进它的相关应用开展。

方法

上中背部的皮肤，避开脊椎旁沟部位，是最适合进行光斑贴试验的部位。双份测试品通过小的铝制小室（Finn 小室 Scanpor, Hermal, Reinbekbei Hamburg）贴附于皮肤上，其中之一加以光照，另一份作为对照。斑贴在皮肤上停留24或者48小时才能取下。不进行光照的斑贴组作为对照，以排除非光敏性、纯粹的接触性过敏。整个试验过程中，测试部位应该避免日光或者人工紫外线光源等非试验光照（表17.1）。

表17.1 光斑贴试验的具体操作过程

参数	试验方案
测试部位	背部
测试品	使用 Finn 小室（scanpor），停留24或48小时
UV 光源	荧光灯泡（Philips TL 09 N, 320~400nm）
UV 剂量	$5J/cm^2$ UVA（<MED UVA）
结果读取	基本：光照前、光照后即刻以及48小时后
	可增加：光照后24、72、96小时后
对照	未光照的斑贴试验

和斑贴试验类似，不应该在大片范围，特别是测试部位，存在活动性炎症时进行光斑贴试验操作。为了避免"愤怒背综合征"（angry back syndrome）效应，建议测试部位在测试前两周内都是临床正常的。在常规的斑贴试验中，应该告

知患者在测试过程中发生致敏的可能风险,取得其知情同意。在给患者的信息页中,应该告知他们在激发试验中发生严重结果的可能性。

在测试前 3 周内避免外用皮质类固醇激素和接受强烈的 UV 暴露。系统性的皮质类固醇激素和抗组胺药物应该在测试前 1 周停药。此外,同时使用系统性或者外用的免疫抑制剂或者组胺阻断剂都可能导致假阴性结果;此时的阳性结果仍然是有效的。

测试品

表 17.2 列出了德国光斑贴试验工作组最近提出的标准光斑贴试验测试品。尽管欧洲市场已经禁用水杨酰苯胺,但第三世界国家的化妆品仍然可能含有这种成分。去这些地区旅游或者使用这些地区进口的产品仍然有致敏的可能风险。六氯酚、硫双二氯酚、磺胺类、盐酸异丙嗪和硫酸奎尼丁都有光致敏的可能,并且目前也在使用。因此德国工作组认为这些成分都应该作为测试品。香料混合物的检测有争议,因为它很少造成光敏性皮炎。如果患者自带产品有光致敏的可能性,也都应该进行测试。

表 17.2 光斑贴试验测试品(德国光斑贴试验工作组提出[10])

测试品	浓度[a]
5-溴-4′-氯水杨酰苯胺	1%
六氯酚	1%
硫双二氯酚	1%
磺胺	5%
盐酸异丙嗪	0.1%
硫酸奎尼丁	1%
香料混合物	8%
4-氨基苯甲酸	10%
2-乙基-4-二甲基-氨基苯甲酸酯	10%
苯甲酮-4(磺异苯酮)	10%
4′-叔丁基-4-甲氧基二苯酰甲烷	10%
4-对甲氧基肉桂酸异戊酯	10%
2-乙基己基-4-甲氧基肉桂酸酯	10%
3-(4-甲基苄烯)-樟脑	10%
2-苯基-5-苯并咪唑磺酸	10%
二苯酮-3	10%

[a] 测试品溶解在石油中
AlmirallHermal GmbH(Trolab Patch Test Allergens),D-21462 Reinbek,Germany 有售

兽医和农民可能会接触盐酸氯丙嗪和喹乙醇。这两种物质历史悠久光致敏原，当出现持续性的光敏感，病因检测应该考虑这两种物质。在特定的情况下，硫脲类也可能有光致敏性。但这些物质的应用范围非常有限。

欧洲专家工作组认为上述所有的传统光致敏原对目前仅有历史意义。其中包括抗菌剂水杨酰苯胺、磺胺类和强镇静剂。因此欧洲版的测试品删除了以上成分。但是人们越来越多地认识到有机防晒剂成为光接触变态反应的常见原因。因此，欧洲光斑贴试验推荐涵盖了所有主要的 UV 吸收剂。在大多数欧洲大陆南部，非甾体类抗炎药物常以外用制剂使用。这样，它们是已知较强的光致敏原[21]，如果患者有使用过，应该在光斑贴试验中加入这些检测。在表 17.3 中，列出了欧洲专家工作组推荐的光斑贴试验测试品。

表 17.3　光斑贴试验测试品（欧洲光斑贴试验专家工作组提出[7]）

防晒剂（国际化妆品成分命名委员会[International Nomenclature of Cosmetic Ingredients, INCI]）	浓度a	CAS 号
石油（对照）		800274-2
甲氧基肉桂酸辛酯（甲氧基肉桂酸乙基己酯，Parsol MCX，Eusolex 2292）	10%	5466-77-3
二苯酮-3（羟基苯酮，Oxybenzone，Eusolex 4360）	10%	131-57-7
戊烷基二甲对胺基苯甲酸（Escalol 507，Eusolex 6007）	10%	21245-02-3
PABA（对氨基苯甲酸）	10%	150-13-0
丁基甲氧基二苯甲酰基甲烷（Par-sol 1789，Eusolex 9020）	10%	70356-09-1
4-甲基苄亚基樟脑（Eusolex 6300，Mexoryl SD）	10%	36861-47-9
二苯酮-4（Uvenyl MS-40）	10%	4065-45-6
p-甲氧基肉桂酸异戊酯（Neo Heliopan，E1000）	10%	7617-10-2
苯基苯并咪唑磺酸（Eusolex 232）	10%	27503-81-7
非甾体类抗炎药物（需要在室内制备）		
萘普生	5%	
布洛芬	5%	
双氯芬酸	1%	
酮洛芬	2.5%	

a 所有的测试品溶解于石油中
AlmirallHermal GmbH（Trolab Patch Test Allergens），D-21462 Reinbek，Germany 或者 Chemotechnique Diagnostics，P. P. Box 80，s320 Malmo，sweden 有售

光照和剂量测量

宽谱 UVA 灯管最适合作为光照光源。应该注意使用的灯管类型,因为这对结果有影响[17]。首选 PUVA 荧光灯(例如 Philips TL 09 N 320~400nm),因为购买方便、光谱可重复性好以及光照均匀。虽然也可以使用金属卤素灯,但是不同类型的灯管发射的光谱有差异,光照也不均匀,因此不适合用于检测。汞蒸气灯、单色光和日光模拟器不推荐用于常规的光斑贴试验。

文献报道的 UVA 剂量均有不同。这个剂量需要足以诱发光变态反应,但又不能产生假阳性结果或者光毒性反应。测试异丙嗪时,$5J/cm^2$ 的剂量优于 $10J/cm^2$[4]。因此推荐 $5J/cm^2$ 作为常规光斑贴试验的光照剂量。慢性光化性皮炎的患者对 UVA 高度敏感,他们在进行光斑贴试验时,应该采用低于个人最小红斑量的 UVA 剂量。

结果读取

根据德国工作组提出的试验方案,应该在光照前、光照后即刻以及 24、48、72 小时后评估测试部位。移除斑贴后即刻以及 24、48 小时后读取对照部位的结果。如果对照部位斑贴仅仅贴附 24 小时,推荐在 72 小时后读取结果。测试反应的分级和标准斑贴试验有少许区别。如果仅有光照过的斑贴部位出现轻微红斑(+),正如国际斑贴试验标准推荐的:不应遗漏这一反应,而应该认为这是阳性反应。评判的第二步,应该记录下阳性反应,下文中会具体讨论这些阳性反应。表 17.4 列出了测试反应的分级。

表 17.4 光斑贴试验反应分级(根据德国光斑贴试验工作组编写[10])

分级	反应
+	红斑
++	红斑和浸润
+++	红斑、浸润、丘疹水疱
++++	糜烂、大疱

和常见的斑贴试验不同,光斑贴试验的结果分级主要基于形态学标准,而没有定量分析。每日评估一次反应,持续四天,可以判定反应类型。不同的类型可以帮助区分光毒性反应和光变态反应[13]。典型的光毒性反应主要为在起始阶段最为严重,之后的 24~72 小时反应程度持续下降。典型皮损为红斑和浸润,

可以加重出现大疱。一些光毒性物质可以导致即刻红斑和风团，伴有烧灼不适感（刺痛感，"smarting"）。测试煤焦油、氯丙嗪或者苯噁洛芬时可以出现这种反应。光毒性反应机制还可以导致另一种反应类型，表现为测试后24小时迟发的仅有红斑和浸润，病程持续类似"平台期"。这种导致迟发持续"平台期"的例子有吩噻嗪、卡洛芬和噻洛芬酸。光变态反应类似接触性变态反应，表现为迟发但进行性加重的过程。形态学改变包括红斑、浸润和丘疹水疱。瘙痒常见。对可疑病例可以进行组织病理学检查，有助于鉴别光变态反应和光毒性反应。

未光照的对照部位出现超过红斑(+)的测试反应提示单纯的接触性反应。在这种情况下，无论光照部位出现何种反应，都无需理会，诊断还是接触性过敏。同时出现接触性和光接触性反应，以及存在光照加重现象，根据德国光斑贴试验工作组的指南都是无需理会的。他们认为现有的证据不足以针对这种特殊情况的评估制定标准。

欧洲光斑贴试验专家工作组提出另一方案，其在结果读取时间点和测试反应分级上有所不同。这一方案遵循了国际接触性皮炎研究工作组（International Contact Dermatitis Research Group, ICDRG）的结果读取方法和评分系统（表17.5）。结果读取的时间点为光照前、光照后即刻和光照后48小时。可以增加光照后72和96小时的时间点，但不是强制的。欧洲专家组认为在亚临床的UVA效应下，假阳性结果可以是弱刺激性/变应性反应。专家组还认为对光变应原和光照的阳性反应，当"接触性"和"光照"对照都是阴性结果时，高度支持光变态反应的存在，特别是阳性结果随着时间记录点推移表现为越来越强的反应。

表17.5 光斑贴试验反应分级（根据欧洲光斑贴试验专家工作组编写[7,22]）

分级	反应
? +	可疑反应（仅有淡红斑）
+	弱阳性反应（红斑、浸润、可能有丘疹）
++	强阳性反应（红斑、浸润、丘疹、水疱）
+++	极强阳性反应（严重红斑、浸润、聚合性水疱或者大疱）
IR	刺激性反应
NT	未测试

专家组还指出，非光照测试部位的阳性结果可能是刺激性/变应性反应，或者刺激性/变应性反应的光加重性反应（在光照部位），以及光毒性反应，此外还可能存在技术性误差，这些原因都应该进行仔细判定和记录。为了阐述这些开

放性问题,应该应用欧洲光斑贴试验专家工作组使用的方法学[7]。

结果相关性

鉴别光毒性反应和光变态反应,以及判断阳性结果的临床相关性是判定光斑贴试验结果中最常见的问题。诊断光敏性疾病时,患者接触相关致敏物质的病史是必要条件。但是通过模式分析诊断为光变态反应的患者,并没有测试物质致敏的病史也很常见。这种假阳性结果的一个典型例子有,对硫柳汞有接触性过敏的患者可以表现为对吡罗昔康的阳性光变态反应[12]。这些案例中,吡罗昔康的光衍生物在光照下和硫柳汞有交叉反应。

假阴性结果可见于检测系统性药物时。对这些病例,应该调整测试过程。如果问题在于测试品不能穿透皮肤角层,使用测试品前可以采用胶带粘贴剥脱角层,或者选用光搔抓或者挑刺试验来获得阳性结果[16,18]。如果药物的代谢产物才是真正的光致敏原,此时只有系统性光激发试验才能确定光致敏物质[8,9]。

针对临床医生的总结

光斑贴试验是判定外用光变应原时的选择。最常见的光变应原包括防晒剂中的 UV 吸收剂(特别是在南欧国家)和外用的非甾体类抗炎药物。测试系统用的物质会产生不一致的结果,对应困难病例需要采用系统性光激发试验。试验包括使用双套测试品,作为对照来排除单纯的接触性过敏。斑贴在背部皮肤保留 48 小时,之后使用 $5J/cm^2$ 宽谱 UVA 照射。照射前、照射后即刻、照射后 48 小时必须读取结果。为了区别变态反应性或者非变态反应性机制的反应,可以进一步增加照射后 72 小时和 96 小时读取结果,通过反应模式判断。鉴别光毒性反应和光变态反应较为困难。对于患者来说,评估阳性反应结果和临床相关性非常重要。

(陈荃 译,肖常青 周欣 校,朱慧兰 审)

参考文献

1. British Photodermatology Group (1997) Workshop Report—photopatch testing—methods and indications. Br J Dermatol 136:371–376
2. Burckhardt W (1941) Untersuchungen über die Photoaktivität einiger Sulfanilamide. Dermatologica 83:63–68
3. Calnan CA, Harmann RRM, Wells GC (1961) Photodermatitis from soaps. Br Med J 11:1266
4. Duguid C, O'Sullivan D, Murphy GM (1993) Determination of threshold UVA elicitation dose in photopatch testing. Cont Derm 28:192–194
5. Epstein S (1939) Photoallergy and primary photosensitivity to sulfanilamide. J Invest Derma-

tol 2:43–51
6. Epstein S, Rowe RJ (1957) Photoallergy and photocross-sensitivity to phenergan. J Invest Dermatol 29:319–326
7. European Taskforce for Photopatch Testing (2004) Photopatch testing: a consensus methodology for Europe. JEADV 18:679–682
8. Ferguson J, Johnson BE (1993) Clinical and laboratory studies of the photosensitizing potential of norfloxacin, a 4-quinolone broad-spectrum antibiotic. Br J Dermatol 128:185–195
9. Galosi A, Przybilla B, Ring J, Dorn M (1984) Systemische Photoprovokation mit Surgam. Allergologie 7:143–144
10. Hölzle E, Neumann N, Hausen B, Przybilla B, Schauder S, Hönigsmann H, Bircher A, Plewig G (1991) Photopatch testing: the 5-year experience of the German, Austrian and Swiss photopatch test group. J Am Acad Dermatol 25:59–68
11. Jansen CT, Wennersten G, Tystedt I, Thune P, Brodthagen H (1982) The Scandinavian standard photopatch test procedure. Contact Dermatitis 8:155–158
12. Ljunggren B (1989) The piroxicam enigma. Photodermatology 6:151–154
13. Neumann N, Hölzle E, Lehmann P, Benedikter S, Tapernoux B, Plewig G (1994) Pattern analysis of photopatch test reactions. Photodermatol Photoimmunol Photomed 10:65–73
14. Neumann NJ, Hölzle E, Plewig G, Schwarz T, Panizzon RG, Breit R, Ruzicka T, Lehmann P (2000) Photopatch testing: the 12-year experience of the German, Austrian, and Swiss Photopatch Test Group. J Am Acad Dermatol 42:183–192
15. Osmundsen PE (1969) Contact photoallergy to tribromsalicylanilide. Br J Dermatol 81:429–434
16. Przybilla B (1987) Phototestungen bei Lichtdermatosen. Hautarzt 38:23s–28s
17. Przybilla B, Holzle E, Enders F, Gollhausen R, Ring J (1991) Photopatch testing with different ultraviolet A sources can yield discrepant test results. Photodermatol Photoimmunol Photomed 8:57–61
18. Schauder S (1990) Der modifizierte intradermale Test im Vergleich zu anderen Verfahren zum Nachweis von phototoxischen und photoallergischen Arzneireaktionen. Z Hautkr 65:247–255
19. Schulz KH, Wiskemann K, Wolf K (1956) Klinische und experimentelle Untersuchungen über die photodynamische Wirksamkeit von Phenothiazinderivaten, insbesondere Megaphen. Arch Klin Exp Dermatol 202:285–298
20. Thune A, Jansen C, Wennersten G, Rystedt I, Brodthagen H, McFadden N (1988) The Scandinavian multicenter photopatch test study 1980–1985: final report. Photodermatology 5:261–269
21. Veyrac G, Paulin M, Milpied B, Jolliet P (2002) Results of a French nationwide survey of cutaneous side effects of ketoprofen gel reported between September 1996 and August 2000. Therapy 57:55–64
22. Wahlberg JE (2001) Patchtesting. In: Rycroft RJG, Menné T, Frosch PF, Lepoittevim J-P (eds) Textbook of contact dermatitis, 3rd ed. Springer, Berlin, pp 939–968
23. Wilkinson DS (1961) Photodermatitis due to tetrachlorsalicylanilide. Br J Dermatol 73:213–219
24. Wilkinson DS (1962) Patch test reactions to certain halogenated salicylanilides. Br J Dermatol 74:302–306

第18章 荧光诊断

C. Fritsch, K. Gardlo, T. Ruzicka

内容

引言和历史回顾	341
应用 ALA/MAL 诱导的卟啉进行荧光诊断	343
已经研究的皮肤病	345
荧光诊断的操作	346
荧光诊断下表现的特点	347
讨论	354
结论	360
总结	362

引言和历史回顾

皮肤科使用各种检查方法来评估不同类型的皮肤病。皮肤镜检查主要用于评估皮肤色素性病变;超声波可以显示淋巴结的病理,测量皮损的厚度,如硬皮病或肿瘤疾病。然而,组织病理学检查是皮肤科确诊任何皮肤病临床诊断的最重要的诊断程序。

我们想向大家介绍一种新的诊断程序,主要用于肿瘤的检测和指导任一肿瘤的治疗:用 δ 氨基酮戊酸(ALA)或其酯化物诱导产生的内源性卟啉进行荧光诊断(fluorescence diagnosis,FD)。此诊断方法首先可以检测亚临床或小的表皮皮肤癌,其次可以划定肿瘤及炎症组织(例如银屑病皮损)与周围正常皮肤的边界。在荧光诊断时,应用卟啉前体 ALA 或甲酯氨基酮戊酸(MAL)后,病变皮肤(如肿瘤)产生并积累大量的卟啉。当用伍德灯[紫外线(UV)光]照射时,卟啉富集的组织会显示特定的红色荧光。

肿瘤组织对光敏剂的显著摄取及其在随后光照后被选择性的摧毁[光动力疗

法的原理(PDT)]是一个绝佳但非创新的主意。早在1900年,Raab[50]就提到几种染料(如吖啶)具有使某些微生物(如草履虫)致敏而随后被光照摧毁的能力。那时,人们也意识到,上述的反应取决于氧气,因此它被称为"光动力作用"或"光动力效应"[61]。在1903年,这种光动力作用被用来治疗不同的皮肤疾病(如扁平湿疣,寻常狼疮和皮肤肿瘤)。其他经测试的光动力作用的适应证包括单纯疱疹,传染性软疣,花斑癣和寻常型银屑病[30,60]。早期,曙红被用作光敏剂,而照射则采用白光。

为了优化和标准化治疗,随后几年测试了不同的光敏物质,特别是卟啉。在1911年,人们首次进行了血卟啉光敏剂实验.至今卟啉仍然是PDT中最有趣的,最有效的,被测试最多的物质。

关于卟啉分子的诊断潜力,在1924年,人们首次使用血卟啉诊断肿瘤[49]。在紫外线照射下,血卟啉在肿瘤组织引发了明亮的红色荧光。在20世纪40年代,在实验诱导的肉瘤和乳腺癌中,通过典型的红色荧光测定,进一步检验证实了血卟啉与肿瘤组织的亲和力[12]。20世纪50年代,在癌症患者的静脉内应用血卟啉后,卟啉优先在肿瘤组织中的累积。这再次证实卟啉在紫外光照射期间出现的特征性红色荧光[51]。注射化学纯化的血卟啉,与注射未纯化的血卟啉相比,在肿瘤组织中选择性较差[48]。

在1960年,利普森等提供的血卟啉衍生物(HpD),是由大约10种卟啉衍生物,双血卟啉酯和双血卟啉醚组成的混合物[40]。HpD在鳞状细胞癌和腺癌中优先富集[27]。静脉内应用HpD,随后使用光纤装置照明,可以有效地检测和治疗膀胱癌和肺癌[10,34]。直到20世纪80年代,HpD一直是PDT中最重要的光敏剂。

由于避免了系统使用光敏剂引起的普遍光敏反应,人们对局部应用光敏剂兴趣越来越大。在1990年,由加拿大研究人员Kennedy等提出的"非光敏"的ALA的局部应用,即通过"肿瘤选择性"光敏可以克服这个缺点[33]。这个最重要的卟啉前体使卟啉优先在肿瘤和快速增生组织中增加产生。外源性的卟啉前体绕过了血红素生物合成的限制步骤,即ALA合成酶的限制(图18.1)。

在过去的10年中,不同的研究小组证实了局部施用ALA/MAL PDT对浅表皮肤肿瘤的有效性[8,17,18,20,21,57,63]。此外,有零星报道,在动物实验和临床治疗中,全身应用ALA成功治疗或缓解支气管癌,胃肠道肿瘤和膀胱癌的症状[36,41,45]。最后,这个新光敏剂前体药物ALA诱导的卟啉荧光可被用于检测肿瘤。通常,在荧光检测技术中所使用的"肿瘤标志物"是卟啉的混合物,如HpD或光敏素[1,6,37]。虽然这些物质可诱发荧光,例如在尿路上皮肿瘤,他们却有很多缺点,比如对肿瘤选择性低。除此之外,卟啉混合物在组织中诱发的荧光量是相当低的,因而需要昂贵的光学技术来检测肿瘤内的荧光。此外,如光敏剂Photofrin的全身应用,总是有光毒性皮肤反应的风险,即使只使用含该物质20%的溶液。

PDT在皮肤科的最新药物的进展是甲基氨基酮戊酸(methylaminooxopenoat, MAL, MAOP, Metvix®)。局部应用的MAL,经由血红素途径转化成光活性卟啉,

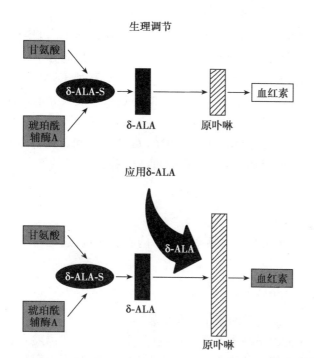

图 18.1 血红素生物合成示意图。琥珀酰辅酶 A 和甘氨酸二者合成 δ-ALA。局部或系统性应用 δ-ALA 绕过了 δ-ALA 合成酶,卟啉合成的限速步骤。因此,大量的卟啉,特别是原卟啉,作为有效的光敏剂被合成

经适当波长的照明后从而发挥治疗效果(例如,破坏肿瘤细胞)[47]。

目前在欧洲、美国和澳大利亚,MAL 经批准可用于日光性角化病(AK),以及结节性和浅表 BCC 的治疗。也有报道显示它治疗鲍温病(BD)非常有效。基于 MAL 的 PDT 既有高治愈率,又有最佳的美学效果[28,53,62]。

局部使用 ALA,特别是 20% 的混合物乳膏,在皮肤科肿瘤组织的检测中具有显著的优势:周围健康的皮肤对光的敏感性几乎不会增加,并且没有全身性的副作用。在过去的几年中,使用光敏剂及其在 UV 光下的荧光对肿瘤的进行检测,被称为"光动力学诊断"(photodynamic diagnosis,PDD)。然而,这个术语并不很适合,因为在荧光检测技术中没有光动力反应必需的反应性物质。因此,我们决定引入更合适的术语 FD。

应用 ALA/MAL 诱导的卟啉进行荧光诊断

FD 荧光的物理背景

荧光检测是 FD 的主要基础。因此,我们想向大家解释荧光及其属性的物理本质。荧光是一种沉降光,由原子或分子在吸收能量后激发发射的。

光的吸收。当光射入介质,它的一部分被反射,一部分被介质吸收,还有一

部分则穿过介质。所吸收的光将被转移成热量或另一种形式的能量[10]。

电子的半稳定条件。 一般而言,材料可以通过电、光或无线电频率的刺激而转化到较高的能级或受刺激的电子级(半稳定的水平)。分子与其他分子的碰撞导致其脉冲能量快速地传输(约 10^{-11} 秒)到周围的分子。分子(处于被刺激的电子状态)的重点逐步移回地面状况。该电子刺激的时间足以自发荧光地发射能量(约 10^{-8} 秒)。通过这一机制,分子变成比基本水平(Frank-Condon 原理)更高的脉冲水平。荧光 $I\alpha$ 的强度通常正比于入射辐射的 Io 的强度和荧光物质 C 的浓度。根据 Lambert-Beer 定律,物质吸收辐射的强度 $\Delta I\alpha$ 律,是:

$$\Delta I\alpha(\nu) = \alpha(\nu) Io(\nu) \Delta x$$

如 $\Delta I\alpha$ 小于 Io。

Δx 代表厚度,$\alpha(\nu)$ 是物质在入射辐射频率为 ν 时的吸收系数,这是物质所含 C 的浓度成比的:

$$\alpha(\nu) = \varepsilon(\nu) C$$

其中,$\varepsilon(\nu)$ 为在光频率 ν 时的物质的摩尔消光系数[7]。

发射。 电磁辐射是由分子回归至基本水平而释放(发射)。通用术语发光涵盖了所有这些发射过程。如果在其受激状态时的分子浓度非常高,或者无辐射失活的速度相对于辐射的速度较低,则该分子的辐射或发射可以容易地表现出来。如果光吸收后发光迅速减弱($10^{-9} \sim 10^{-3}$ 秒),光吸收取决于波长,这种发光被称为荧光。与此相反,如果是磷光,发光时间更长,典型的可以延续到吸收后几秒钟。

在室温下,大多数液体和溶液的辐射失活过程如此之快,以致荧光或磷光无法观察。然而,也有溶液,比如荧光素溶液,表现出明显的荧光。荧光发射是浓度的线性函数,因此可以用来测定相应物质的浓度。下面的列表举例说明使用荧光进行光度测定:测定牛乳中核黄素(维生素 B_6),肉和谷物中硫胺素(B_1),空气中的多环芳香族化合物,以及卟啉、酶、雌激素和组氨酸在血液或尿液中的浓度。荧光存在于电磁波谱的所有部分。荧光遵循 Stock 规则,即所发射的辐射不可能比激发光的波长更短。

18 既往 FD 的适应证

临床使用 ALA 诱导卟啉荧光进行肿瘤检测首次在泌尿科报道。将 ALA 溶液滴注入膀胱(50ml $NaCO_3$ 中含有 1.5g ALA;0.17mol/L)后,荧光膀胱镜检查可检测膀胱癌。406.7nm 波长的紫色激光,可直接观察泌尿道上皮肿瘤组织中 ALA 生物转化成卟啉的量的增加[35,36,54]。这种技术为肿瘤检测和泌尿道上皮肿瘤的治疗后的监测提供了很大的便利,因为白光内镜往往无法检查到平坦的黏膜病变,如发育不良或原位癌。

局部应用 ALA 后,荧光强度定量分析显示,在恶性组织中的荧光强度是相邻正常组织的 10 倍。荧光分析表明,内源性形成的卟啉,特别是原卟啉的积累,具有肿瘤选择性。因此,FD 似乎是早期检测泌尿道上皮肿瘤的一个可靠和易于操作的技术。

浅表膀胱癌的复发率和进展率,取决于肿瘤切除后黏膜中残余的癌前或恶性细胞数量,因此早期诊断可疑肿瘤组织对于患者的预后非常重要。

我们分别对支气管癌和结肠癌的卟啉水平,以及离体的肿瘤周围正常组织的卟啉水平进行了生化学的研究。这里,我们也发现了肿瘤中卟啉水平是正常组织的 1.5~2 倍(数据未发表)。

FD 在皮肤科的运用

过去的 10 年,已经进行了应用 ALA PDT 治疗不同皮肤病的研究,尤其是日光性角化病,也用于鲍温病,角化棘皮瘤,基底细胞癌(浅表和实体型),鳞状细胞癌,蕈样肉芽肿和银屑病[8,17,18,21,38,63]。我们自己的经验表明,局部应用 ALA 和随后的红光(570~750nm)或绿光(540~550nm)照射,只能治愈浅表皮肤肿瘤,主要是浅表性基底细胞癌和早期的鳞状细胞癌,和皮肤癌前病变,尤其是日光性角化病[18]。

我们局部应用 ALA 或者 MAL 处理各种组织,并用 Wood 灯照射来检查卟啉的累积规律。因此,我们有机会收集,在外用 ALA/MAL 后皮肤病荧光数量和质量的详细数据[2,16,17,20,21]。迄今为止,还没有对肿瘤或健康皮肤诱导荧光的精确分布的系统检查。对肿瘤组织卟啉荧光的严格定位,将优化外科治疗或其他治疗策略(CO_2 激光,冷冻手术,放射治疗)的规划。为了证明这一理论,我们用 FD 研究了不同的皮肤病,切除荧光皮肤区域,并进行了组织病理学检查。接下来的部分将综述其特征及可能性。

已经研究的皮肤病

FD 运用于不同皮肤病和(或)下列情况:
- 临床和组织学诊断为癌前病变或皮肤肿瘤
- 临床上怀疑肿瘤但未经组织学证实
- 缺乏清晰临床分界的癌前病变或皮肤肿瘤
- 肿瘤复发
- 其他快速增生的组织,如银屑病样皮损

以下皮肤病可用 FD 进行研究:
- 皮肤肿瘤
  - 基底细胞癌(固体和浅表型)
  - 鳞状细胞癌

- 恶性黑色素瘤
- 蕈样肉芽肿
- 佩吉特氏病（乳腺外型）
- 卡波济氏肉瘤
- 日光性角化病
- 鲍温病
- 恶性雀斑样痣
- 其他组织
  - 银屑病
  - 寻常疣
  - 痣细胞痣
  - 红斑狼疮斑块

此外，我们研究了身体各个部位，如躯干、面部、头皮、腹股沟、腋窝等区域健康皮肤的卟啉荧光。此外，还选择了不同的 ALA 应用时间。

荧光诊断的操作

PDT 采用了含有 10%～20% ALA（（Merck，Darmstadt，德国）浓度的软膏（Neribassalbe，schering Berlin，德国）。10% 的混合物足以治疗日光性角化病，而 20% 是用于治疗浅表性基底细胞癌或鳞状细胞癌的最佳浓度。在 FD 中，取决于临床诊断和身体部位，ALA 浓度（10%～20%）被证明可有效地诱发典型荧光的呈现。在 Metvix 有的情况下，该药物是 16% 的乳膏。我们进行了 FD，过程如下所述：

用 Dibromol 液将皮肤清洁杀菌。在病变皮肤区域，及其周围大约 1cm 健康皮肤上局部应用 ALA 或 MAL。每 $1cm^2$ 皮肤区域大约用 0.2 克总量的乳膏（20～40mg ALA/cm^2 或 0.1g Metvix/cm^2）。将处理过的区域用防光绷带（Tegaderm®，纱布，铝箔，Fixomull®）覆盖，以避免光漂白，并使之最大限度地渗透。封包最多 3～4 小时后，用伍德灯（Fluolight；370～405nm，saalmann 有限公司，德国）进行 FD。

将 FD 的荧光强度与荧光标准（不断发荧光塑料条带）对比，以进行半定量测量：0，无荧光；+，轻微的荧光；++，中等强度的荧光；+++，强荧光。

运用摄相是非常难以捕捉荧光量的细微差异的。让老年患者保持足够长时间的静止尤其困难。然而，长的曝光时间是获取最佳的轻微荧光图像必不可少的。我们很幸运能够拍摄记录众多皮肤疾病的组织荧光。精选照片位于图 18.2 至 18.10。临床和荧光照片一并呈现。我们可以根据荧光图案来估计病变的大小和边界，及其恶性程度。

荧光诊断下表现的特点

所有得到的荧光强度的结果示于表 18.1。所有的上皮性肿瘤,在应用 MAL 或 ALA 后三至四小时,在伍德光下可呈现强烈的红色荧光:如基底细胞癌(图 18.2,图 18.9 和图 18.10),鳞状细胞癌,鲍温病(图 18.3),日光性角化病(图 18.4 至图 18.6),以及乳房外 Paget 病。在伍德光下呈现中等强度荧光的有:Kaposi 肉瘤,红斑狼疮的病变,皮肤 T 细胞淋巴瘤(蕈样肉芽肿)的斑块。色素性良性或恶性皮肤病变呈轻微荧光或无荧光,如痣细胞痣,恶性雀斑样痣,和恶性黑色素瘤。所检查的寻常疣(图 18.7)没有呈现任何荧光。在银屑病皮损可检测出中等至强度荧光,但荧光规律往往非均一(图 18.8)。

表 18.1　局部运用 ALA 后各种皮肤肿瘤的荧光强度(10%/20%)

皮肤病(正常皮肤部位)	n	应用时间(h)	荧光强度	边界
BCC-表浅型	16	6	+++	锐利
BCC-实体型	12	6	+++	锐利
SCC	6	6	+++	锐利
鲍温病	6	6	+++	锐利
日光性角化病	24	6	++/+++	锐利
Paget 病	3	6	+++	锐利
蕈样肉芽肿	4	6	++	锐利
Kaposi 肉瘤	5	6	+/++	锐利
恶性黑色素瘤	8	6	−	不适用
恶性雀斑样痣	4	6	−	不适用
痣细胞痣	12	6	−	不适用
脂溢性角化病	8	6	−	不适用
寻常疣	8	6	−	不适用
红斑狼疮	5	6	++	锐利
银屑病斑块	8	6	++/+++	锐利
正常皮肤(躯干)	8	3	−	不适用
	8	6	+	不适用
	8	12	+	不适用
	8	24	+/++	不适用
正常皮肤(面部)	8	3	+	不适用
	8	6	+/++	不适用
	8	12	++/+++	不适用

续表

皮肤病（正常皮肤部位）	n	应用时间（h）	荧光强度	边界
正常皮肤（腹股沟，腋部）	8	24	++	不适用
	4	3	+	不适用
	4	6	+/++	不适用
	4	12	++	不适用
	4	24	++	不锐利

-无荧光，+轻微的荧光，++中等强度的荧光，+++强荧光

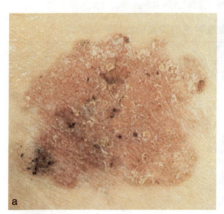 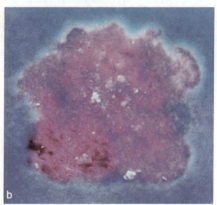

图 18.2　鲍温病。**a.** 红色斑块，大约 12cm×10cm，多环的和相对锐利的边界，部分有鳞屑和出血性的痂皮。**b.** FD（ALA20%，6 小时）：强烈的红色荧光，是极为有限的，与病变的临床扩展有关

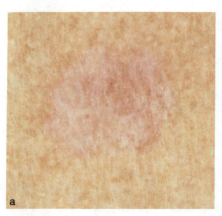 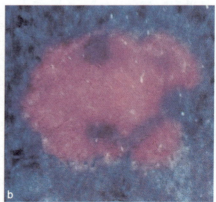

图 18.3　表浅型基底细胞癌。**a.** 临床上区别病变的边界是不可能的。**b.** 用 FD（ALA20%，6 小时）可以清晰地看到肿瘤，可以确切的划定肿瘤的边界

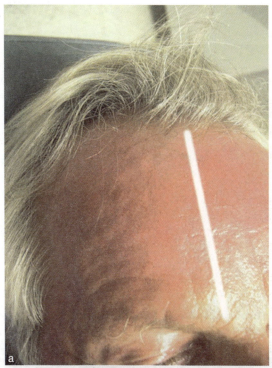

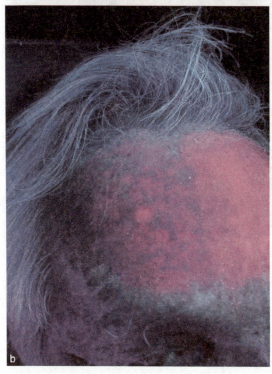

图18.4 a. 日光性角化病（前额，男性，82岁）白线代表了应用区域的边界。b. FD在左侧应用10% ALA，在右侧应用MetvixL 3小时。左侧前线出现均匀的亮红色荧光，而右侧显示了参差不齐的荧光模式。这张图片非常清楚地显示，与ALA相比，MAL引起的卟啉的富集更具有选择性

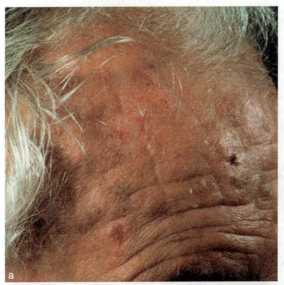
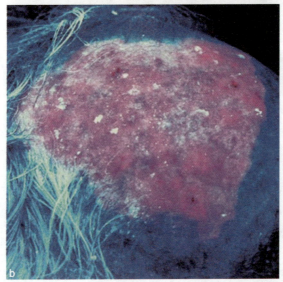

图 18.5　**a.** 日光性角化病。**b.** FD(ALA 10%,6 小时):多个荧光斑点表明为日光性角化病。相比之下,在临床上,病变的数量似乎较少

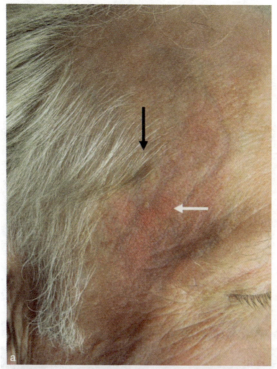
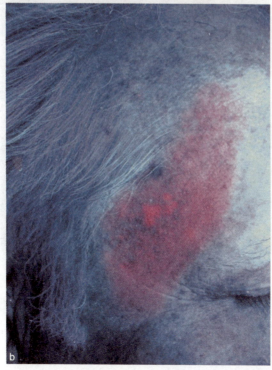

图 18.6　a. 脂溢性角化病和日光性角化病(左颞部,男,72 岁)。脂溢性角化病处(黑色箭头),卟啉没有增加,而日光性角化病处(白色箭头)显示出明亮的荧光 (b)(Metvix® 16%,3 小时)

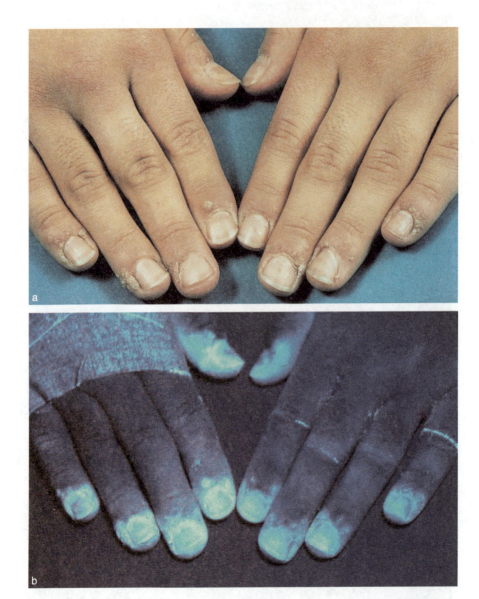

图 18.7　a. 寻常疣(女,12 岁)。b. FD(ALA 20%,6 小时):疣呈现为白色斑点而没有任何卟啉荧光

第 18 章　荧光诊断　　353

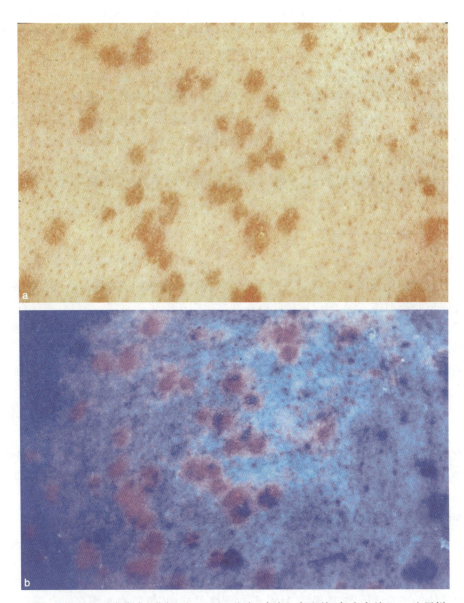

图 18.8　**a.** 银屑病病变(背部,女,38 岁)临床:多个红色斑块,每个大约 2cm,边界锐利,部分融合,部分有鳞屑。**b.** FD(ALA 20%,6 小时):银屑病病变为红色荧光岛屿,可以与周围的正常皮肤相区别

组织病理学检查发现,肿瘤,癌前病变,或快速增殖的组织,如银屑病皮损的组织,呈现中等强度和强荧光(++到+++)。荧光区域与临床上边界明确的肿瘤以及与临床边界不清的皮损的组织病理学边界相关。在面部,头皮,腹股沟和腋窝区域,肿瘤和癌前病变的荧光划界似乎比其他位置更困难。这里,肿瘤特异性荧光被正常组织轻微但可见度良好的荧光包围并部分覆盖。此背景荧光的产生可能部分是由于在这些部位细菌(如丙酸杆菌)增多。然而,区分正常皮肤与肿瘤仍然是可能的,因为肿瘤组织荧光的强度比正常皮肤较高。此外,可以通过减少 ALA 的封包时间至 2 小时,或者通过使用 MAL,来改善在这些身体区域的肿瘤分界(图 18.4)。

Metvixe 与游离酸的 ALA 相比,FD 显示的卟啉荧光更具有选择性(图 18.4)。

讨论

最近几年,PDT 已发展为一种新的治疗浅表性皮肤肿瘤和癌前病变的技术。卟啉或卟啉前体 ALA 的应用使卟啉在肿瘤组织中的优先富集。至今,才仅有几例 ALA 诱导卟啉荧光可有效检测和描绘肿瘤的报道。有许多应用 ALA 诱发卟啉进行 PDT 的研究,经常提到肿瘤存在高荧光强度[8,18,20,38,63]。此外,生化研究证明了增加的荧光强度与在肿瘤组织中所提取的卟啉浓度相关[22,26,29]。然而,有关 FD 的报告,至今只报道了膀胱癌[35,54]和脑肿瘤[56]的经验。

本文研究的所有皮肤肿瘤(基底和鳞状细胞癌,Bowen 病,日光性角化病,佩吉特氏病),在局部应用 ALA 6 小时后,在 Wood's 灯下呈现密集,强烈,边界清晰的红色荧光。甚至在银屑病皮损,我们发现了典型强烈的 ALA 诱发的卟啉荧光。然而,在色素性病变如恶性黑素瘤或痣中,则无荧光出现。这些结果表明,肿瘤和银屑病斑块与相邻的"正常"的皮肤相比,生物合成的卟啉有所增加。增加的卟啉生物合成,似乎是依赖于肿瘤或炎症过程中角质层的损伤和组织细胞的增殖率增加。在寻常疣(图 18.7)、脂溢性角化病(图 18.6)或痣细胞痣中,未见 ALA 诱发卟啉荧光。

在恶性黑色素瘤中只见轻微的强度的荧光,可能有几个方面原因。一方面,通过体外实验已证实,如果将 ALA 添加到培养基中,黑色素瘤细胞能合成高水平的卟啉[5]。但是,恶性黑色素瘤通常表皮完整的,与表皮层被损坏的基底细胞癌相比,可能会限制 ALA 的渗透。物理因素也可能参与恶性黑色素瘤的 FD 的发生:黑色素减少了卟啉荧光的激发或发射。这些因素也可能是卡波西肉瘤荧光微弱的原因。

正常皮肤,取决于身体部位,显示出不同的荧光动力学。头部,腹股沟,及腋下,与其他皮肤区域相比,荧光显示更强,更密集。这种差异可能是由生产卟啉的细菌(如丙酸杆菌)更多定植引起。在施用 ALA 24 小时后,我们证实了在这些部位有中等强度的荧光。这里,肿瘤和健康的皮肤之间的对比,可以通过减少 ALA 的作用时间而得到改善。另一种细菌,微小棒状杆菌,是红癣的致病因子,也可产生大量的原卟啉。因此,未经治疗的红癣病变,可以呈现类似于 FD 中的红色荧光。痤疮患者在 Wood's 灯照射下,呈现明亮的聚集在毛孔周围的荧光[42]。

卟啉在皮肤中的代谢

目前为止,针对人类皮肤中卟啉生物合成进行的研究并不多[3,25,45]。这些研究主要用来解释卟啉症的病理机制,但现在它们越来越多地被用于测量 ALA 诱发卟啉进行 PDT 的效果。

在体外研究,在不同的细胞培养(K562 白血病细胞,内皮细胞,HaCaT,成纤维细胞,sk-Mel 23,sk-Mel 28,Bro,HepG2)应用 ALA,则呈现卟啉合成的特定的增加。合成的卟啉量与细胞系的"恶性程度"无关[39,43](未发表的研究结果)。

在正常人组织(肝,脂肪组织,皮肤)中,基础卟啉水平是低的,$0.2 \sim 1.2 nmol/g$[25]。基础卟啉浓度在人类肿瘤,如支气管癌和胃肠道癌(未发表数据),或皮肤表皮肿瘤,如基底和鳞状细胞癌[22],或癌前病变,如日光性角化病[19]也是低的,$<1 nmol/g$。皮肤肿瘤和正常皮肤样本显示基础卟啉水平相近。此发现反驳了肿瘤可能已经改变了血红素相关酶活性这一理论。

用外源的 ALA 处理活体外或活体内的皮肤组织,都导致卟啉合成的增加。在有机培养模型中,证实了卟啉生物合成的增加,并具有部分肿瘤特异性的卟啉代谢物规律(主要是原卟啉或粪卟啉,取决于肿瘤)[15]。局部应用 ALA 于在体皮肤表皮肿瘤和银屑病病损,表明卟啉合成具有时间依赖性,基底细胞癌或鳞状细胞癌 $1 \sim 4$ 小时达最高水平($50 \sim 60 nmol/g$ 蛋白质),而银屑病病损则在 6 小时达到($90 nmol/g$ 蛋白质)[22]。正常皮肤的卟啉合成是相当低的(在 6 小时:$12 nmol/g$ 蛋白质);然而,应用 ALA 后 24 小时内仍然有增加(24 小时:$15 nmol/g$ 蛋白质)。

总结现有的数据,我们必须假设,在实验性肿瘤和不同的人类皮肤组织中,存在有一种特定的卟啉代谢,产生了不同程度的卟啉代谢物的累积。

肿瘤对 ALA/MAL 的吸收

作者以及文献中使用的 ALA 的浓度和载体,都在 FD 和 PDT 中显示了充分的疗效。仍然没有明确哪些机制使得 ALA 渗透到皮肤中。角质层是局部应用于皮肤的物质的主要障碍。由于浅表皮肤肿瘤和癌前病变的角质层发生病理改变,ALA 能够迅速渗透到那些病变中,而相比之下,正常皮肤由于表面屏障完整,对 ALA 的摄取较低[32,47,58]。另一提示 ALA 渗透与角质层相关性的证据是,通过用二甲基亚砜(DMSO)处理皮肤,导致皮肤屏障破坏,可强化 ALA 或 ALA 诱发卟啉的吸收[47]。

这些实验结果目前为止无法判定:相比正常细胞,皮肤中的肿瘤细胞是积累更多的 ALA,还是卟啉的生物合成增多。从 ALA 是由甘氨酸和琥珀酰-CoA 合成的假设出发,作为一个如同氨基酸这样相对小分子,它可以穿透细胞膜。最近检查显示,有主动和被动的运输机制参与 ALA 的细胞摄取,某些氨基酸可通过竞争限制其转运[44]。也许,在 FD 和 PDT,不仅氨基酸在细胞的接收是限制性和选择性的步骤,而且在肿瘤细胞中卟啉合成和优先的积累是极为相关的。虽然 ALA 具有良好的价值诊断,但它对皮肤深层的渗透是有限的[19,46]。与 ALA 相比,MAL 由于亲脂性更高,具有更好的穿透性,从而增加了光活性卟啉的形成。此外,与 ALA 相比,MAL 还拥有较高的组织特异性,卟啉优先在皮损内富集,这使得它在荧光诊断中占据更重要的地位(图 18.4)[20]。

肿瘤组织中的卟啉代谢

许多作者推测,在应用 ALA 后肿瘤对卟啉优先积累的原因,与卟啉的生物合成相关的酶活性有关。线粒体亚铁螯合酶催化铁插入原卟啉,其障碍可降低血红素浓度,降低的负反馈。这可以证明原卟啉在肿瘤组织中的积累,类似于红细胞生成性原卟啉症(EPP,铁螯合酶的先天性缺陷)患者的成纤维细胞[4]或淋巴细胞。血红素生物合成相关酶与卟啉在皮肤上聚集的相关性,可通过测试数种卟啉症患者的皮肤组织活检表明:急性间歇性卟啉病(AIP,尿卟啉原脱羧酶缺陷)与健康人相比,卟啉在皮肤中的形成呈明显减少,约 50%。与之相反,在迟发性皮肤卟啉病(PCT,尿卟啉原脱羧酶常染色体显性遗传缺陷)患者的皮肤,被发现基卟啉和卟啉的生物合成在应用的 ALA 后量增加(相比与健康人或皮肤 AIP 病人)[3]。因此,可以想到的是,对血红素的生物合成,从而导致了血红素前体(如,卟啉)的积累是一种或几种酶的缺陷。卟啉的生物合成的其他酶,如 ALA 脱水酶,它被认为在肿瘤(小鼠乳腺癌,人乳腺腺癌),及肿瘤携带动物的肝脏中含量是减少,由此改变了卟啉在肿瘤的生产[9,45,59]。ALA 合成酶目前认为是血红素生物合成的唯一限速酶[31,55]。仍然存在的问题是,为什么肿瘤细胞得到更多的 ALA,为什么肿瘤细胞主要是转化积累的 ALA 到卟啉,而为什么不将卟啉代谢成血红素?

红细胞中,有一个影响因素限制了 ALA 合成酶和亚铁螯合酶。红细胞提供特殊环境。在这里,一个位于 X 染色体的基因调节 ALA 合成酶,但在所有其他细胞是位于 13 号染色体的基因表达不同的 ALA 合成酶控制着血红素的生物合成[31]。虽然红细胞和肿瘤细胞是非常不同的,但有一点可以假设,在肿瘤细胞或快速增殖细胞的 ALA 合成酶和亚铁螯合酶的调节也受限。荧光和生化研究的结果提示,在肿瘤模型(体内,体外)出现原卟啉富集[26,58]。此外,至少在某些特殊的观察存在铁螯合酶活性的减少。

进一步的研究集中在这个问题上,为什么局部或全身应用 ALA 后,肿瘤细胞的卟啉增加,部分还有特殊的卟啉代谢模式形成,导致卟啉的富集。

FD 的参数

ALA

目前,ALA 是进行 FD 最合适的物质。需要进一步的临床和生化研究证明,是否其他卟啉前体,卟啉产品,ALA 酯类,甚至合成的物质(比如,porphycenes),可以在将来被用于标记肿瘤组织。此外,还必须澄清,局部应用 ALA 的不同载体,是否可以增加卟啉的生物合成或 ALA 的渗透能力。在这种情况下,用二甲基亚砜预处理似乎提高 FD 和 PDT 的效力[47]。虽然 ALA 具有良好的价值诊断,它难以渗透至皮肤深层[19,46]。与 ALA 相比,MAL 因为亲脂性高从而增加了光活性卟啉的形成,因而具有更好的穿透性。此外,与 ALA 相比,MAL 还拥有更高的组织特异性,使卟啉优先富集于皮损,这使其在荧光诊断中发挥更大的作用(图 18.4)[20]。ALA 和 MAL 的差异显现在不同的荧光比率——比较 BCC 卟啉电阻与正常皮肤的卟啉电阻;使用 MAL 的卟啉比例远高于使用 ALA 的。最近的一项研究[19]比较应用 MAL 或 ALA,日光性角化病(SK)病变和相邻正常皮肤上皮的卟啉。发现应用 MAL 比应用 ALA 后,SK 病变与邻近的正常皮肤相比,卟啉比率更高。

ALA/MAL 浓度

进行皮肤肿瘤和癌前病变的 FD,已证明有效的 ALA 浓度是 10% ~ 20%,总剂量为 40mg/cm^2。

ALA 混合物/Metvix® 的应用时间

在 FD 和 PDT,已证明 ALA/MAL 应用时间是中间的 3 ~ 4 小时最好,因为此时肿瘤中所检测的卟啉荧光标记与调整后的正常组织相比最显著。所检测的卟啉荧光,仅反映积累在皮肤表层而不是皮肤深层的卟啉。卟啉渗透的荧光显微镜研究显示更深真皮层的卟啉荧光,在 ALA 应用 3 ~ 6 小时后并不均质,但在稍后的时间点(24 ~ 48 小时)变得可见且部分均质[47,58]。FD 对病变的深度不感兴趣。FD 可以评估肿瘤的表浅的大小,但 FD 不能提供特定病变浸润深度的信息。然而,对于 PDT,为保证治疗的成功,了解肿瘤是否已完全卟啉致敏是很重要的;否则,在曝光时肿瘤的深部将无法得到治疗。在结节状或外生性组织情况下,以获得最佳的 FD 和 PDT 结果,就必须除去(刮匙,手术切除)特定肿瘤的外生部(图 18.9)。

358　　第 5 篇　临床实践中的光诊断学

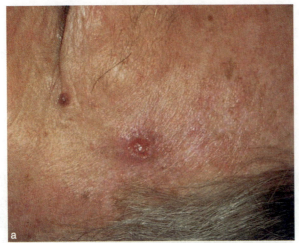

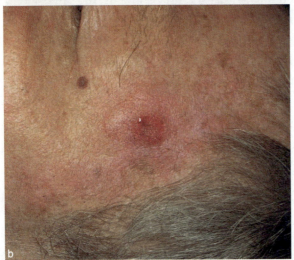

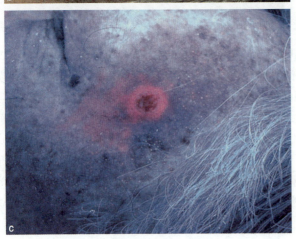

图 18.9　**a.** 左侧颞区的结节型 BCC。**b.** 这些外生型的肿瘤部分被刮匙去除。**c.** 应用 Metvix 用 3 小时后，肿瘤表现出一个明亮的红砖色的荧光。该 BCC 经过 3 次的 PDT 治疗，已被成功治愈

ALA/Metvixa® 的应用方法

FD 和 PDT 大多通过局部应用 ALA 进行。如前所诉,肿瘤组织通过卟啉的增敏只限于浅表皮肤层。因此,只有表浅肿瘤组织可以通过局部外用 ALA 进行 PDT。根据病变所处的身体部位(脸,腋窝,腹股沟),减少应用时间可利于优化肿瘤组织和正常组织的 FD 对比度。

有趣的是,起初报告的结果显示,全身应用 ALA 能使较深部位的肿瘤得到更好、更均匀的增敏。口腔内鳞状细胞癌的患者,口服 30~60 毫克/公斤的 ALA[26]。ALA 应用后 24 小时内,进行数次肿瘤活检,并显微镜评估荧光强度。ALA 应用后 4 至 6 小时荧光最强,肿瘤组织荧光比周围组织高一倍。荧光是在所有肿瘤中均匀分布。色谱分析分析经 ALA 预处理的肿瘤样本,显示原卟啉是卟啉的主要代谢物。在治疗 24 小时后,活检就再没有卟啉荧光。这表明,在这种情况下,即使全身应用相对高剂量的 ALA 不会导致长期的光敏性。其他报告表明,直肠癌、十二指肠癌、食道癌和膀胱癌患者口服 30~60 毫克/千克 ALA 进行 PDT,副作用包括如眩晕、恶心、呕吐、头痛、循环不稳定,以及转氨酶和光敏的暂时增加(Goetz 等[14])。因此,由于结果矛盾,有必要在口服及静脉使用 ALA 后测量其药物动力学。在未来几年中进一步的研究,应着眼于 ALA 的全身性使用。

辐射源

要获得对卟啉最有效的荧光刺激,必须用其最大吸收波长 405nm(索瑞波段)照射。Saalmann's Fluolight(UVA,380~405nm)荧光光源,大幅提高了 ALA 诱导的卟啉荧光。虽然在市场上有很多手提灯发 Wood's light,通常它们的强度太低,不能诱发足够的卟啉荧光。此外,许多可用的紫外光源常含过多的可见光,从而因覆盖频谱而减少了荧光的效果。这种诊断技术被越来越多地应用于,术前确定边界不清的肿瘤的边界,和控制肿瘤疗法(PDT,冷冻手术,外科手术)的功效。DyaDerm 科目前为可视化的荧光提供了最有效的技术。该计算机单元是由 Biocam (Regensburg,Germany;http://www.bio-cam.de)提供,并包括一个高灵敏度的 CCD 照相机系统,和可数秒内检测和划界皮肤癌病变的特别软件。另外,西班牙公司 Digimed(http://www.digimedsys.com)拥有一个可相媲美,但小的多的设备 Clearstone® CUV-DA,可用于 FD 以及用于早期检测太阳斑,黑斑病,皮肤老化和痤疮。

副作用

在过去的 7 年中,我们已经应用局部 ALA 治疗大约 1000 例病人。观察到极少(<2%)病人出现意味着毒性和过敏性接触性皮炎的皮肤刺激。除了轻微的刺痛,患者在 Wood's 灯照射过程中(FD)没有任何不适。与此不同,在应用

ALA 后进行红光照射（PDT），则部分会导致中等甚至强烈的疼痛。如果治疗的病变范围大（如前面的多个日光性角化病或大的基底细胞癌），或有多处病变，这种疼痛则特别强烈。持续进行的实验表明，将 ALA 减量（10%）[20]，应用稍弱强度的光照，并用绿光代替红光照射[23]，疼痛感将显著减弱。

在局部应用 ALA 后，患者血液或尿液中的卟啉或卟啉前体未见增加。这表明 ALA 局部用量不大可能使卟啉代谢应激或导致全身光敏[24]。因此，ALA PDT 是一种易于操作，快速，无副作用，可以常规和反复使用的方法。

结论

应用 ALA 进行 PDT 和 FD 的有效性是基于肿瘤特异的 ALA 生物转化，但机制未清。FD 诊断程序的方法理论基础已让人满意。FD 不是一种组织学检查，它不能确定肿瘤或皮肤变化是良性或恶性。

FD 的主要重要性在于可标明肿瘤和正常皮肤间的边界，可更好地规划进一步治疗。应用 MAL 进行 FD 既简单，且对肿瘤组织有高选择性，因而成为诊断和控制 NMSC 的极佳技术。临床研究表明，与手术，冷冻疗法，和局部施用 5-氟尿嘧啶或咪喹英特等其他治疗相比，患者更愿接受 MAL PDT，这基于其优异的美容效果和耐受性[13,19,20,52]。制定相应病变的治疗方法：或手术切除，或冷冻手术，或二氧化碳激光治疗，或 PDT，或放射疗法，应该取决于 FD 的结果。除此之外，FD 可以检测术后（或肿瘤其他方法治疗后）是否还有任何肿瘤残留（图18.10：FD-控制的肿瘤治疗）。在 FD 的帮助下，手术，冷冻术和光动力治疗开展的肿瘤治疗和肿瘤术后护理更有保障。

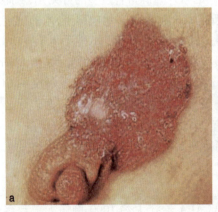 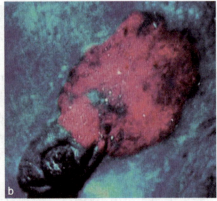

图 18.10　a. 表浅型基底细胞癌（乳房，女，55 岁）该病例经过 FD 引导而反复进行 PDT 治疗。在 PDT 之前，右侧乳房有一个特征性的、有裂缝的大的红色斑块。b. 用 FD，肿瘤完整的显现荧光

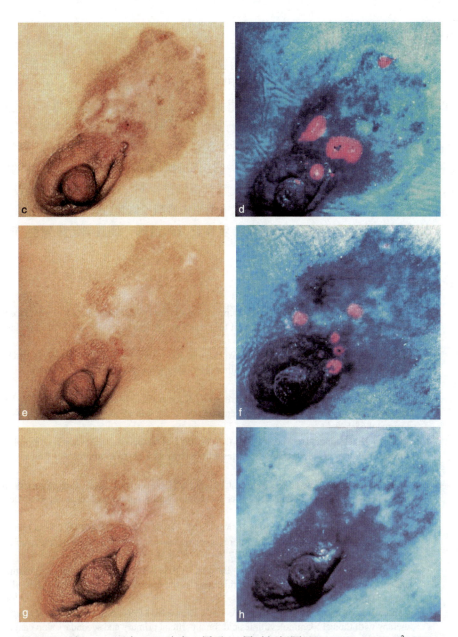

图 18.10(续) c. 两次 PDT 治疗 5 周后(3 周时间间隔;20% ALA;180J/cm², 570~650nm)肿瘤的主要部分已被治愈。d. 用 FD,显示仍然有几个密集的荧光区域,提示有剩余的肿瘤组织。肿瘤组织仍部分浸润乳头乳晕复合体。e. 第三次 PDT 治疗 4 周之后。f. 用 FD,发现只有一些荧光斑点,仍然浸润乳头乳晕复合体。斑点明显,切除,缺陷是覆盖旋转皮瓣,重建乳头。反复的 PDT 治疗 5 周后,手术切除肿瘤的剩余部分,无论是临床(g)或用 FD(h)怀疑有任何的肿瘤组织。该肿瘤病人 4 年之内都没有任何的肿瘤

总结

光动力疗法(PDT)主要应用卟啉药物。在1990年,卟啉前体δ氨基酮戊酸(ALA)首次用于PDT,现在越来越频繁地用于器官浅表肿瘤的治疗。ALA的应用,诱导卟啉首选在肿瘤组织中生物合成。卟啉累积的组织在伍德灯光照下可见红色荧光。该原理称为应用ALA诱导的卟啉进行荧光诊断(FD)。这种新技术在肿瘤检测中的适应证和有效性主要在膀胱癌和脑肿瘤提到。在过去的几年中,FD与皮肤科日益相关。最终检查表明,FD在受损皮肤肿瘤组织的检测和划定临床界限不清的肿瘤,是非常有用的方法。本文就应用ALA及其甲酯进行FD,对于皮肤肿瘤,皮肤癌前病变,炎症性皮肤病,以及皮肤色素性病变的临床诊断价值和适应证,进行了讨论。

(罗育武 译,孟珍 周欣 校,朱慧兰 审)

参考文献

1. Baumgartner R, Fuchs N, Jocham D, Stepp H, Unsöld E (1992) Photokinetics of fluorescent polyporphyrin photofrin II in normal rat tissue and rat bladder tumor. Photochem Photobiol 55:569–574
2. Becker-Wegerich P, Fritsch C, Neuse W, Schulte KW, Ruzicka T, Goerz G (1995) Effektive Kryochirurgie oberflächlicher Hauttumoren unter photodynamischer Diagnostik. H G 70:891–895
3. Bickers DR, Keogh L, Rifkind AB, Harber LC, Kappas A (1977) Studies in porphyria. VI. Biosynthesis of porphyrins in mammalian skin and in the skin of porphyric patients. J Invest Dermatol 68:5–9
4. Bloomer JR, Brenner DA, Mahoney MJ (1977) Study of factors causing excess protoporphyrin accumulation in cultured skin fibroblasts from patients with protoporphyria. J Clin Invest 60:1354–1361
5. Bolsen K, Lang K, Verwholt B, Fritsch C, Goerz G (1996) In vitro incubation of porphyrin biosynthesis in various human cells after incubation with δ-aminolevulinic acid. Arch Dermatol Res 288:320
6. Braichotte DR, Wagnieres GA, Bays R, Monnier P, van den Bergh HE (1995) Clinical pharmacokinetic studies of Photofrin by fluorescence spectroscopy in the oral cavity, the esophagus, and the bronchi. Cancer 75:2768–2778
7. Bruls WAG, Slaper H, van der Leun JC, Berrens L (1984) Transmission of human epidermis and stratum corneum as a function of thickness in the ultraviolet and visible wavelengths. Photochem Photobiol 40:485–494
8. Cairnduff F, Stringer MR, Hudson EJ, Ash DV, Brown SB (1994) Superficial photodynamic therapy with topical 5-aminolevulinic acid for superficial primary and secondary skin cancer. Br J Cancer 69:605–608
9. Denk H, Kalt R, Abdelfattah-Gad M, Meyer UA (1981) Effect of griseofulvin on 5-aminolevulinate synthase and on ferrochelatase in mouse liver neoplastic nodules. Cancer Res 41:1535–1538
10. Doiron DR, Profio E, Vincent RG, Dougherty TJ (1979) Fluorescence bronchoscopy for detection of lung cancer. Chest 76:27–32
11. Dougherty TJ (1987) Photosensitizers: therapy and detection of malignant tumors. Photochem Photobiol 45:879–889

12. Figge FHJ, Weiland GS, Manganiello LOJ (1948) Cancer detection and therapy: affinity of neoplastic, embryonic, and traumatized tissues for porphyrins and metalloporphyrins. Proc Soc Exp Biol Med 68:640–641
13. Freeman M, Vinciullo C, Francis D (2003) A comparison of photodynamic therapy using topical methyl 5 amino-levulinate (Metvix®) with single cell cryotherapy in patients with actinic keratosis: a prospective randomised study. J Dermatol Treat 14:99–106
14. Fritsch C, Abels C, Goetz AE, Stahl W, Bolsen K, Ruzicka T, Goerz G, Sies H (1997) Porphyrins preferentially accumulate in a melanoma following intravenous injection of 5-aminolevulinic acid. Biol Chem 378:51–57
15. Fritsch C, Batz J, Bolsen K, Schulte KW, Ruzicka T, Goerz G (1994) Exogenous δ-aminolevulinic acid induces the porphyrin biosynthesis in human skin organ cultures with different porphyrin patterns in normal and malignant human tissue. SPIE Proc 2371:215–220
16. Fritsch C, Becker-Wegerich PM, Menke M, Ruzicka T, Goerz G, Olbrisch RR (1997) Successful surgery of multiple recurrent basal cell carcinomas guided by photodynamic diagnosis. Aesthetic Plast Surg 21:437–439
17. Fritsch C, Becker-Wegerich PM, Schulte KW, Neuse W, Lehmann P, Ruzicka T, Goerz G (1996) Photodynamische Therapie und Mamillenplastik eines großflächigen Rumpfhautbasalioms der Mamma. Effektive Kombinationstherapie unter photodynamischer Diagnostik. Hautarzt 47:438–442
18. Fritsch C, Goerz G, Ruzicka T (1998) Photodynamic therapy in dermatology. A review. Arch Dermatol 134:207–214
19. Fritsch C, Homey B, Stahl W, Lehmann P, Ruzicka T, Sies H (1998) Preferential relative porphyrin enrichment in solar keratoses upon topical application of δ-aminolevulinic acid methylester. Photochem Photobiol 68:218–221
20. Fritsch C, Ruzicka T (2003) Fluorescence diagnosis and photodynamic therapy of skin diseases. Atlas and handbook. Springer, Wien
21. Fritsch C, Lehmann P, Bolsen K, Ruzicka T, Goerz G (1994) Photodynamische Diagnostik und Photodynamische Therapie von aktinischen Keratosen. Z Hautkr 69:713–716
22. Fritsch C, Lehmann P, Stahl W, Schulte KW, Blohm E, Lang K, Sies H, Ruzicka T (1999) Optimum porphyrin accumulation in epithelial skin tumours and psoriatic lesions after topical application of δ-aminolaevulinic acid. Br J Cancer 79:1603–1608
23. Fritsch C, Stege S, Saalmann G, Goerz G, Ruzicka T, Krutmann J (1997) Green light is effective and less painful than red light in photodynamic therapy of facial solar keratoses. Photodermatol Photoimmunol Photomed 13:181–185
24. Fritsch C, Verwohlt B, Bolsen K, Ruzicka T, Goerz G (1996) Influence of topical photodynamic therapy with 5-aminolevulinic acid on the porphyrin metabolism. Arch Dermatol Res 288:517–521
25. Goerz G, Link-Mannhardt A, Bolsen K, Zumdick M, Fritsch C, Schürer NY (1995) Porphyrin concentrations in various human tissues. Exp Dermatol 4:218–220
26. Grant EW, Hopper C, MacRobert AJ, Speight PM, Bown SG (1993) Photodynamic therapy of oral cancer: photosensitisation with systemic aminolaevulinic acid. Lancet 324:147–148
27. Gregorie HG Jr, Horger EO, Ward JL (1968) Hematoporphyrin-derivate fluorescence in malignant neoplasms. Ann Surg 167:820–828
28. Horn M, Wolf P, Wulf HC, Warloe T, Fritsch C, Rhodes LE, Kaufmann R, De Rie M, Legat FJ, Stender IM, Soler AM, Wennberg AM, Wong GA, Larko O (2003) Topical methyl aminolaevulinate photodynamic therapy in patients with basal cell carcinoma prone to complications and poor cosmetic outcome with conventional treatment. Br J Dermatol. 149:1242–1249
29. Hua Z, Gibson SL, Foster TH, Hilf R (1995) Effectiveness of δ-aminolevulinic acid-induced protoporphyrin as a photosensitizer for photodynamic therapy in vivo. Cancer Res 55:1723–1731
30. Jesionek A, von Tappeiner H (1905) Zur Behandlung von Hautcarcinome mit fluorescieren-

den Stoffen. Arch Klin Med 82:72–76
31. Kappas A, Sassa S, Galbrath RA, Nordmann Y (1989) The porphyrias. In: Scriver CR, Beaudet AL, Sly WS, Volle D (eds) The metabolic basis of inherited diseases, 6th edn. McGraw-Hill, New York, pp 1305–1365
32. Kennedy JC, Pottier RH (1992) Endogenous protoporphyrin IX, a clinically useful photosensitizer for photodynamic therapy. J Photochem Photobiol 14:275–292
33. Kennedy JC, Pottier RH, Pross DC (1990) Photodynamic therapy with endogenous protoporphyrin IX: basic principles and present clinical experience. J Photochem Photobiol 6:143–148
34. Kinsey JH, Cortese DA, Sanderson DR (1978) Detection of hematoporphyrin fluorescence during fiberoptic bronchoscopy to localize early bronchogenic carcinoma. Mayo Clin Proc 53:594–600
35. Kriegmair M, Baumgartner R, Knuechel R, Ehsan R, Lumper W, Hofstetter A (1994) Fluorescence cystoscopy—a new method in diagnosis of bladder cancer. Urology 44:836–841
36. Kriegmair M, Baumgartner R, Knüchel R, Stepp H, Hofstädter F, Hofstetter A (1996) Detection of early bladder cancer by 5-aminolevulinic acid induced porphyrin fluorescence. J Urol 155:105–109
37. Lam S, Palcic B, McLean D, Hung J, Korbelik M, Profio E (1990) Detection of early lung cancer using low dose Photofrin II. Chest 97:333–337
38. Landthaler M, Rück A, Szeimies RM (1993) Photodynamische Therapie von Tumoren der Haut. Hautarzt 44:69–74
39. Lim HW, Behar S, He D (1994) Effect of porphyrin and irradiation on heme biosynthetic pathway in endothelial cells. Photodermatol Photoimmunol Photomed 10:17–21
40. Lipson RL, Baldes EJ, Olsen AM (1961) The use of a derivate of hematoporphyrin in tumor detection. J Natl Cancer Inst 26:1–4
41. Loh CS, Vernon D, MacRobert AJ, Bedwell J, Bown SG, Brown SB (1992) Endogenous porphyrin distribution induced by 5-aminolaevulinic acid and in the tissue layers of the gastrointestinal tract. J Photochem Photobiol B Biol 20:47–54
42. Lucchina LC, Kollias N, Gillies R, Phillips SB, Muccini JA, Stiller MJ, Tranick RJ, Drake LA (1996) Fluorescence photography in the evaluation of acne. J Am Acad Dermatol 35:58–63
43. Malik Z, Lugaci H (1987) Destruction of erythroleukaemic cells by photoactivation of endogenous porphyrins. Br J Cancer 56:589–595
44. Moan J, Bech O, Gaullier JM, Stokke T, Stehen HB, Ma LW, Berg K (1998) Protoporphyrin IX accumulation in cells treated with 5-aminolevulinic acid: dependence on cell density, cell size and cell cycle. Int J Cancer 75:134–139
45. Navone NM, Frisardi AL, Resnick ER, Del C, Battle AM, Polo CF (1988) Porphyrin biosynthesis in human breast cancer. Preliminary mimetic in vitro studies. Med Sci Res 16:61–62
46. Peng Q, Moan J, Warloe T, Iani V, Steen HB, Bjorseth A, Nesland JM (1996) Build up of esterified aminolevulinic-acid-derivative-induced porphyrin fluorescence in normal mouse skin. J Photochem Photobiol B Biol 34:95–96
47. Peng Q, Warloe T, Moan J, Heyerdahl H, Steen HB, Nesland JM, Giercksky KE (1995) Distribution of 5-aminolevulinic acid-induced porphyrins in noduloulcerative basal cell carcinoma. Photochem Photobiol 62:906–913
48. Pimstone NR (1985) Utility of porphyrins and light in the diagnosis and treatment of malignancy (editorial). Hepatology 5:338–340
49. Policard A (1924) Etude sur les aspects offerts par des tumeurs expérimentales examinées à la lumière de Wood. Cr Soc Biol 91:1423–1424
50. Raab O (1900) Über die Wirkung fluorescirender Stoffe auf Infusoriera. Z Biol 39:524
51. Rassmusen-Taxdal DS, Ward GE, Figge FHJ (1955) Fluorescence of human lymphatic and cancer tissues following high doses of hematoporphyrin. Cancer 8:78
52. Rhodes L, de Rie M, Engtrom Y (2002) A randomized comparison of excision surgery and PDT using methyl aminolevulinate in nodular basal cell carcinoma. An Dermatol Venereol

129(S1):1S108
53. Soler AM, Warloe T, Berner A, Giercksky KE (2001) A follow-up study of recurrence and cosmesis in completely responding superficial and nodular basal cell carcinomas treated with methyl 5-aminolaevulinate-based photodynamic therapy alone and with prior curettage. Br J Dermatol 145:467–471
54. Steinbach P, Kriegmair M, Baumgartner R, Hofstädter F, Knüchel R (1994) Intravesical instillation of 5-aminolevulinic acid: the fluorescent metabolite is limited to urothelial cells. Urology 44:676–681
55. Stout AL, Becker FF (1986) Heme enzyme patterns in genetically and chemically induced mouse liver tumors. Cancer Res 46:2756–2759
56. Stummer W, Stocker S, Wagner S, Stepp H, Fritsch C, Goetz C, Goetz AE, Kiefmann R, Reulen HJ (1998) Intraoperative detection of malignant gliomas by 5-aminolevulinic acid-induced porphyrin fluorescence. Neurosurgery 42:518–526
57. Szeimies RM, Abels C, Fritsch C, Karrer S, Steinbach P, Bäumler W, Goerz G, Goetz AE, Landthaler M (1995) Wavelength dependency of photodynamic effects after sensitization with 5-aminolevulinic acid in vitro and in vivo. J Invest Dermatol 105:672–677
58. Szeimies RM, Sassay T, Landthaler M (1994) Penetration potency of topical applied delta aminolevulinic acid for photodynamic therapy of basal cell carcinoma. Photochem Photobiol 59:73–76
59. Tschudy DP, Collins A (1957) Reduction of δ-aminolevulinic acid dehydratase activity in the livers of tumor-bearing animals. Cancer Res 17:976–980
60. von Tappeiner H, Jesionek A (1903) Therapeutische Versuche mit fluoreszierenden Stoffen. MMW 50:2042–2044
61. von Tappeiner H, Jodlbauer A (1904) Ueber die Wirkung der photodynamischen (fluorescierenden) Stoffe auf Protozoen und Enzyme. Arch Klin Med 80:427–487
62. Wennberg AM, Wulf HC, Warloe T (2000) Metvix® photodynamic therapy in patients with basal cell carcinoma at risk of complications and poor cosmetic outcome after conventional therapy. J Eur Acad Dermatol Venereol 15(S2):225
63. Wolf P, Rieger E, Kerl H (1993) Topical photodynamic therapy with endogenous porphyrins after application of 5-aminolevulinic acid: an alternative treatment modality for solar keratoses, superficial squamous cell carcinomas, and basal cell carcinomas? J Am Acad Dermatol 28:17–21

19 第19章 宽谱UVB、窄谱UVB和UVA-1的光疗应用指南，以及PUVA光化学疗法的建议

H. Hönigsmann, J. Krutmann

内容

引言 ·· 367
不使用光敏剂的光疗方案 ··································· 367
光化学治疗（PUVA）方案 ····································· 371

要点

› 紫外线B（UVB）光疗：UVB光疗对中重度银屑病及薄斑块型银屑病治疗高度有效。患者通常需要每周治疗2到5次。在治疗期间，皮肤暴露于UVB，这种光源由特定的灯产生。为了增加UVB射线的渗透，润滑剂经常使用于曝光前。UVB光疗有两种类型：宽谱UVB，窄谱UVB。窄谱UVB已大部分取代了传统的UVB光疗。窄谱UVB治疗几乎与PUVA治疗一样有效而比传统的宽谱治疗更有效。窄谱UVB已经成功运用于许多联合治疗如与系统使用维A酸，局部使用地蒽酚和钙泊三醇联合运用。

› UVA-1：UVA-1光疗对于特应性皮炎，仍然是首先运用的，不断检测其有效性的治疗方式。使用剂量为130J/cm^2，但是近期，正在研究中、低剂量的治疗疗效。UVA-1照射是治疗多种皮肤疾病的良好选择，是硬化性疾病的一线治疗之一，并且可以显著改善患者的瘙痒症状。UVA-1治疗特应性皮炎，硬皮病，硬化萎缩苔藓，慢性苔藓样角化病，结节性痒疹和皮肤T细胞淋巴瘤疗效显著，对部分色素性荨麻疹和环状肉芽肿有效。

第19章 宽谱UVB、窄谱UVB和UVA-1的光疗应用指南，以及PUVA光化学疗法的建议

> **要点**
>
> › 补骨脂素紫外线A(PUVA)：即光化学疗法，PUVA治疗斑块型，点滴状的，和掌跖银屑病有效，且能达到长期缓解。治疗需要患者在照射UVA前口服或局部应用补骨脂，或进行补骨脂素浴。补骨脂素增加皮肤对UVA的敏感性。在口服治疗后，患者暴露于日光下时需配戴阻断UVA的墨镜。在完全皮疹完全清除前在2到3个月内需要约25次治疗。皮肤科医生需对接受PUVA治疗的患者仔细监测。PUVA常用于对其他治疗无反应的银屑病患者或是皮损泛发者。和窄谱一样。PUVA可以联用其他治疗。

引言

本章是回顾作者单位所运用的UV辐射和补骨脂素光化学疗法治疗皮肤疾病指引准则。当然也有其他有效的使用流程。然而，这里提供的指引经过多年的光疗实践被证实安全有效，也可能目标在于通过最优化治疗策略来最小化潜在的短期或长期副作用。

UVB治疗和PUVA作为皮肤病的辅助治疗已被广泛接受。在这一章中，我们探讨非敏感性UV光疗(没有外在光敏剂的光疗)和补骨脂素UV光疗(PUVA)。治疗将首先描述银屑病，这也是UVB和PUVA治疗的最常见的应用，而其他应用只会简短地讨论。

不使用光敏剂的光疗方案

光疗最初是指使用由紫外线灯传输的人工宽谱UVB照射。今天，宽谱和窄谱UVB、UVA和UVB结合均用于光疗。窄谱UVB(311~313nm)光疗在银屑病的清除和缓解时间上优于传统的宽谱UVB。这是由于治疗的需要而调整改善灯管的排放。在欧洲，窄谱UVB已经大部分取代了传统的UVB光疗。在美国，由于部分技术原因，飞利浦TL01灯最近才开始使用。我们和其他人已经观察到窄谱光疗在治疗银屑病上几乎与PUVA等效。窄谱UVB也已经成功用于一系列联合治疗里，如联合系统使用维A酸，局部使用地蒽酚和钙泊三醇。最近，UVA-1照射(340~400nm)已经试验性地用于特定的炎症性皮肤病。

UVB 光疗

安全和有效地使用 UVB 光疗的一般要求

1. 适应证:除了银屑病,UVB 治疗的许多其他适应证,这在本书中将深度讨论。
2. 相对禁忌证:肿瘤病史及光敏性皮肤病史。
3. 告知患者 UVB 治疗的有效性,副作用和潜在的长期风险后签署知情同意。
4. UVB 红斑反应的动力学知识。
5. 定期测量和记录照射光源的输出功率(mW/cm^2),确定照射剂量(J/cm^2;mJ/cm^2)。
6. 测定照射光源的最小红斑量(MED)来确定个体 UVB 敏感性。
7. 对治疗期间患者的持续的监测。

UVB 光疗的实践——放射量测定

由于单纯的皮肤类型常不能反映个体的实际敏感性,建议在光疗之前,使用光测试评估个体的 UV 敏感性。选择非日光暴露区如下背部或臀部区域内 6 个小的模型区域(例如直径1cm的圆圈),逐渐增加照射剂量(10mJ)或增加最低计量的百分比(例如40%)。在表 19.1 中已举例。指出这些剂量很依赖于所使用光源直径。

表 19.1 MED 测试中使用的宽波 UVB 和窄谱 UVB 暴露光源剂(mJ/cm^2),用完整的 UV 直径测量(Waldmann,schwenningen,德国)

宽谱 UVB	20	40	60	80	100	120
窄谱 UVB	200	400	600	800	1000	1200

表 19.2 MED 判读

0	没有红斑
+/−	有尖锐边缘的最小感触红斑
+	粉红色红斑
++	显著的红斑,无水肿和疼痛
+++	显著的红色红斑,轻微水肿,轻微疼痛
++++	紫罗兰色红斑,显著的水肿,强烈地疼痛,部分的起水疱

照射 24 小时后产生最小可测红斑反应的辐射剂量就是最小红斑量（MED）（表 19.2）。应告知患者至少在测试前 24 小时避免日光浴或阳光照射。由于宽波和窄波能量评估存在量级不同，记录用于 MED 测量的灯光类型非常重要。

肉眼可测的 MED 是否是放射量测定的最佳参照指标存在争议。然而，这种评估方式最实际且容易操作，除了光疗设备不需要借助任何仪器。

宽谱 UVB 治疗的指南

初始治疗阶段（治疗直至疾病的清除）。UVB 初始治疗剂量为最小红斑量（MED）的 70%。每周照射 2~5 次。由于高峰 UVB 红斑出现于照射后 24 小时内，每次连续治疗都需要增加剂量。如果每周治疗 5 次，那么建议每次治疗后增加剂量。增加的速度取决于治疗的频率和之前的光暴露。剂量增加的目的是维持最小可见红斑量，后者是最佳计量的临床指示器。例如，一周三次的治疗，如果未产生红斑，则增加 30% 的剂量，而出现轻度红斑则增加 20% 的剂量。如果红斑轻微但是持续，不增加剂量。如果每天照射，增加量分别不超过 30%，15% 和 0%。如果有严重或疼痛性红斑，暂停照射直至症状消失。治疗一直持续到症状完全缓解或者持续光疗不能取得进一步的进展（表 19.3）。

表 19.3 窄谱 UVB 和宽谱 UVB 的治疗方法

第一步	最小红斑量（MED）的测定	24 小时后判读	
第二步	治疗开始	初始治疗剂量	70% MED
第三步	每周三次持续治疗（每日一次）	无红斑	增加 30%
		轻度红斑	两次治疗后增加 20%
		持续无症状红斑	不增加
		疼痛性红斑伴或不伴水肿或大疱	停止治疗直到症状消退
第四步	恢复治疗	症状解决后	末次剂量减至 50%；以后以 10% 增加照射计量

维持阶段。持续治疗能否使患者取得更长时间的缓解尚未达成一致。没有能证实持续光疗的意义的精确数据存在。皮肤 T 细胞淋巴瘤，常维持治疗数月。在持续治疗中症状复发，UVB 剂量和照射频率将再次增加直至皮损消退。

窄谱 UVB 治疗指南

相同的物理单位(J/cm^2)窄谱 UVB 较宽谱 UVB 产生的红斑显著减少。因此,就像上面指出的,计量不同,MED 必须由这些光波长所决定。24 小时后判读红斑。初始治疗剂量不超过 MED 的 70%。

初始治疗阶段和最终的维持治疗阶段与宽谱 UVB 推荐使用的完全一致(见表 19.2)。

宽谱 UVB 到窄谱 UVB 转换,窄谱 UVB 到宽谱 UVB 转换

当患者转移到其他治疗机构,向他们提供患者详细的治疗数据十分重要:光疗机器的类型、初始 MED、最终有效剂量、治疗频率。如果用另外的光源维持治疗,现有的 MED 必须由新光源确定。以此计量的 70% 维持治疗。

UVA-1 光疗

UVA-1 光疗对于特应性皮炎,仍然是首先运用的,不断检测其有效性的治疗方式。$130J/cm^2$ 的的剂量已在运用,但近期,正在研究中低剂量的治疗方法。此部分光疗正在发展,更多的适应证将逐渐纳入。

安全和有效使用 UVA-1 治疗的一般需要

1. 适应证:多中心研究已经确证对严重和急性进行期特应性皮炎治疗有效。
2. 处在试验阶段的适应证:局限性和系统性硬皮病,色素性荨麻疹,早期皮肤 T-细胞淋巴瘤,HIV+患者。
3. 禁忌:皮肤肿瘤病史,光敏性皮肤病和服用光敏感性药物。年龄小于 18 岁,因为长期的危险因素仍不清楚。
4. 用治疗光源测定最小红斑量来确定个体的 UVA-1 敏感性。
5. 在告知患者 UVA-1 治疗的有效性、负作用和潜在长期危害后签订知情同意书。
6. UVA-1 色沉反应的动力学知识。
7. 常规精确的测量和记录照射源的输出功率(mW/cm^2)和剂量的确定(J/cm^2)。
8. 治疗期间患者持续监控。

UVA-1 光疗的实践——放射量测定

UVA-1 光疗的放射量测定由个体的 UVA-1 敏感性而调节。在启动完整的

个体治疗前,排除任何可能在治疗期间被诱发的 UVA-1 敏感的光敏性皮肤病很重要。基于现存的观点,照射的目标是达到最高计量 $130J/cm^2$。MED 测试过程和 UVA 光源基本相同,用递增的 UVA-1 剂量照射 6 个模型区域(表 19.4)。

表 19.4 MTD 测试(J/cm^2)

皮肤类型	UVA-1 测试剂量					
Ⅰ ~ Ⅱ	10	20	40	60	100	130
Ⅲ ~ Ⅳ	20	40	60	80	100	130

色素沉着在 24 小时判读。引起最小可见色素沉着的最小光源被定义为 MTD(表 19.5)。另外,记录如红斑、丘疹、水疱等严重不良反应。MTD 的确定并不是作为初始治疗剂量的指标,而是为了获得个体 UVA-1 敏感性的信息。

表 19.5 MTD 判读

0	无色素沉着
+/-	最小可见境界清楚的色素沉着
+	轻微的色素沉着
++	明显的色素沉着
+++	显著色素沉着

高剂量 UVA-1 治疗指南

初始治疗阶段(治疗直至疾病清除)。对于特应性皮炎和局限性硬皮病,每日照射 $130J/cm^2$(周六日休息),不增加剂量。特应性皮炎的治疗 15 次,硬皮病治疗 30 次。对于色素性荨麻疹,治疗起始用 $60J/cm^2$ 照射体表四分之一面积,然后增加到 $130J/cm^2$,然后改为全身 $60J/cm^2$ 照射,2 ~ 3 次,最终 $130J/cm^2$ 直至 15 次治疗结束。

复发的治疗。如果复发,UVA-1 可以重复治疗。然而,由于长期风险等不确定因素,限定每年两个治疗周期。

光化学治疗(PUVA)方案

安全有效使用 PUVA 的一般要求

1. 适应证:PUVA 被用于治疗多种严重的皮肤疾病,特别是严重的银屑病和皮肤 T-细胞淋巴瘤和其他在本书中提及的皮肤病。

2. 相对的禁忌证:有肿瘤病史及光敏性皮肤病史,和使用光敏性药物(补骨脂素除外)。

3. 告知患者 PUVA 治疗的有效性,副作用和潜在的长期风险后签署知情同意书。

4. 光毒性 PUVA 红斑反应的动力学知识。

5. 补骨脂素的光动力学知识。

6. 准确测量和记录照射光源输出功率(mW/cm^2),确定 UVA 剂量(J/cm^2)。

7. 通过测定最小光毒量(MPD)来确定个体敏感性。

8. 治疗期间对患者的持续监测。

PUVA 的实践方面

口服 PUVA 和药浴 PUVA 是 PUVA 使用的两种主要形式。最近,PUVA 霜剂被推荐使用于限定的皮肤区域(手和足,头和颈)。这三种类型使用的一般原则相同,然而实际运用有所不同,尤其是放射量测定。

光敏剂

口服 PUVA。8-甲氧补骨脂(8-MOP,Oxsoralen)或 5-甲氧补骨脂(5-MOP,Geralen)已用于 PUVA 治疗。5-MOP 目前仅在少数欧洲国家使用。两种补骨脂素的用量需根据体重来确定。基于两种物质的不同的药代动力学,为了达到最高组织浓度,8-MOP 需在照光前 1 小时使用,5-MOP 需在照光前 2 小时使用。

- 8-MOP(Oxsoralen)0.6mg/kg 体重
- 5-MOP(Geralen)1.2mg/kg 体重

PUVA 浴。对于 PUVA 浴,8-MOP 和 4,5′,8-三甲基补骨脂素(TMP)在使用。斯堪的纳维斯半岛目前多采用 TMP 浴 PUVA。在局部应用后,TMP 诱导了较高的光敏感性,使用的浓度低于 8-MOP。由于实际的原因,我们在这里只讨论 8-MOP。8-MOP 溶解于洗澡水中以达到 1.0mg/L 的最终浓度。这通过溶于储存的沐浴水(0.5% 8-MOP 于 96% 乙醇)中获得(1:5000),或者,换一句话说,20ml 储存溶液溶于 100L 洗澡水中。患者在洗澡水中浸泡 15~20 分钟,然后迅速照射 UA。由于光敏剂衰减迅速,维持时间短于 4 小时,故沐浴和照射的间隔时间不能超过 15 分钟。

PUVA 霜剂。PUVA 霜剂使用的是 8-MOP。用于全身治疗的是浓度为 0.0006% 8-MOP。若所选区域已经过治疗,推荐浓度加倍。霜剂使用后 30 分钟,获得最佳光敏性。

辐射量的测定

我们常规的治疗与欧洲方案一致。草案要求治疗初期需测定个体 MPD。MPD 测试与 MED 测试相同。连续不同剂量的 UVA 照射下背部或臀部皮肤(在口服摄取补骨脂或补骨脂药浴后)。为了避免严重的反应,根据皮肤类型给予不同的 UVA 测试剂量(表 19.6)。由于 PUVA 沐浴诱导了更明显的光敏性,测试剂量必须相对低一些(表 19.7)。而对于 UVB 光试验,尽可能地的选择非曝光区皮肤。

表 19.6 用口服和 PUVA 霜剂时,MPD 测试的照射剂量(J/cm^2)

皮肤类型 Ⅰ~Ⅳ						
UVA 剂量(8-MOP)	0.5	1	2	3	4	5
UVA 剂量(8-MOP)	1	2	4	6	8	10

表 19.7 PUVA 沐浴测试时 MPD 的暴露剂量(J/cm^2)

皮肤类型 Ⅰ~Ⅱ						
UVA 剂量(8-MOP)	0.25	0.5	1	1.5	2	2.5
皮肤类型 Ⅲ~Ⅳ						
UVA 剂量(8-MOP)	0.5	1	2	3	4	5

迟发的光毒性红斑反应在 72 小时后被评估(不晚于 96 小时)。使患者出现最小的、境界清楚的红斑的最小能量代表了 MPD(表 19.8)。

表 19.8 MPD 判读

0	无红斑
+/-	最小可见境界清楚的红斑
+	粉红色红斑
++	显著的红斑,无水肿,无疼痛
+++	鲜红色红斑,轻度水肿,轻度疼痛
++++	紫罗兰色的红斑,显著的水肿,强烈地疼痛,局部的大疱

PUVA 治疗指南

初始治疗阶段(治疗直至疾病清除)。PUVA 红斑在 72~120 小时前达不到高峰。因此,在 MPD 测试后 72 小时后才能开始治疗。口服 PUVA 安全的初始治疗剂量是 70% MPD(最近的研究显示 50% MPD 对银屑病的治疗常常就已足够有效)。PUVA 浴的起始剂量仅仅可采用 30% MPD,因为 MPD 在开始治疗后的第一天就能够减少 50% 以上。这可能由于持续的补骨脂单体经曝光后相互交联。

UVA 初始剂量:
- 口服 PUVA:50%~70% MPD
- PUVA 浴:30% MPD
- PUVA 霜剂:50%~70% MPD

每周最多照射四次,每周提高照射计量不超过 2 次,(至少间隔 72 小时)在治疗的第一周不要提高计量,以免迟发性皮肤光毒性作用累积。出现可见红斑提示达到了足够照射计量,尽管它不是成功治疗所必需的。对于剂量增加没有严格的规定,剂量调节的主要标准是疾病对治疗的反应和色素沉着的程度。

一般情况下,如果未出现红斑,UVA 剂量同时在口服 PUVA 和 PUVA 沐浴中增加 30%。(表 19.9)

表 19.10 中显示 PUVA 放射量测定的一个例子(每周四次)。由于出现红斑和或明显的治疗反应,一些患者在持续治疗期间不需调整剂量。

表 19.9 口服 PUVA 和 PUVA 沐浴的治疗时刻表

			PUVA 类型 口服 PUVA	PUVA 沐浴	PUVA 霜
第一步	最小光毒剂量(MPD)的测定	72 小时后判读			
第二步	治疗开始	初始治疗剂量	50%~70% MPD	30% MPD	50%~70% MPD
第三步	治疗持续,每周 2~4 次	无红斑,好的反应	每周增加 30%	每周增加 30%	每周增加 30%
		无红斑,无反应	增加 30%	增加 30%	增加 30%
		最小红斑	不增加	不增加	不增加
		持续的无症状红斑	不增加	不增加	不增加
		疼痛性红斑有或无水肿或大疱	不治疗直至症状减弱	不治疗直至症状减弱	不治疗直至症状减弱
第四步	治疗恢复	症状缓解后	最后治疗剂量减 50%;如果很好耐受,进一步减少 10%	最后治疗剂量减 50%;如果很好耐受,进一步减少 10%	最后治疗剂量减 50%;如果很好耐受,进一步减少 10%

表 19.10　口服/霜剂 PUVA 和 PUVA 沐浴的放射量测定

	日期															
	1	2	3	4	5	6	7	8	9	10	11	12	13	14	15	16
口服/霜剂 PUVA(J/cm^2)	2	2	0	2	2	0	0	2.6	2.6	0	3.4	3.4	0	0	4	4
PUVA 沐浴(J/cm^2)	1	1	0	1	1	0	0	1.3	1.3	0	1.3	1.3	0	0	1.7	1.7

维持阶段。维持治疗推荐使用于复发较早的特定人群。包括运用清除期的末次治疗剂量,每周治疗 2 次,治疗 1 个月,接下来每周 1 次,治疗 1 个月。参照英国皮肤医师协会的推荐,只有为避免迅速复发才考虑维持治疗。尽管迄今使用 PUVA 已超过 25 年,而维持治疗是否能防止银屑病的早期复发仍存在争议。许多机构建议对皮肤 T 细胞淋巴瘤采取某种形式的长期维持治疗。然而,由于缺乏前瞻性研究,目前仍旧不能给予有效建议,也许每月一次的治疗比较可行。

维持阶段轻度复发可临时增加治疗频率;严重的复发病例,必须重新使用原先清除阶段的治疗方案直到皮疹再次清除。

(杨艳 译,周欣　孟珍 校,朱慧兰 审)

参考文献

1. American Academy of Dermatology Committee on Guidelines of Care (1994) Guidelines of care for phototherapy and photochemotherapy. J Am Acad Dermatol 31:643–648
2. British Photodermatology Group (1994) British Photodermatology Group guidelines for PUVA. Br J Dermatol 130:246–255
3. German Guidelines at http://leitlinien.net/
4. Halpern SM, Anstey AV, Dawe RS, Diffey BL, Farr PM, Ferguson J, Hawk JL, Ibbotson S, McGregor JM, Murphy GM, Thomas SE, Rhodes LE (2000) Guidelines for topical PUVA: a report of a workshop of the British photodermatology group. Br J Dermatol 142:22–31
5. Hönigsmann H, Szeimies R-F, Knobler R (2008) Photochemotherapy and photodynamic therapy. In: Wolff K, Goldsmith LA, Katz SI, Gilchrest BA, Paller AS, Leffell DJ (eds) Fitzpatrick's dermatology in general medicine, 7th edn. McGraw-Hill, New York, pp 2249–2262
6. Ibbotson SH, Bilsland D, Cox NH, Dawe RS, Diffey B, Edwards C, Farr PM, Ferguson J, Hart G, Hawk J, Lloyd J, Martin C, Moseley H, McKenna K, Rhodes LE, Taylor DK; British Association of Dermatologists (2004) An update and guidance on narrowband ultraviolet B phototherapy: a British Photodermatology Group Workshop Report. Br J Dermatol 151:283–297
7. Krutmann J, Morita A (2008) Therapeutic photomedicine: phototherapy. In: Wolff K, Goldsmith LA, Katz SI, Gilchrest BA, Paller AS, Leffell DJ (eds) Fitzpatrick's dermatology in general medicine, 7th edn. McGraw-Hill, New York, pp 2243–2249
8. Lebwohl M, Drake L, Menter A, Koo J, Gottlieb AB, Zanolli M, Young M, McClelland P (2001) Consensus conference: acitretin in combination with UVB or PUVA in the treatment of psoriasis. J Am Acad Dermatol 45:544–553

9. Morison WL (2005) Phototherapy and photochemotherapy of skin disease, 3rd ed. Taylor & Francis Group, Boca Raton
10. Rombold S, Lobisch K, Katzer K, Grazziotin TC, Ring J, Eberlein B (2008) Efficacy of UVA1 phototherapy in 230 patients with various skin diseases. Photodermatol Photoimmunol Photomed 24:19–23
11. Taylor DK, Anstey AV, Coleman AJ, Diffey BL, Farr PM, Ferguson J, Ibbotson S, Langmack K, Lloyd JJ, McCann P, Martin CJ, Menage Hdu P, Moseley H, Murphy G, Pye SD, Rhodes LE, Rogers S; British Photodermatology Group (2002) Guidelines for dosimetry and calibration in ultraviolet radiation therapy: a report of a British Photodermatology Group workshop. Br J Dermatol 146:755–763

第 20 章　技术及设备

R. Mang, H. stege

内容

紫外线疗法·· 377
激光疗法·· 378
光动力疗法·· 378
光疗设备清单·· 379

要点

› 准分子激光治疗设备和激光器的市场发展变化迅速。其互联网的存在为获得一个可用的产品提供了很好的可能性。

紫外线疗法

20 世纪初，Finsen 开始使用人工紫外线治疗皮肤病。起初，紫外线治疗设备只能小范围照射。虽然紫外线治疗卓有成效，但到 1958 年才把全身人工紫外线光疗引进临床常规治疗。1958 年，Zimmermann 报道称，拥有八个灯泡和一个计时器构造的轻型柜机式仪器可以进行全身光线疗法。现代橱柜式设备就是在此基础得到突破，常利用高达 48 个金属卤化物灯泡或灯柱。光疗至关重要的发展，包括不同的紫外光谱可提供特定的治疗效果，另外，工业上灯泡类型的进化也带来了这些特殊紫外线光谱的变化。

Finsen 碳弧灯由含有微量金属的双碳电极组成，其电力的流动产生光和热。碳弧灯可发出类似于阳光的连续发射光谱。由于其产生烟雾、气味和可变的辐射输出，碳弧灯被密闭的汞蒸气弧灯取代。汞蒸气弧灯由封闭在石英（二氧化硅)中的汞蒸气组成,它允许波长大于 180nm 的光谱传输。汞蒸汽灯发出的不连续光谱主要在紫外线区域。低压水银蒸汽弧光灯,也被称为"冷石英",产生的波长主要为 253.7nm,因此主要用于杀菌。热石英灯(高压汞)产生 UVB 和 UVA 范围内的不连续光。这些设备被广泛应用于治疗银屑病。然而,其中不足之处是照射范围小,对于大面积治疗不切实际。

现代光疗设备中,荧光灯最为常用。它们由一个在涂有荧光粉的长玻璃管中封闭的低压汞排放源组成。发生的波长取决于涂层荧光粉的类型。荧光灯发生的光谱通常是连续的。有不同的商业"Max"荧光灯——"日光"(D)、"蓝光"(B)和"特别蓝"(BB)灯用于新生儿黄疸光疗。用于皮肤病光疗的专用荧光灯包括发出 60% 的 UVB(270~390nm)的太阳灯(Fs),发出 20% UVA(320~340nm)和少于 3% UVB 的早期紫外线灯,和发出约 30% UVA(320~340nm)和 8% UVB 的 UVA/UVB 灯。新发展包括不同类型的窄谱 UVB 辐射,其具有特殊定点的发光管或管,例如,低剂量紫外线 A1 辐射(340~400nm)。荧光灯的优点是具有均一的辐射、相对较低的成本、最低限度的产热及约 200 小时的寿命。

根据顾客的需要,机柜可以配备不同类型灯管。发射窄谱 UVB(311nm)管联合 UVA 发射管较常见,其提供了一个广泛的临床应用范围。应连续测定辐射剂量。

激光疗法

窄谱 UVB 治疗采用的是菲利普斯 TL-01 荧光灯。一项 UVB 光疗新进展是使用氯化氙(XeCl)激光发射 308nm 波长的 UVB 进行针对性的治疗。2001 年 3 月 1 日,XeCl 激光器、™XTRAC 准分子激光(PhotoMedex)得到了美国食品药品管理局(FDA)的批准,用于治疗轻度至中度银屑病和白癜风。FDA 批准的"510(k)"不需要相关的临床疗效数据,因为 XTRAC 准分子激光被认为是一项产生紫外线辐射的不同技术,因此 XTRAC 装置被认为可以提供的一种窄谱 UVB 治疗。XTRAC 装置的独特之处在于它可以手持操作。这个装置的独特方面有利与否有待商榷。该手持设备的优点包括对病变部位的精确定位,减少对周围非皮损皮肤的暴露,与光箱相比它能允许更高的剂量,并且最终使用更少的治疗就可产生效果。一般情况下,XeCl 准分子激光治疗主要用于局部银屑病患者,即皮肤的受累面积小于皮肤体表面积的 10%。

光动力疗法

光动力疗法(PDT)是一种专业性很高的光疗,特别是治疗(皮肤)癌。与其他方案相比,PDT是微创的,因其较少产生瘢痕或无瘢痕,而达到比较好的美容效果。最近,PDT被证明可用于治疗炎症性皮肤病。

光动力疗法是利用光和光活性染料(光敏剂),优先定位于代谢增强的细胞(例如,肿瘤)而非正常、健康的细胞。

几种光敏剂已被确定为PDT光敏剂;有些已获得FDA和EMEA批准使用或目前正在科研中。Δ-氨基乙酰丙酸(ALA)是常用的光敏剂。在德国或其他欧洲国家,ALA是一种未被批准的药物,含有ALA成分的软膏产生于皮肤科医生办公室中。在美国,一个FDA批准的含ALA配方,即所谓的Kerastick,治疗光线性角化病使用氨基乙酰丙酸(ALA)和蓝光是光动力疗法最常见的皮肤病指征。FDA批准的蓝光来源系统包括Blu-U和ClearLight系统。甲基氨基酮戊酸(MAL),一种(丙氨酸酯)ALA酯,已在欧洲、澳大利亚和新西兰及美国获得批准。除了蓝光,PDT也可在红光或绿光下进行。一些公司使用红光作为PDT光源。目前只有Curelight系统是FDA批准的。然而,Aktilite是欧洲使用最广泛的设备系统。

通过适当的波长激活,光敏剂可代谢转化成卟啉。卟啉光敏剂或与四吡咯结构相关的光敏剂显示一个典型的吸收光谱,其最大吸收波长为405nm,即所谓的soret带。此外,在长波区域有几个Q带,其中一个在635nm处。虽然吸收峰值小于405nm,但由于能更深地渗透到皮肤中,因此优选的发射光源在红光光谱范围内。此外,也有白光或绿光应用于PDT中。然而,一项对比研究表明短波光源治疗鲍温病疗效不如同等剂量的长波光源。因此,对于皮肤肿瘤的PDT治疗,只有红光被推荐应用。红光可以治疗厚度达2~3mm的非黑色素皮肤癌,但是较厚的病变组织仍需要术前行组织消融术。PDT可采用非相干光源或激光进行。尽管脉冲激光发射的波长与卟啉化合物的吸收光谱并不完全相符,但是使用发射585nm或595nm的脉冲激光治疗光线性角化病的疗效与使用非相干光和非均一光源的疗效相当。

激光的特定的优势如相干性,PDT则不要求;其治疗可以采用非相干性光源进行。非相干性光源是可靠的、更易获得、更便宜,通常与照明激光一样有效。市售的非相干光源有卤素灯(例如,PDT 1200L, Waldmann Medical Technology, Villingen-schwenningen)或LEDs(发光二极管)(例如, Aktilite,™ Galderma, Dusseldorf and Omnilux PDT,™ Photo Therapeutics, England)。这些设备可允许同时照明较大的区域,而且它们发射的光谱与ALA或MAL诱导卟啉的吸收光谱相匹配。

光疗设备清单

在这本书第1版中,我们提到了一系列用于光(化学)治疗的辐照设备,在欧洲（特别是德国、奥地利和瑞士市场）和美国市场上均有销售。我们的目标是提出一个完整而真实的概述。图书出版后，我们发现要实现这个目标几乎是不可能的。市场变化迅速，特别是在美国存在大量的家庭护理。已发布的设备目录也不能完全涵盖当前所有设备。因此，我们决定给读者提供一个生产光疗设备的公司清单。

紫外线疗法：

- www. cynosure. com
- www. daavlin. com
- www. drhoenle. de
- www. houva. com
- www. medisun. de
- www. saalmann. net
- www. sellamed. de(UVA-1)
- www. waldmann. com

光动力疗法：

- www. daavlin. com
- www. houva. com
- www. hydrosun. de
- www. medisun. de
- www. photocure. no
- www. phototherapeutics. com
- www. saalmann. net
- www. waldmann. com

激光疗法/IPL：

- www. aerolase. com
- www. aldermna. com
- www. asclepion. com
- www. candelalaser. com
- www. cooltouch. com
- www. conbio. com
- www. cutera. com
- www. cynosure. com
- www. dermamedusa. com
- www. lumenis. com
- www. palomarmedical. com

- www. sciton. com
- www. syneron. com
- www. wavelight. com

Photophersis：

- www. therakos. com

在欧洲和美国,关于辐照设备系统治疗应用的法律现状是不同的。一般说来,我们建议皮肤科医生应要求生产商或供应商提供法律声明,表明其供应设备系统的治疗用途符合当地的法律法规。

（罗权 译,林玲 周欣 校,朱慧兰 审）

参考文献

1. Amatiello H, Martin CJ (2006) Ultraviolet phototherapy: review of options for cabin dosimetry and operation. Phys Med Biol 51:299–309
2. Anderson RR (2000) Lasers in dermatology—a critical update. J Dermatol 27:700–705
3. Asawanonda P et al (2000) 308-nm excimer laser for the treatment of psoriasis: a dose-response study. Arch Dermatol 136:619–624
4. Calzavara-Pinton PG, Venturini M, Sala R (2007) Photodynamic therapy: update 2006. Part 1: photochemistry and photobiology. J Eur Acad Dermatol Venereol 21:293–302
5. Calzavara-Pinton PG, Venturini M, Sala R (2007) Photodynamic therapy: update 2006. Part 2: clinical results. J Eur Acad Dermatol Venereol 21:439–451
6. Grossweiner L, Grossweiner JB, Rogers G, Jones L (2005) The science of phototherapy: an introduction. Springer, Heidelberg
7. Jekler J, Diffey B, Larko O (1990) Ultraviolet radiation dosimetry in phototherapy for atopic dermatitis. J Am Acad Dermatol 23:49–51
8. Kollner K et al (2005) Comparison of the 308-nm excimer laser and a 308-nm excimer lamp with 311-nm narrowband ultraviolet B in the treatment of psoriasis. Br J Dermatol 152:750–754
9. Kraemer CK, Menegon DB, Cestari TF (2005) Determination of the minimal phototoxic dose and colorimetry in psoralen plus ultraviolet A radiation therapy. Photodermatol Photoimmunol Photomed 21:242–248
10. Mackenzie LA (1985) UV radiometry in dermatology. Photodermatol 2:86–94
11. Schneider LA et al (2007) Examples for the importance of radiophysical measurements in clinical phototherapy. J Dtsch Dermatol Ges 5:384–389
12. Schooneman F (2003) Extracorporeal photopheresis technical aspects. Transfus Apher Sci 28:51–61
13. Szeimies RM, Karrer S (2006) Towards a more specific therapy: targeting nonmelanoma skin cancer cells. Br J Dermatol 154(Suppl 1):16–21
14. Trehan M, Taylor CR (2002) High-dose 308-nm excimer laser for the treatment of psoriasis. J Am Acad Dermatol 46:732–737
15. Warshaw JB, Gagliardi J, Patel A (1980) A comparison of fluorescent and nonfluorescent light sources for phototherapy. Pediatrics 65:795–798
16. Wilson BC (1989) Photodynamic therapy: light delivery and dosage for second-generation photosensitizers. Ciba Found Symp 146:60–73; discussion 73–77

索引

308 nm 氙激光 177
5-MOP 142,372
5-甲氧补骨脂 71,372
5-甲氧补骨酯素 142
5-甲氧基补骨酯素 308
8-MOP 142,372
8-甲氧补骨脂 71,372
8-甲氧补骨酯素 142
β-胡萝卜素 310

A

ALA 211
ATMPn 228
氨基酮戊酸(ALA) 211,341

B

BB-UVB 177
白癜风 130
斑秃 186
瘢痕疙瘩 268
半胱氨酸 311
鲍温病 221,223,233
苯并卟啉衍生物单环 225
扁平苔藓 177,253
表儿茶素没食子酸酯 310
表没食子儿茶素-3-没食子酸酯(EGCG) 310,311
波长 5
卟吩姆钠 210,221,223
补骨脂 70,72
补骨脂光化学(PUVA) 66

补骨脂光化学疗法 70,177

C

CAT 198
CTCL 116,248
长波红外线 9
长波紫外线 276
长波紫外线辐射 10
长末端重复序列 198
成像光学 11
持续性虫咬反应 189
持续性色素黑化 298
出汗障碍性湿疹 180
出口区 12
穿通性皮肤病 189
传播速度 5,6
传统白炽灯 23
次要组织相容性抗原 160

D

DAPT 333
Darier 征 183
DHA 308
DNA 光损伤 288
DNA 修复酶 309
单-L-天冬酰胺二氢卟吩 E6 225
单纯性痒疹 189
单探测器狭窄出口 12
胆汁淤积性瘙痒症 185
德国光斑贴试验工作组 333
低压水银灯 27

电磁波能量　7
电磁辐射　4
淀粉样变性　189
动谱曲线　43
短波红外线　9
短波紫外线　276
短波紫外线辐射　10
短弧汞灯　29
短暂性棘层松解性皮炎　188
多发性硬化症　253
多形性日光疹　103,324
多足蕨属提取物　310

肥厚性瘢痕　268
分散设备（棱镜或光栅）　11
辐射度　16
辐射功率 φ_e　16,17
辐射光谱　10
辐射率 L_e　16,18
辐射能 Q_e　16,17
辐射曝量 H_e　16,19
辐射强度 I_e　16,17
辐射效率 η_e　16,17
辐照度 E_e　19
复发性转移性乳腺癌　221

E

ECP　247
恶性黑素瘤　284
二羟丙酮　308
二羟基丙酮　134
二酰基甘油　308

G

Goeckerman 疗法　279
Grover 病　188
GvHD　160
干扰素　120
肝炎相关瘙痒症　185
高压水银灯　27
骨髓增生异常综合征　185
固态紫外辐射源　34
光斑贴试验　324,327
光变态反应　327,339
光动力疗法　209,378
光毒性反应　339
光防护　294
光分离置换疗法　247
光（化疗）治疗　54
光化性类网状细胞增多症　111
光化性痒疹　108
光化学辐射计　16
光化学治疗（PUVA）　371
光激发试验　104
光老化　285,312
光免疫学　54
光敏剂　213,379
光谱仪　10
光搔刮　328

F

FDA　296
FD　341
发光二极管　34
发射　344
泛发型脓疱型银屑病　74
防护系数　299
防晒剂　294
防晒系数　296
防水　300
放电灯　25
非常防水　300
非黑色素瘤皮肤癌　221
非黑素瘤皮肤肿瘤　313
非黑素皮肤癌　280
肥大细胞白血病　183
肥大细胞瘤　183
肥大细胞增多症　183

光生物学 61
光试验 324
光挑刺试验 328
光稳定性 306
光线性角化病 233
光氧化反应 218
光抑制 109
光致癌 279
光致敏原 324,336
光子能量 8
国际接触性皮炎研究工作组 338

H

HIV 性瘙痒症 186
HLA 160
黑素瘤 313
黑素细胞移植 136
红斑狼疮 188,268,329
红皮病型银屑病 74
红外辐射 4,9
红外线 8
红细胞生成性卟啉病 325
化学性 UV 吸收剂 294
环状肉芽肿 182
回旋形线状鱼鳞病 188

I

ICDRG 338
IFN 120
IPD 298

J

基底细胞癌 221,224,313
激发性光试验 324
即刻色素黑化 298
急性 GvHD 161,165
急性苔藓样糠疹 178
剂型 299
甲基氨基酮戊酸 342

甲萎缩 189
甲酯氨基酮戊酸(MAL) 341
角化型湿疹 180
结缔组织病 264
结节性痒疹 188
金属卤化物灯 28
进行性系统性硬化症 249
局限性硬皮病 181,264
巨大色素颗粒 306
聚合酶链反应 198

K

Köbner 现象 132
KUVA 143
卡波西肉瘤 224
凯林(Khellin) 142,143
可见光 8
可见光辐射 9
刻晒黑,IPD 324
宽谱 UVB 67,177,367
宽谱防晒剂 295

L

LED 34
LTR 198
LyP 179
L-苯丙氨酸 142
类风湿性关节炎 250
类脂质渐进性坏死 188
连续光谱 13,14
联合治疗 70
淋巴瘤样丘疹病 178,179
鳞癌 223
鳞状细胞癌 221,313
卤素白炽灯 24
氯化氙(XeCl) 378
氯霉素乙酰转移酶 198

M

MED 69,104,138

Mel-5　131
MPD　142,373
MTD　324,371
mTHPC　225
MUD　109
慢性 GvHD　164
慢性斑块型银屑病　69
慢性光化性皮炎　111,326
慢性皮肤型 GvHD　161
慢性苔藓样角化病　181
慢性苔藓样糠疹　178
毛发红糠疹　268
玫瑰糠疹　179
美国食品药品管理局　296
门区　11
嘧啶二聚体　67
免疫抑制　289

N

NB-UVB　177,276
NMSC　280
Npe6　225
尿毒症性瘙痒症　185

O

Ofuji 丘疹性红皮病　188
Ofuji 嗜酸性脓疱性毛囊炎　185

P

PAUVA　143
PCR　198
PDT　209
PLA　178
PLC　178
PPD　298
PpIX　211
PUVA　70,89,93,164,177,367
PUVASol　145
PUVA 霜剂　372

PUVA 浴　372
PUVA 浴疗　166
PUVA 浴治疗　74
疱疹样皮炎　189
皮肤 T 淋巴细胞瘤　224
皮肤 T 细胞淋巴瘤(CTCL)　116,247,261
皮肤型轻型 GvHD　161
频率　5
频谱　10

Q

浅表性基底细胞癌　233
青石莲提取物　310,311

R

RePUVA　76
热辐射器　21
人类白细胞抗原　160
人类免疫缺陷病毒(HIV)　185,198
人乳头状瘤病毒(HPV)　234
日光　40
日光性荨麻疹　109,326
乳腺癌皮肤转移　224

S

SCT　159
SnET　225
SPF　294,296
SPRG　333
Sézary 综合征　116
三甲补骨脂内酯　142
色素性荨麻疹　183,263
色素性紫癜　181
晒伤　288
嗜酸性粒细胞增多性皮肤病　185
嗜酸性脓疱性毛囊炎　186
手部慢性过敏性接触性皮炎　180
手部湿疹　268
霜剂-PUVA 光化学治疗　96

水源性瘙痒 185
斯堪纳维亚光敏性皮炎研究工作组 333
四苯基卟啉磺酸盐 227

T

tetra(m-hydroxyphenyl)chlorin 225
TMP 142
TPPS 227
苔藓样糠疹 178
蕈样肉芽肿 224,233
特发性光线性皮肤病 103
特应性皮炎 87,260
体外光化学免疫疗法 89,166
体外光免疫化学疗法 247
透射率 37

U

UV 53
UVA-1 10,177,259,367
UVA1 光疗 168
UVA-1 光疗 89,90,370
UVA-2 10
UVA 276
UVA/UVB 光疗 95
UVB 10,276
UVB 光疗 168
UVC 10,276
UVED 34
UVR 276
UV 保护因子 311

V

VitC 309
VitE 309

W

外光化学免疫疗法 93
外用 PDT 228
外用 PUVA 74

外用光化学疗法 144
微色素颗粒 306
维 A 酸 76,120
维持治疗 69
维替泊芬 225
伍德灯 130,341
物理 UV 滤光剂 294
物理性防晒剂 294

X

系统光动力疗法 221
系统性肥大细胞增生症 183
系统性光化学疗法 142
系统性光激发试验 328
系统性红斑狼疮 252
系统性硬化症 266
氙短弧灯 31
鲜红斑痣 226
线谱 14
香豆素补骨脂素 142
像素探测器 12
选择性紫外光治疗 69
血卟啉衍生物 210
寻常痤疮 187
寻常型天疱疮 249
寻常型银屑病 234
蕈样肉芽肿 116

Y

移植物抗宿主病 160,251
异源干细胞移植 159
银屑病 225
吲哚美辛 311
英国光皮肤病学工作组 333
荧光灯 32,378
荧光诊断 341
硬斑病 181
硬化效应 104
硬化性黏液性水肿 184

硬化性苔藓　269
硬皮病　181
用太阳光线进行光化学疗法　145
阈剂量　49
原卟啉　211

Z

窄谱 UVB　168,177,276,367,369
窄谱 UVB 光疗　95
掌跖脓疱病　180
掌跖银屑病　180
照相检测器　12
真性红细胞增多症　185
脂溢性皮炎　179
脂溢性皮炎型银屑病　69
痣细胞痣　313
中波红外线　9

中波紫外线　276
中波紫外线辐射　10
种痘样水疱病　107,326
准分子308nm 激光　139
紫外辐射　4,53
紫外线　8
紫外线辐射　9,276
紫外线辐射器　19
紫外线滤光剂　301
组织细胞增多症 X　184
最小光毒量(MPD)　277
最小红斑量(MED)　69,104,138,277,324,368,369,
最小荨麻疹量　109
最小晒黑量　324
作用光谱　68
作用谱　43